BIOPSY INTERPRETATION SERIES

BIOPSY INTERPRETATION

OF THE THYROID

BIOPSY INTERPRETATION SERIES

Series Editor: Jonathan I. Epstein, M.D.

BIOPSY INTERPRETATION
OF THE THYROID

Scott L. Boerner, MD
Head, Division of Cytopathology
Laboratory Medicine Program
University Health Network
Associate Professor, Department of Laboratory
Medicine and Pathobiology
University of Toronto
Toronto, Ontario, Canada

Sylvia L. Asa, MD, PhD
Pathologist-in-Chief and Medical Director
Laboratory Medicine Program
University Health Network
Senior Scientist, Ontario Cancer Institute
Professor, Department of Laboratory
Medicine and Pathobiology
University of Toronto
Toronto, Ontario, Canada

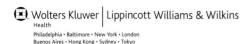
Wolters Kluwer | Lippincott Williams & Wilkins
Health
Philadelphia · Baltimore · New York · London
Buenos Aires · Hong Kong · Sydney · Tokyo

Senior Executive Editor: Jonathan W. Pine, Jr.
Product Manager: Marian Bellus
Vendor Manager: Alicia Jackson
Senior Manufacturing Manager: Benjamin Rivera
Senior Marketing Manager: Angela Panetta
Creative Director: Doug Smock
Production Service: Aptaracorp

Printed in the People's Republic of China

Library of Congress Cataloging-in-Publication Data

Boerner, Scott L.
  Biopsy interpretation of the thyroid / Scott L. Boerner, Sylvia L. Asa.
      p. ; cm. — (Biopsy interpretation series)
  Includes bibliographical references and index.
  ISBN 978-0-7817-7204-4 (alk. paper)
  1. Thyroid gland—Biopsy.   I. Asa, Sylvia L., 1953-   II. Title.
III. Series: Biopsy interpretation series.
  [DNLM: 1. Thyroid Neoplasms—diagnosis.   2. Thyroid
Neoplasms—pathology.   3. Biopsy.   4. Diagnosis, Differential.   WK 270
B671b 2010]
  RC655.49.B64 2010
  616.4'40758—dc22

                                                        2009023157

Care has been taken to confirm the accuracy of the information presented and to describe generally accepted practices. However, the authors, editors, and publisher are not responsible for errors or omissions or for any consequences from application of the information in this book and make no warranty, expressed or implied, with respect to the currency, completeness, or accuracy of the contents of the publication. Application of the information in a particular situation remains the professional responsibility of the practitioner.

The authors, editors, and publisher have exerted every effort to ensure that drug selection and dosage set forth in this text are in accordance with current recommendations and practice at the time of publication. However, in view of ongoing research, changes in government regulations, and the constant flow of information relating to drug therapy and drug reactions, the reader is urged to check the package insert for each drug for any change in indications and dosage and for added warnings and precautions. This is particularly important when the recommended agent is a new or infrequently employed drug.

Some drugs and medical devices presented in the publication have Food and Drug Administration (FDA) clearance for limited use in restricted research settings. It is the responsibility of the health care provider to ascertain the FDA status of each drug or device planned for use in their clinical practice.

To purchase additional copies of this book, call our customer service department at (800) 638-3030 or fax orders to (301) 223-2320. International customers should call (301) 223-2300.

Visit Lippincott Williams & Wilkins on the Internet: at LWW.com. Lippincott Williams & Wilkins customer service representatives are available from 8:30 am to 6 pm, EST.

10 9 8 7 6 5 4 3 2

RRS1003

CONTENTS

PREFACE

The thyroid gland is a site of frequent and common pathological processes that result in clinical manifestations. Because of its location in the anterior neck, pathological processes that result in glandular enlargement create masses than can be palpable or even visually conspicuous. The functional effects of hormone hyper- or hyposecretion create clinical scenarios that prompt investigation. The increasing application of ultrasound as a noninvasive, office-based, low-risk technique has increased the prevalence of clinically detected thyroid lesions. Moreover, thyroid cancer is one of the few malignancies that is increasing in incidence. For all of these reasons, the interpretation of thyroid biopsies is becoming an increasingly important and complex area of diagnostic pathology.

In this text, we review the classification of thyroid pathologies to identify the various changes that confront the diagnostic pathologist. In different practices, cytologic and histologic biopsies are performed; each has advantages and disadvantages that are reviewed. There are a number of ancillary tools that can be applied to improve the accuracy of diagnosis; these include special histologic stains, immunohistochemical localization of antigens, flow cytometric studies to classify cell types and to determine ploidy, molecular diagnostics to identify gene mutations and rearrangements, and electron microscopy. The indications and applications of these various techniques are discussed. The diagnostic approach to each morphologic pattern of disease is reviewed in detail.

We hope that the reader will find this book to be a practical and accessible educational tool to guide the practicing diagnostic pathologist through the interpretation of biopsies of thyroid that can be challenging and complex.

Scott L. Boerner, MD
Sylvia L. Asa, MD, PhD

1

INTRODUCTION TO THYROID PATHOLOGY

The thyroid gland is a butterfly-shaped gland in the anterior inferior neck. It is readily palpable and even visible in the slender patient. It is a source of common pathology. The most common problems that develop in the thyroid include the following:

- Hypothyroidism
- Hyperthyroidism
- Thyroiditis
- Goiter
- Thyroid nodules

An estimated 27 million Americans have thyroid disease, and more than half are undiagnosed. Women are at the greatest risk, developing thyroid problems seven times more often than men. A woman faces as high as a one-in-five chance of developing thyroid problems during her lifetime, a risk that increases with age and for those with a family history of thyroid problems [1,2].

The majority of patients with hypo- or hyperthyroidism have functional disease that is not the subject of biopsy. These patients are diagnosed with biochemical tests, and treated accordingly. However, knowledge of the functional status of the thyroid is critical to the correct interpretation of biopsies, since the changes that underlie the functional alterations impact on the structure of the gland.

The majority of biopsies are used to classify nodules in the gland. These may arise in the setting of nodular goiter or thyroiditis, or they may be solitary neoplasms.

Thyroid nodules are extremely common in the general population; it has been estimated that about 20% of the population has a palpable thyroid nodule and approximately 70% has a nodule that can be detected by ultrasound [3]. The prevalence of thyroid nodules is greater in women than in men, and multiple nodules are more common than solitary nodules.

The differential diagnosis of the thyroid nodule includes numerous entities, nonneoplastic and neoplastic, benign and malignant [4–7]. The pathologist has an important role to play in their evaluation through biopsy. But what exactly constitutes a "biopsy" of the thyroid? Historically, this consisted of a lobectomy or hemithyroidectomy. Certainly, a number of lobectomies and hemithyroidectomies are required for definitive classification of a thyroid nodule of clinical suspicion. However, fine needle aspiration (FNA) and needle core biopsy have taken prominent roles in the preoperative assessment of thyroid lesions prior to surgical resection. Therefore, our discussion will attempt to explore the pathological findings seen in each of these samples: FNA, needle core biopsy, and surgical resection specimens.

While some of these entities are readily diagnosed on the basis of specific features seen in a routine slide stained with conventional dyes, the morphologic evaluation of many of these lesions is fraught with controversy and diagnostic criteria are highly variable from pathologist to pathologist [8,9]. Nevertheless, histology remains the gold standard against which we measure outcomes of cytology, intraoperative consultations, molecular and other studies, and it represents the basis on which we determine patient management and the efficacy of various therapies. Unfortunately, no current morphologic criteria provide adequate information to predict outcome for many follicular nodules of thyroid. However, the diagnosis of most other lesions is accurate and plays an important role in determining appropriate management and outcome.

Advances in our understanding of the molecular basis of thyroid cancer allow more accurate characterization of specific subtypes of neoplasia and malignancy even on single cells obtained at FNA biopsy. This should further enhance the usefulness of this technique and better guide the management of patients with a thyroid nodule. The new knowledge has also provided novel targets for therapy and predictive genetic screens for patients with genetic predisposition to certain endocrine neoplasia syndromes.

REFERENCES

1. Wang C, Crapo LM. The epidemiology of thyroid disease and implications for screening. *Endocrinol Metab Clin North Am* 1997;26:189–218.
2. Vanderpump MP, Tunbridge WM, French JM, et al. The incidence of thyroid disorders in the community: a twenty-year follow-up of the Whickham Survey. *Clin Endocrinol (Oxf)* 1995;43:55–68.
3. Ezzat S, Sarti DA, Cain DR, et al. Thyroid incidentalomas. Prevalence by palpation and ultrasonography. *Arch Intern Med* 1994;154:1838–1840.
4. DeLellis RA, Lloyd RV, Heitz PU, et al. Pathology and genetics of tumours of endocrine organs. *WHO Classification of Tumours.* Lyon: IARC Press, 2004.
5. LiVolsi VA. *Surgical pathology of the thyroid.* Philadelphia: WB Saunders, 1990.
6. Murray D. The thyroid gland. In: Kovacs K, Asa SL, eds. *Functional endocrine pathology.* Boston: Blackwell Science, 1998:295–380.
7. Rosai J, Carcangiu ML, DeLellis RA. Tumors of the thyroid gland. In: *Atlas of tumor pathology.* 3rd series, fascicle 5. Washington, DC: Armed Forces Institute of Pathology, 1992.
8. Lloyd RV, Erickson LA, Casey MB, et al. Observer variation in the diagnosis of follicular variant of papillary thyroid carcinoma. *Am J Surg Pathol* 2004;28:1336–1340.
9. Elsheikh TM, Asa SL, Chan JK, et al. Interobserver and intraobserver variation among experts in the diagnosis of thyroid follicular lesions with borderline nuclear features of papillary carcinoma. *Am J Clin Pathol* 2008;130:736–744.

2

THE NORMAL THYROID

The normal adult thyroid gland weighs 16 to 25 g and is composed of two lateral lobes and an isthmus (Fig. 2.1, e-Fig. 2.1). Because it derives from an evagination of the base of the tongue and migrates down the anterior neck, there is usually a thin remnant of the track of descent known as the pyramidal lobe at the superior end of the isthmus [1]. In the normal mature gland, each lobe has a pointed superior pole and a blunt, rounded inferior pole. Each lobe measures approximately 4 cm in the superoinferior plane, 2.5 cm in the mediolateral plane, and 2 cm in the anteroposterior plane [2]. The isthmus is more variable in size; it usually measures from 1 to 2 cm mediolaterally, but can vary from 0.5 to 2 cm in the superoinferior plane. There are usually several small lymph nodes around the isthmus. The dominant node is known as the "Delphian node" because of its prophetic role in patients with thyroid cancer.

Lobules of thyroid parenchyma are composed of follicles. The lobulation is subtle but the fibroconnective tissue that defines the lobules is important to recognize (Fig. 2.2, e-Figs. 2.2–2.4), since they are lost in neoplastic proliferations and they can be accentuated in inflammatory lesions.

The follicles of the normal gland are lined by follicular epithelial cells that are heterogeneous. They are mainly cuboidal cells (Fig. 2.3, e-Figs. 2.5–2.6); the most active are columnar cells with basal nuclei and some follicles have areas of flat attenuated epithelium. The follicular cells maintain adhesion to the basement membrane surrounding the follicle. The follicles contain thyroglobulin that is usually stored as pale and homogeneous colloid. Colloid often retracts from the surrounding tissue during fixation, but when it is being actively resorbed for thyroid hormone synthesis, the proteolytic cleavage induced by the resorbing cell causes a peculiar scalloping effect (Fig. 2.4, e-Figs. 2.7–2.8).

Scattered within this parenchyma at the junction of the upper third and lower two-thirds of each lateral lobe are the C cells that produce calcitonin [3,4]. C cells are so called because they have clear cytoplasm and because they make calcitonin. These neuroendocrine cells are difficult to recognize on routine sections stained with hematoxylin and eosin but are readily identified by calcitonin immunohistochemistry (Fig. 2.5, e-Figs. 2.9–2.11). They are usually isolated as single cells within the basement

3

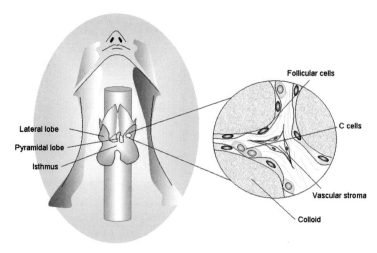

FIGURE 2.1 The normal thyroid gland. The normal gland is composed of a left and right lobe connected by an isthmus from which a variably sized pyramidal lobe may take origin. The gland itself is subdivided into ill-defined lobules by a fine fibrovascular stroma (inset and Fig. 2.2). Microscopically, the lobules are composed of follicles filled with colloid and lined by a single layer of follicular epithelial cells (inset). C cells (or parafollicular cells) are difficult to identify on routine hematoxylin and eosin staining, but lie adjacent to the basement membrane of follicles in the middle third of the right and left lobes (see Fig. 2.5). (Illustration by Sonia Cheng, University Health Network)

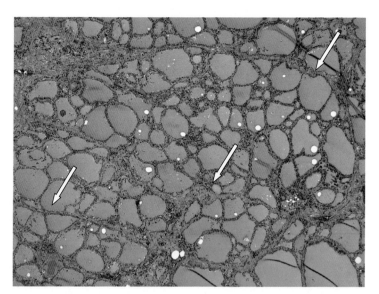

FIGURE 2.2 Normal lobular architecture of the thyroid gland. The normal thyroid gland is divided into lobules composed of variably sized follicles separated by delicate bands of fibrovascular tissue (*white arrows*). These fibrovascular septae are lost in neoplastic proliferations and are frequently exaggerated in inflammatory lesions (hematoxylin, phloxine, & saffron stain).

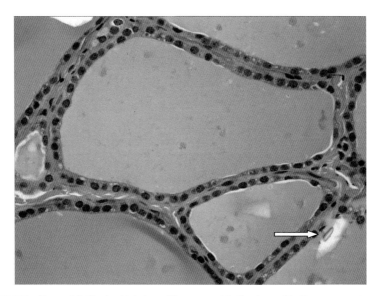

FIGURE 2.3 Normal follicular histology. The normal follicular epithelium presents as a single layer of cells closely apposed to their basement membrane with a central pool of colloid. The epithelium may have a variety of appearances. Commonly, the epithelium is seen as cuboidal cells as in this illustration, but when active, the epithelial cells are columnar with basally oriented nuclei; when atrophic, they are flattened, attenuated epithelium. Notice the presence of calcium oxalate crystals within the colloid (**white arrow**) (hematoxylin & eosin stain).

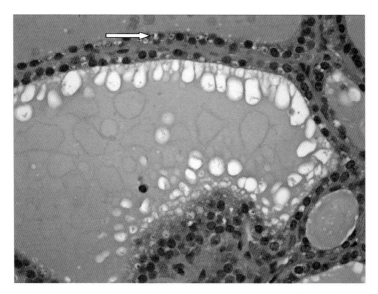

FIGURE 2.4 Scalloping of colloid. Proteolytic cleavage of the colloid by resorbing epithelial cells generates a peculiar scalloped effect on the adjacent colloid. Notice the presence of lipofuscin in the cytoplasm of a number of the epithelial cells (**white arrow**) (hematoxylin & eosin stain).

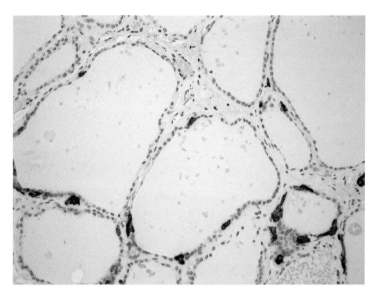

FIGURE 2.5   C cells (parafollicular cells) in the normal thyroid gland. The C cells of the normal thyroid are difficult to appreciate on routine staining. In this immunohistochemical stain for calcitonin, the C cells are highlighted and their position adjacent to the basement membrane of the follicles becomes apparent (calcitonin stain).

membrane of a follicle, but they may form a small cluster of two or three cells. They are not usually found in the isthmus or lower poles of the lobes.

Also found at the junction of the upper pole and lower two-thirds of each lobe are other vestigial remnants of the ultimobranchial body, known as "solid cell nests" or "ultimobranchial body rests" (Fig. 2.6, e-Figs. 2.12–2.14) [5–9]. These solid nests and cords are composed of polygonal, epidermoid, or transitional cells with focal cystic areas that may contain eosinophilic material. Occasionally, there is evidence of mucin production. They can be confused with papillary microcarcinomas and their importance is in recognition to avoid a false diagnosis of malignancy.

Other structures that can be found in the thyroid include parathyroid glands and tissue, normal thymus, salivary gland remnants, and occasional teratomatous elements such as cartilage. The gland is richly vascularized but only weakly innervated, mainly around vascular channels, with the exception of the recurrent laryngeal nerve that is embedded in the posterior surface of the gland.

The subject of the thyroid capsule is an important one that rarely receives attention. Surgeons often refer to the thyroid capsule when dissecting the gland and reference is made to invasion of the thyroid capsule in discussions of thyroid malignancies. However, there is no anatomical

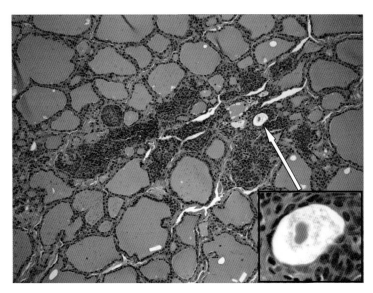

FIGURE 2.6 Solid cell nests. Solid cell nests represent vestigial remnants of the ultimobranchial body. The cells are frequently have squamoid or transitional morphology with focal cyst formation containing eosinophilic material (**white arrow** with inset). They may exhibit mucin production. It is important to distinguish these structures from microcarcinomas (hematoxylin & eosin stain).

structure that could be construed as a capsule of the gland. As indicated above, the lobules of thyroid are separated by fibroconnective tissue and this fibroconnective tissue at the periphery of the gland creates an anatomical plane for dissection. However, as evidenced by the pathology of sporadic nodular goiter, there are usually many embryological rests of thyroid tissue throughout the soft tissue of the neck, and often along the path of descent from the base of tongue to the mediastinum [10]. These are not surrounded by a capsule and are usually separate from the gland itself, disproving the hypothesis of a "thyroid capsule."

REFERENCES

1. Hoyes AD, Kershaw DR. Anatomy and development of the thyroid gland. *Ear Nose Throat J* 1985;64:318–333.
2. LiVolsi VA. *Surgical pathology of the thyroid*. Philadelphia: WB Saunders, 1990.
3. Wolfe HJ, DeLellis RA, Tashjian AH Jr. Distribution of calcitonin-containing cells in the normal adult human thyroid gland: a correlation of morphology with peptide content. *J Clin Endocrinol Metab* 1974;38:688–694.
4. DeLellis RA, Wolfe HJ. The pathobiology of the human calcitonin (C)-cell: a review. *Pathol Annu* 1981;16:25–52.
5. Janzer RC, Weber E, Hedinger C. The relation between solid cell nests and C cells of the thyroid gland. An immunohistochemical and morphometric investigation. *Cell Tissue Res* 1979;197:295–312.

6. Harach HR. Histological markers of solid cell nests of the thyroid. With some emphasis on their expression in thyroid ultimobranchial-related tumors. *Acta Anat* 1985;124: 111–116.

7. Williams ED, Toyn CE, Harach HR. The ultimobranchial gland and congenital thyroid abnormalities in man. *J Pathol* 1989;159:135–141.

8. Beckner ME, Shultz JJ, Richardson T. Solid and cystic ultimobranchial body remnants in the thyroid. *Arch Pathol Lab Med* 1990;114:1049–1052.

9. Harach HR, Vujanic GM, Jasani B. Ultimobranchial body nests in human fetal thyroid: an autopsy, histological, and immunohistochemical study in relation to solid cell nests and mucoepidermoid carcinoma of the thyroid. *J Pathol* 1993;169:465–469.

10. Spinner RJ, Moore KL, Gottfried MR, et al. Thoracic intrathymic thyroid. *Ann Surg* 1994;220:91–96.

3

CLASSIFICATION OF THYROID PATHOLOGY

The classification of thyroid pathology includes congenital, inflammatory, and neoplastic disorders. These are listed in Table 3.1. Many of these are diagnosed on the basis of clinical and biochemical features and do not require biopsy. In general, biopsy plays a key role in the diagnosis of nodular disease. However, biopsies of nodules may contain nonnodular thyroid tissue with variable pathologies.

Congenital aplasia and hypoplasia and enzymatic disorders give rise to hypothyroidism that is usually detected by screening early in life. When enzymatic deficiency results in subclinical disease and goiter ensues, the patient develops diffuse hyperplasia, known as dyshormonogenetic goiter; nodules may arise in this setting [1]. The commonest congenital lesion is the thyroglossal duct cyst that presents as a mass; this entity is discussed in Chapter 7.

Inflammatory lesions of the thyroid include infectious and autoimmune disorders. Infections give rise to acute and subacute or granulomatous inflammation. Autoimmune disease is usually characterized by a chronic lymphocytic process, but the granulomatous inflammatory process known as de Quervain's thyroiditis is thought to be of autoimmune etiology. These lesions are reviewed in Chapter 8.

Hyperplasia can be diffuse, as in compensatory goiters of patients with thyroid hormone deficiency due to any cause (congenital, endemic, or chemically induced). In areas of iodine deficiency, endemic goiter is common, but in many parts of the world this entity is disappearing due to the use of iodized salt. In places where dietary iodine is sufficient, the most common form of diffuse hyperplasia is Graves' disease, an autoimmune disorder characterized by stimulating antibodies directed at the TSH receptor. Unlike other autoimmune lesions, inflammation is scant and the disorder is mainly characterized by papillary hyperplasia; this is discussed in Chapter 9.

Sporadic nodular goiter is a common nodular proliferation of thyroid follicular epithelium. The follicular proliferations have been considered to be hyperplastic on the basis of morphologic features, but molecular studies have suggested that there may be a neoplastic component. The distinction

TABLE 3.1	Classification of Thyroid Pathology

Congenital lesions
  Aplasia
  Hypoplasia
  Enzymatic defects resulting in goiter
  Thyroglossal duct cyst and other aberrant thyroid nodules
Inflammatory lesions
  Acute
    Infections
  Granulomatous (subacute)
    Infections
    de Quervain's thyroiditis
  Chronic
    Chronic lymphocytic thyroiditis
Hyperplasia
  Diffuse
    Compensatory goiter
    Graves' disease
  Nodular
    Sporadic nodular goiter
Benign Neoplasms
  Follicular adenoma
  Intrathyroidal parathyroid adenoma
Primary Malignant Neoplasms
  Well-differentiated carcinoma of follicular epithelium
    Papillary carcinoma
    Follicular carcinoma
  Poorly differentiated carcinoma of follicular epithelium
    Insular carcinoma
    Trabecular carcinoma
  Anaplastic carcinoma
  Medullary carcinoma
  Mixed and composite follicular and medullary carcinomas
  Mucoepidermoid carcinoma
  Thymic carcinoma
  Intrathyroidal parathyroid carcinoma
  Sarcomas
  Lymphomas
Metastatic Malignancy

between hyperplasia and neoplasia is not clear and it may be that there is progression from hyperplasia to clonal adenomas. This interesting, common, and diagnostically challenging disorder is discussed in Chapter 10.

There is only one benign thyroid neoplasm recognized: the follicular adenoma. This lesion has several morphological variants; the majority with follicular patterns are discussed in Chapter 10. One variant has papillary architecture and is reviewed in Chapter 9.

The critical objective of thyroid biopsy is the diagnosis, classification, and management of malignancy. The vast majority of thyroid malignancies derive from thyroid follicular epithelium. These are the most common malignancy of endocrine organs [2–4]. Age-adjusted global incidence rates vary from 0.5 to 10 cases per 100,000 population [5]. Thyroid cancer incidence rates have steadily increased over the last decades [6]. This represents one of the most challenging biopsy diagnoses [7] and the controversies in this field are clearly important, given the fact that these cancers frequently affect patients 20 to 50 years of age, and the disease is two to four times more frequent in females than in males, giving them high impact to health-care programs and society in general as well as the affected individuals. Radiation exposure, iodide intake, lymphocytic thyroiditis, hormonal factors, and familial history are putative causative factors for thyroid carcinoma [8] and the recognition of specific mutations implicated in the various subtypes is providing novel diagnostic markers as well as targets for individualized therapies [8].

Malignancies derived from thyroid follicular epithelium are classified on the basis of their degree of differentiation as well-differentiated, poorly differentiated, or anaplastic carcinomas. Well-differentiated thyroid carcinoma includes papillary and follicular types. Although initially defined by architectural criteria, the histologic diagnosis of papillary thyroid carcinoma rests on a number of nuclear features that predict the propensity to lymphatic spread [5]. The diagnosis of this most frequent type of thyroid malignancy (85% to 90%) has been increasing, possibly due to changing recognition of morphologic nuclear criteria. On the other hand, follicular thyroid carcinoma is characterized by hematogenous spread and the frequency of its diagnosis has been declining [9]. Fortunately, these cancers have been treated with the first and, to date, the most successful form of targeted therapy—radioactive iodine. Accordingly, most well-differentiated thyroid cancers, even when already metastatic, behave in an indolent manner and have an excellent prognosis.

In marked contrast, undifferentiated thyroid carcinoma is a highly aggressive and lethal tumor [5]. The presentation is dramatic with a rapidly enlarging neck mass that invades adjacent tissues. There is currently no effective treatment and death usually ensues within 1 year. Poorly differentiated thyroid carcinomas are morphologically and behaviorally intermediate between well-differentiated and undifferentiated thyroid carcinomas [5].

The theory of sequential progression of well-differentiated thyroid carcinoma through the spectrum of poorly differentiated to undifferentiated thyroid carcinoma is supported by the presence of pre- or coexisting well-differentiated thyroid carcinoma and the common core of genetic loci with identical allelic imbalances in coexisting well-differentiated components [10,11].

Other rare malignancies arise in the thyroid gland. These include neoplasms arising from the thyroid C cells that produce calcitonin, lesions derived from other ultimobranchial tissues such as thymus and parathyroid, and malignancies derived from stromal elements. Metastases to thyroid occur in patients with disseminated malignancy. The criteria used to distinguish these various entities are discussed throughout the chapters of this book.

REFERENCES

1. Murray D. The thyroid gland. In: Kovacs K, Asa SL, eds. *Functional endocrine pathology*. Boston: Blackwell Science, 1998:295–380.
2. Hundahl SA, Fleming ID, Fremgen AM, et al. A National Cancer Data Base report on 53,856 cases of thyroid carcinoma treated in the U.S., 1985–1995 [see comments]. *Cancer* 1998;83:2638–2648.
3. Landis SH, Murray T, Bolden S, et al. Cancer statistics, 1998. *CA Cancer J Clin* 1998;48:6–29.
4. Parkin DM, Bray F, Ferlay J, et al. Global cancer statistics, 2002. *CA Cancer J Clin* 2005;55:74–108.
5. DeLellis RA, Lloyd RV, Heitz PU, et al. *Pathology and genetics of tumours of endocrine organs*. WHO Classification of Tumours. Lyons: IARC Press, 2004.
6. Liu S, Semenciw R, Ugnat AM, et al. Increasing thyroid cancer incidence in Canada, 1970–1996: time trends and age-period-cohort effects. *Br J Cancer* 2001;85:1335–1339.
7. Lloyd RV, Erickson LA, Casey MB, et al. Observer variation in the diagnosis of follicular variant of papillary thyroid carcinoma. *Am J Surg Pathol* 2004;28:1336–1340.
8. Kondo T, Ezzat S, Asa SL. Pathogenetic mechanisms in thyroid follicular-cell neoplasia. *Nat Rev Cancer* 2006;6:292–306.
9. LiVolsi VA, Asa SL. The demise of follicular carcinoma of the thyroid gland. *Thyroid* 1994;4:233–235.
10. van der Laan BFAM, Freeman JL, Tsang RW, et al. The association of well-differentiated thyroid carcinoma with insular or anaplastic thyroid carcinoma: evidence for dedifferentiation in tumor progression. *Endocr Pathol* 1993;4:215–221.
11. Hunt JL, Tometsko M, LiVolsi VA, et al. Molecular evidence of anaplastic transformation in coexisting well-differentiated and anaplastic carcinomas of the thyroid. *Am J Surg Pathol* 2003;27:1559–1564.

4

CYTOLOGIC APPROACH TO DIAGNOSIS OF THYROID PATHOLOGY

FINE NEEDLE ASPIRATION OF THE THYROID

On superficial examination, FNA appears to be an exceedingly simple procedure. The target lesion is fixed in position with one hand. Using the other hand and often a syringe holder with syringe and attached needle, the needle is inserted through the skin into the lesion. Suction is applied by drawing back on the plunger of the attached syringe and the needle is moved back and forth within the lesion. After a number of these needle strokes, the suction is released and the needle is withdrawn to distribute the collected sample for examination. This would appear to be a simple procedure. However, one of the greatest problems in fine needle aspiration (FNA) of the thyroid is that of unsatisfactory samples [1–3]. If FNA is not a difficult procedure, why are there so many unsatisfactory FNA samples of thyroid?

Although the procedure seems simple, obtaining an optimum sample requires practice and the abandonment of some myths. The predominant factor that leads to unsatisfactory FNA specimens is the misplaced belief that the suction of aspiration is responsible for collection of the sample. Moreover, reliance on large bore needles, aggressive aspiration techniques, and failure to control hemostasis in a highly vascular gland result in specimens that are either markedly hemodiluted or frankly unsatisfactory due to the failure to recover any thyroid tissue. So how does one obtain an adequate FNA of the thyroid gland?

First, it will help if the aspirator abandons the myth that it is the suction from aspiration that generates the sample. The ability to obtain an adequate specimen of the thyroid without aspiration is proof that suction is not necessary. Many publications have shown that FNA of thyroid can be performed with either aspiration or nonaspiration techniques [4–9]. Although the procedure's name, "fine needle aspiration," may perpetuate the myth that the aspiration is responsible for the generation of the sample, in fact the aspiration component of the procedure helps to retain the collected sample, potentially generating a better yield, but can actually result in the collection of a hemodiluted and unsatisfactory sample.

13

Physics dictates that with suction alone, the only material that will enter the needle is the material with the least resistance to flow. In FNA of solid organs, the materials with the least resistance to flow are tissue fluid, blood, and possibly inflammatory cell populations if present. Even with inflammatory cell populations, collection through aspiration alone will meet with limited success unless the inflammation is in the form of an abscess, since even inflammatory cells have attachment, albeit weak, to the surrounding stroma. Tissue is structured and the tissue elements are anchored in place. The only way by which tissue can be collected during FNA is to disrupt the tissue structure, thereby liberating the component elements from their surroundings and allowing them to enter into the bore of the needle.

The disruption of the tissue occurs as the sharpened beveled edge of the needle cuts through the tissue during the forward movement of the needle. A single thrust (or stroke) of the needle into the tissue dislodges a minute quantity of the tissue including both epithelial and stromal elements that is then forced into the bore of the needle. It is during the backward movement of the stroke that the suction comes into play, for a portion of the dislodged material would be lost from the needle if suction were not present upon the backward movement of the needle. The suction does not generate any sample. Actually, suction can be counterproductive. As already stated, suction will tend to draw in any fluid that is present in the aspiration bed. Blood generated by the disruption of the capillaries during the needle stroke will enter into the needle preferentially. Thus, two keys to solve the mystery of unsatisfactory FNA are revealed; there must be a minimization of bleeding and it is the strokes of the needle that will generate a good FNA sample.

Each thrust of the needle through the lesion, also referred to as a "needle stroke," generates a minute quantity of dislodged tissue fragments that are forced into the bore of the needle. It should be noted that the ease at which tissue is liberated will influence the quantity of sample collected. FNA is successful because the vast majority of lesions that we sample are predominantly epithelial in nature and these epithelial components are easily dislodged from their surroundings. In neoplastic epithelial lesions, the epithelial elements appear to be even more readily separated from their surroundings. However, stromal elements are much more difficult to dislodge and this in part explains why stromal elements are less well represented in FNA specimens than one would see in equivalent tissue sections, for example in core needle biopsies. Furthermore, lesions rich in connective tissue elements, such as sclerotic tumors, do not provide good FNA samples. The aspirator is often aware of this situation when it arises, because the lesion appears to grip the needle, making the strokes difficult to perform and feeling "gritty."

As aspiration is not necessary in order to collect the sample for FNA, a very pure sample may be obtained by simply using a needle alone without an attached syringe. One disadvantage of the needle-alone approach is that the sample collected may be so pure that the production of direct smears may be difficult due to the viscosity of the sample. However, the reason for avoidance of the needle-alone approach for FNA of thyroid lesions is the frequency of cystic lesions and those containing abundant colloid. Once the needle is first inserted into the lesion, aspiration is applied to evacuate any cystic fluid contents. If no fluid contents are present, either aspiration may be maintained and the needle strokes initiated or the aspiration may be released and then the needle strokes performed.

After multiple needle strokes, the collected material actually fills the needle bore and is forced into the hub of the needle where the sample becomes visible to the aspirator; this is referred to as the "flashback" of the sample. At this stage, the needle strokes should be terminated. If there is an immediate flashback, then it would mean that the FNA has been traumatic as the aspiration bed is now flooded with blood and the possibility of obtaining an adequate sample from that needle is very low. If this occurs, the aspiration should be stopped with pressure applied to the aspiration site in order to establish hemostasis. Hemostasis is important not only to prevent the development of a hematoma, but also to prevent contamination of the aspiration site with blood, with the hope that immediate repeat aspiration will more likely be successful.

Although any gauge of needle could be used for FNA, the principle of minimizing bleeding dictates that the smallest possible needle gauge be chosen. The optimal needle size for biopsy of a palpable lesion is 27G or 25G; the latter has the advantage of greater rigidity with less bending of the needle during the aspiration procedure. Another myth that must be dispelled is that a bigger needle is better, based perhaps on the idea that a fine gauge needle will be too small to collect tissue fragments. Although the needles are of very small caliber, they are sufficiently large to collect abundant material; intact papillary structures can be recovered from papillary carcinoma with 27G or 25G needles. Such fine needles also receive high patient acceptance and reduce discomfort, if only because of the psychological impact of telling the patient that the needle being used is much smaller than the one used to collect a blood sample. In practice, many aspirators use 21G or 22G needles that certainly can collect good quality samples, but increase bleeding and may result in marked hemodilution of the samples.

Lesion immobilization is also important for obtaining adequate FNA samples. If the lesion is able to move during the procedure, as a needle is advanced, the lesion moves away from the force so that the net movement of the needle within the lesion is reduced substantially. As the movement of the needle through the lesion is critical for obtaining the sample, if the lesion moves with the needle there is no cutting action and the effect is to blockade sample acquisition.

Multiple needle strokes are required to fill the needle bore with sample, but multiple passes are likely to be required in order to obtain sufficient tissue for evaluation and to ensure representation of the lesion cytologically. A pass is the complete process of collecting one sample with the use of one needle and multiple strokes. Each pass is repetition of the aspiration with a new needle, hopefully positioned within the lesion, but somewhat away for the site of first aspiration. The repositioning is intended to avoid the bloody field elicited by the first pass and to ensure that different portions of the lesion are sampled. Some lesions are notorious for appearing deceptively bland and benign in one focus and then definitively diagnostic in another focus. The exact number of passes required to ensure representation of the lesion is a matter of debate and will be influenced by the experience of the aspirator, the quality of sample recovered, the size and nature of the lesion, and the availability of immediate evaluation of sample quality or assessment or adequacy. Using very broad generalization, two or three passes will likely generate an adequate and representative sample under most circumstances, but five to six passes may be necessary for some lesions [10–13].

There is no question that ultrasound-guided FNA of the thyroid has allowed better visualization and needle placement into increasing smaller thyroid lesions and surrounding structures [14–17]. There is actually little difference in the overall technique whether there is direct visualization or palpation alone. It must be remembered that FNA sampling has two components, the first of which is target fixation and penetration by the needle and the second is tissue collection. Although direct visualization allows confirmation of needle placement, it does nothing to assist in sample acquisition. The best-placed needle will not collect any material of diagnostic value unless the aspiration procedure is correctly applied. "I'm in the lesion" is a battle cry of many imagers, but this is only half of the maneuver. Now the aspirator must get the lesion onto the slide for the cytologist to examine.

Cytologic Preparation and Sample Distribution

The optimum processing and slide preparation for FNA of thyroid is a matter of debate. Although there have been attempts to determine the optimum preparatory procedures, there is actually little scientific evidence to support one method over another, as all such studies suffer from interpretation bias. We learn to interpret the artifacts with which we have had to live and we choose those artifacts as the "optimum" even though they may not be so. Trying to determine which processing and slide preparation protocol is optimum is tantamount to trying to ascertain which language is optimal for expression of complex thoughts. It is evident that each person would choose their native language to communicate, and the same is true for choice of processing of FNA specimens. Combine this with the inherent problems of sample diminution that occur in any attempt to study more than one processing method in parallel, and it becomes apparent that the answer to the dilemma of optimal processing and slide preparation protocol is likely to remain elusive.

A critical aspect of this discussion is that each processing and preparatory protocol induces slightly different artifacts. Therefore, one must be cognizant of the processing artifacts found in the sample under examination and realize that the cytologic features described in a sample processed and prepared by an alternative technique may not be evident, or not as clearly evident as in the sample under consideration. For example, the incidence of nuclear grooving and intranuclear inclusion not only may vary from lesion to lesion but may also be influenced by how the sample has been prepared [18]. The optimum processing and preparatory techniques are those that result in the greatest diagnostic accuracy. As a result, each laboratory should analyze its outcomes and use the technique that yields the highest degree of accuracy that is at least comparable to, if not greater than, that of their peers and the literature. Furthermore, there is no single processing method that will encompass all variations in samples. As in other aspects of pathology, the pathologist must demonstrate a degree of flexibility and alter the processing technique chosen given the material received to optimize recovery of diagnostic information.

The preparation of direct smears, both air dried and wet fixed in alcohol, gives the greatest amount of information about background constituents and appearance, stromal fragments and their epithelial relations, and intact epithelial structures with minimization of the trauma induced on these structures. However, direct smears are interpretable only when the smears are properly prepared. Sample maldistribution, excessive obscuring blood, profound hemodilution, overly thick smearing, and improper air drying or wet fixation will ruin a sample. If direct smears cannot be properly prepared, then a liquid preparation should be employed.

To produce a good-quality direct smear, a single droplet of the FNA sample should be placed on a glass slide 3 cm from the top of the label end and in the center between the two edges. The sample droplet deposited on the glass "sample" slide should have a diameter that does not exceed 2 or 3 mm (Fig. 4.1, e-Fig. 4.1). With a sample droplet of appropriate size, the sample slide is taken up in one hand and held with the thumb on the surface of the label end with the fingers distributed along the length of the back of the slide to support the entire length (Fig. 4.1, e-Fig. 4.2). With the second hand, the center of a second "spreading" slide is brought over top of the droplet with the spreading slide perpendicular to the sample slide (Fig. 4.2, e-Fig 4.3). The spreading slide is gently lowered toward the sample slide, and when the spreading slide contacts the sample droplet, it spreads underneath the spreading slide, mainly by capillary action with very gentle pressure applied. The spreading slide is then drawn down away from the label end along the length of the sample slide, distributing the sample into an oval shape of approximately 3 cm in length without the sample reaching either side of the slide or the end of the sample slide (Fig. 4.3, e-Fig 4.4). During the smearing process, very gentle pressure is applied from the spreading slide. The sample is not to be crushed and the motion of the spreading slide should be a single direct linear stroke. If done correctly, the sample droplet should exhaust before the spreading slide reaches the end of the sample slide and the spreading slide should have

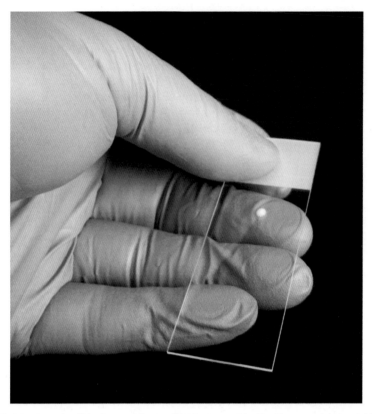

FIGURE 4.1 Sample slide for making a direct smear. Ideally, the sample should be deposited on the microscope slide 2 to 3 cm from the top of the label end and in the center between the two side edges of the slide. The sample droplet should not exceed 2 or 3 mm in maximum diameter and preferably is 1 to 2 mm. To smear the sample, the sample slide is taken up in one hand and held with the thumb on the surface of the label end with the fingers distributed along the length of the back of the slide to support the entire length of the slide.

virtually no material left on it, with all of the sample deposit onto the sample slide.

How does one generate the sample droplet of 2 to 3 mm on the sample slide from the FNA sample held within the needle bore? Prior to commencing the aspiration procedure, approximately 2 mL of air is drawn into the syringe. After the FNA strokes are completed, release of the plunger should result in the plunger returning to its starting position with approximately 2 mL of air within the syringe. This amount of the air in the syringe allows gentle pressure to be applied to the plunger, generating the force to expel a small drop of sample at the end of the needle. This can then be lightly touched to the sample slide to generate a sample of appropriate size. Since a larger quantity of material will be present in the needle bore, it is best to have multiple sample slides laid out on a tray and simply

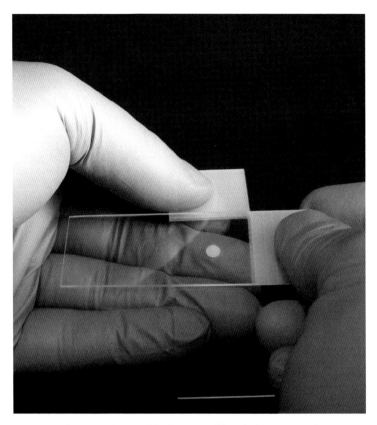

FIGURE 4.2   Smearing technique. With the second hand, the center of a second "spreading' slide is brought over top of the droplet with the spreading slide perpendicular to the sample slide. The spreading slide is gently lowered toward the sample slide and when the spreading slide contacts the sample droplet, it spreads underneath the spreading slide, mainly by capillary action with very gentle pressure applied. The spreading slide is then drawn down away from the label end along the length of the sample slide, distributing the sample into an oval shape of approximately 3 cm in length (Fig. 4.3).

touch one drop to each slide to produce a number of direct smears. Many illustrations of the aspiration procedure recommend that after completion of the aspiration, the needle be detached from the syringe and the syringe be filled with air to expel the material. This is unnecessary if the syringe is preloaded with 2 mL of air to allow expulsion of the sample. Furthermore, when the syringe is fully filled with air, which is pressurized for expulsion, this generates tremendous force behind the sample which usually results in large quantity of material being squirted onto the slide all at once and exceeding the amount that should be on the slide for direct smears. This situation is worsened if there is any clotting of the sample within the needle prior to expulsion, as greater air pressure will be generated by the aspirator in attempts to get the sample out.

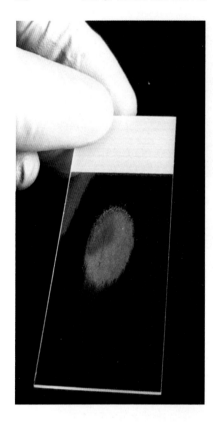

FIGURE 4.3 Direct smear slide. During the smearing process, very gentle pressure is applied from the spreading slide. The sample is not to be crushed and the motion of the spreading slide should be a single direct linear stroke. If done correctly, the sample droplet should exhaust before the spreading slide reaches the end of the sample slide and the spreading slide should have virtually no material left on it, with all the sample deposit onto the sample slide.

If in exuberance the aspirator has generated a sample droplet that is too large, the material may be redistributed to multiple slides using a "touch off" procedure. For a "touch off," the sample slide is held as if to smear the sample. A second sample slide is held as if to smear the sample. Rather than smearing, the second sample slide is brought down to contact the surface of the sample and by capillary action a small quantity of sample will be transferred or "touched off" onto the second slide (Fig. 4.4, e-Figs. 4.5–4.6). This will usually result in a sample droplet that is of appropriate size to allow smearing and "touch offs" can be performed repetitively to distribute the sample. The "touch off" slides are then smeared as previously described.

Clearly direct smearing is not applicable to samples in which a large volume of fluid sample has been collected. These samples must be processed as liquid-based preparations or centrifuged with the sediment used for direct smearing once back in the laboratory.

For air-dried smears, a Romanowsky stain is utilized. There are several variants, including Diff Quik, Hemacolor, Field's stain, and May–Grunwald–Giemsa. All of the variants have slightly different staining characteristics, but are similar in many aspects and the choice of one over another is based on personal preference, rapidity of staining, and costs.

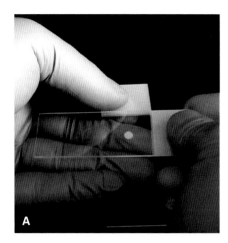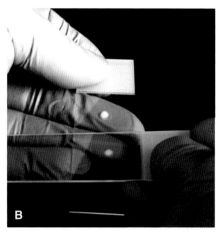

FIGURE 4.4 Producing a "touch off slide." If excessive sample is deposited on the sample slide, a "touch off" slide may be produced. A second sample slide is held as if to smear the sample. Rather than smearing, the second sample slide is brought down to contact the surface of the sample **(A)** and by capillary action, a small quantity of sample will be transferred or "touched off" onto the second slide. This will usually result in a sample droplet that is of appropriate size to allow smearing **(B)** and "touch offs" can be performed repetitively to distribute the sample. The "touch off" slides are then smeared.

Wet fixation can be combined with immediate erythrolysis using a modified Carnoy's solution, a combination of 95% ethanol in varying ratios with a small amount of glacial acetic acid. The acetic acid is an effective erythrolytic agent for unaltered red blood cells introduced into the sample during acquisition, but does not destroy old erythrocytes that are indicative of previous hemorrhage. There are variations on wet fixation with some preferring spray fixative and some preferring air drying with rehydration. Again each approach has its own artifact, and some artifacts are touted to have benefits over others. The wet-fixed direct smears are stained using a modified Papanicolaou stain, which again is quite variable from formulation to formulation and laboratory to laboratory.

Even after making direct smears, there is typically some residual sample in the bore of the needle. This is collected by inserting the needle into a fluid, drawing the fluid into the syringe, and expelling the contents into the container. The rinse procedure may be repeated to clear the sample from the needle. The entire FNA sample may also be placed into the needle rinse, particularly when a large volume of fluid is recovered. The fluid used for a needle rinse may be a balanced salt solution, tissue culture media, or fixative. The choice of the rinse solution is dictated by how the needle rinse will be used. If cytomorphologic evaluation is required, then a fixative solution may be chosen; many fixatives have the added advantage of containing an erythrolytic agent to help reduce contaminating blood. A variety of processing techniques are available to allow cytomorphologic examination of the needle rinse including cytocentrifugation, ThinPrep [18–25], direct smears from the centrifuged sentiment, filtration methods [26], and preparation of a paraffin cell block [27,28]. The variations and permutations of these techniques are too large to be detailed here and the reader is directed to the literature listed in the references for more details.

The needle rinse is a highly valuable commodity as it is the substrate upon which ancillary testing can be performed. On a basic level, a formalin-fixed paraffin-embedded cell block produced from the needle rinse can be employed for immunoperoxidase studies. As another example, the needle rinse from an FNA showing an abnormal lymphoid population may be collected into a sterile salt solution and becomes an ideal cell suspension for immunophenotyping by laser scanning or flow cytometry. Finally, the needle rinse either fresh in a salt solution or recovered from a fixative may be used for molecular analysis. It is evident, therefore, that the ideal handling of a specimen should include capture of this material.

Evaluation of a Thyroid FNA

ADEQUACY OF THE SAMPLE. In the preceding sections, we reviewed the process of obtaining and preparing an adequate specimen. The importance of this cannot be overemphasized. No matter how great the interpretive skills of the pathologist, if the sample obtained is inadequate, or has been grossly perturbed, no accurate interpretation will be possible. Thus, no discussion of interpretations can be undertaken without consideration of the determination of sample adequacy.

There are few areas in cytology that engender as much controversy as the assessment of adequacy of a thyroid FNA by pathologic criteria. Here we emphasize the qualifying statement of pathologic criteria. Unquestionably, the assessment of adequacy goes beyond the simple pathologic features that are evident on the slides. However, many situations arise where the pathologist is not the aspirator, or is unable to obtain the clinical or imaging information, and the pathologist is left with no choice but to use pathologic criteria to determine if the sample is adequate. The pathological assessment of adequacy is tremendously flawed. Every assessment of every pathologic sample begins with the determination of whether or not the sample is representative of the lesion in question. Yet, it is impossible to determine if a sample is adequate pathologically unless one can definitively diagnose a pathologic lesion and this lesion is sufficiently unique in its characteristics so that reasonable differential diagnoses can be removed from consideration. Thus, when abnormal cells are present in the sample, some degree of adequacy is assured. But when one is faced with relatively bland follicular epithelial cells, the assessment of adequacy becomes problematic. How does one determine if the benign follicular epithelium is representative of the targeted lesion and how much of this epithelium must be assessed to assure a level of clinical significance to the sample?

In general, we acknowledge that if there are no cells present in the sample (acellular), a pathologic interpretation cannot be rendered. Clearly, when there is abundant cellular material, most pathologists feel relatively confident that this lesion has likely been sampled and the interpretation is likely to be representative of the lesion. But somewhere in between, a sample is probably becoming inadequate when the cellularity is low. This is the premise behind the concept of epithelial quantitation as a means of determining sample adequacy [29]. But where this premise fails is that no one has established, nor will anyone ever be able to establish, how much epithelium is really required to assess the nature of the lesion. Furthermore, some would argue that epithelium itself is not always required to assess adequacy. For example, the identification of constituents of a cystic lesion, including proteinaceous material, possible blood, and macrophages, both regular and hemosiderin-laden, is indicative of a cystic lesion and therefore provides diagnostic information. Clearly, this is true; however, we know that cystic lesions of the thyroid may be benign or malignant. The aspiration procedure itself is often indicative of that the lesion is cystic by the recovery of some significant volume of fluid and thus the sample has been sent for pathologic evaluation not to determine if it is a cystic lesion, but to ascertain whether it is a benign cyst or a malignant cystic tumor. The distinction between these two entities depends on examination of the epithelium that lines the cystic lesion. Therefore, we are back to an evaluation of a number of epithelial cells to determine if the sample is adequate. Several definitions have been employed using different cutoff points for epithelial quantitation [10,29–33]. As none of these definitions has adequate scientific investigation or proof behind them, we leave it to the reader to review this material on their own and establish what constitutes an adequate sample. It must be remembered that epithelial quantitation will fail in a number of benign lesions such as a colloid nodule, in which it has been recommended that no minimum number of epithelial cells is required to consider a sample adequate [13].

In an effort to improve sample adequacy, many laboratories provide immediate evaluation of the sample during the time of acquisition [34–40]. This on-site assessment is achieved by the use of direct smears, most commonly air dried and Romanowsky stained or alternatively alcohol fixed with a rapid Papanicolaou stain. The presence of on-site assessment of adequacy is particularly useful with novice aspirators by providing immediate feedback on each pass to inform the aspirator which modifications in technique successfully increase sample yield and those that fail. Thus, it is not surprising that on-site assessment appears less beneficial for experienced aspirators [41].

INTERPRETATION OF EPITHELIAL STRUCTURES. The indication for aspiration of the thyroid is the presence of one or more nodules, be they palpable or detected sonographically. Statistically, the vast bulk of these nodules will be epithelial based. Therefore, it is natural that the assessment of a thyroid FNA focuses on the evaluation of epithelial structures. This is not to overlook the fact that nodules may have a variety of origins and may be composed of elements that are nonepithelial, including lymphoma and mesenchymal tumors, and they may also have deposition of amorphous material such as amyloid. However, the nonepithelial nodules are typically immediately apparent on cytologic examination and it is actually the evaluation of epithelial structures that becomes the most significant problem faced by the pathologist. The fact that most thyroid neoplasms are well differentiated complicates the evaluation of follicular epithelium, since the bulk of FNAs of the thyroid present the pathologist with relatively innocent-appearing follicular epithelial cells, even when malignant. This is in contrast to many other organs wherein the malignant cells are grotesquely abnormal in comparison to their normal counterparts. Thus, strict cytologic features of malignancy are often absent in thyroid FNA, and in many cases the classification of the lesion is based on the presence of abnormal epithelial architectural arrangements and specific nuclear alterations found in papillary carcinoma.

Those less familiar with FNA of the thyroid may think that the process of aspiration and deposition of the material on the cytologic slides eradicates any or at least most of the architectural information about the lesion. This opinion is false. The epithelial structures seen in FNAs have distinct architecture arrangements and it is the evaluation of this architecture that is paramount in the evaluation of the FNA. Epithelial architecture may be divided into five appearances seen in FNA. These include the following:

1. Monolayered sheets
2. Syncytial epithelial aggregates
3. Epithelial clusters with transgressing vessels
4. Microfollicular structures
5. Papillary structures

The most common architecture seen is that of monolayered sheets. The normal thyroid is composed of variably sized follicles, many of which are large. These macrofollicles are lined by a single layer of follicular epithelial cells and filled with colloid. These follicles are so large that they cannot be aspirated intact. The rupture of a macrofollicle during aspiration releases the colloid to form lakes of proteinaceous fluid in the background of the cytology slide and generates sheets of epithelial cells that have a single layer (Fig. 4.5, e-Figs. 4.6–4.7); thus, the term "monolayered sheets." As the follicles vary in size, and the FNA procedure disrupts these epithelial fragments into unequal fragments, the monolayered sheets are of variable size and may be large, including thousands of cells, but more typically are composed of tens to hundreds of cells. Since the supporting stroma investing the follicles and microvasculature is too fine and delicate, most of the monolayered sheets arising from macrofollicles will appear devoid of capillaries and stroma and are seen as naked sheets. Thus, one

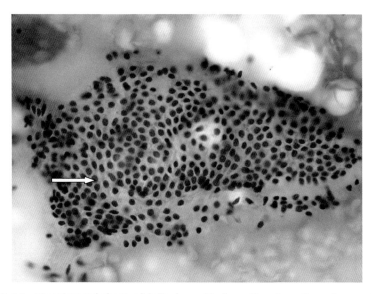

FIGURE 4.5 Monolayered sheet of follicular epithelium. The disruption of macrofollicles during the process of aspiration and slide preparation releases the colloid as a thick proteinaceous fluid seen in the background of the picture. The epithelium lining the macrofollicle is composed of a single cell layer that is deposited as a single sheet of epithelial cells on the slide. Note the wave or gully in the epithelium (*white arrow*) generated by partial folding of the sheet when the slide was smeared (direct smear, Papanicolaou stain).

interpretation of monolayered sheets in cytologic samples is that they represent a macrofollicular architecture seen in the thyroid. Unfortunately, monolayered sheets may also be seen in a neoplastic growth pattern, so simply seeing monolayered sheets is not enough, and specimens must be scrutinized for further architectural features.

When scrutinized, the monolayered sheets often preserve a honeycomb arrangement to the cells where cell boundaries can often be resolved (Fig. 4.6, e-Fig. 4.8). The resolution of the cell boundaries is important as it indicates cells of low nuclear/cytoplasmic (N/C) ratio and maintenance of an ordered arrangement to the epithelium, both features suggestive but not diagnostic of nonneoplastic thyroid. The nuclei of the sheets of macrofollicles are quite round and regular and will be evenly spaced with cytoplasm separating each nucleus, again reflecting a low N/C ratio. The chromatin pattern of these cells is fine with a small, relatively indistinct nucleolus (Fig. 4.6). It must be remembered that any sheet can be folded upon itself. A simple monolayered sheet may, in the process of aspiration and deposition on the glass slide, fold upon itself and thus appear complex by having multiple layers (Fig. 4.7, e-Fig. 4.9). Folding beyond one or two layers is relatively uncommon, and if the observer simply changes the plane of focus, it is usually quite obvious that the structure is a folded monolayered sheet by resolving the presence of

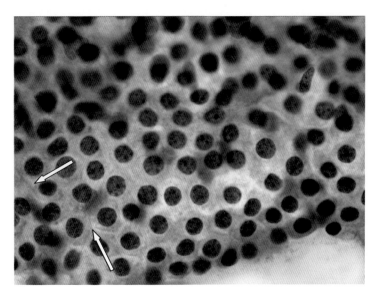

FIGURE 4.6 Honeycomb arrangement. The monolayered sheets of normal or hyperplastic thyroid maintain evenly and well-spaced nuclei allowing the cell boundaries to be partially resolved (**white arrows**) and resulting in a "honeycomb" like appearance to the epithelium. This is an important indicator of a low nuclear/cytoplasmic ratio and thus a nonneoplastic fragment of epithelium. Note the nuclei are round, regular, and contain finely granular chromatin with inconspicuous nucleoli (direct smear, Papanicolaou stain).

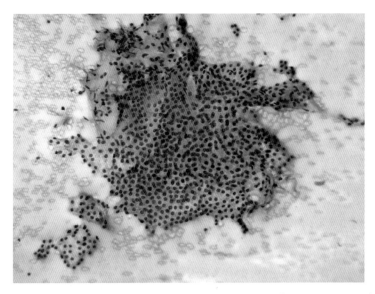

FIGURE 4.7 Folded monolayered sheets of follicular epithelium. Large monolayered sheets have a tendency to fold upon themselves. This appears to increase the complexity of the structure as multiple nuclei become superimposed upon one another and the monolayered nature of the epithelium is less evident. However, by changing the focal plane, it is possible to discern two distinct levels of nuclei and along the edge the monolayered nature of the sheet becomes indisputable (direct smear, Papanicolaou stain).

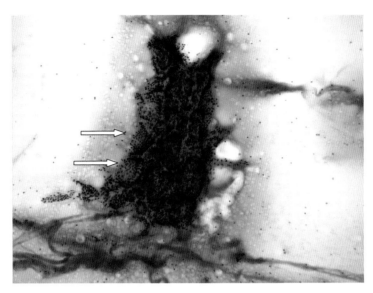

FIGURE 4.8 Macrofollicles with supporting fibrovascular stroma. Intact tissue fragments of thyroid parenchyma may be aspirated in which the macrofollicular structures are still evident and are invested by their supporting fibrovascular stroma. This may appear complex in structure and its thickness makes the evaluation of the epithelium more difficult. However, along the edge of the fragment, partially ruptured follicles are appreciated where the lining epithelium is revealed to be a simple monolayered sheet (*white arrows*) (direct smear, Papanicolaou stain).

the nuclei in distinct planes as opposed to haphazardly arranged within the mass of cytoplasm. Therefore, it is important to evaluate thicker epithelial fragments to ascertain whether or not they are structured and represent a folded monolayered sheet or if they are disordered syncytial aggregates of cells.

Occasionally, monolayered sheets may become more complex in appearance if some supporting stroma and vasculature are aspirated with the sample (Fig. 4.8, e-Fig. 4.10). The delicate fibrovascular stroma of the normal thyroid is typically inapparent in cytologic preparations. However, in hyperplastic conditions, there may be fibrosis of the intervening stroma and the vasculature may become more complex. In this situation, fibrovascular stroma may be aspirated and remained attached to the follicular epithelium. The significance of these structures is that they may be misidentified for more complex epithelial structures. It may make the monolayer sheets appear complex and may even be mistaken for the fibrovascular stalks of papillary structures. If the epithelium is examined carefully with consideration of the three-dimensional nature of the tissue, usually it can be determined that the epithelium is still simple in structure (Fig. 4.8). The thin delicate nature of the vasculature of normal or hyperplastic epithelium and the absence of blunt ends containing capillary

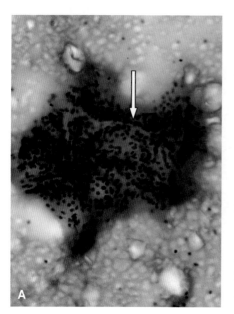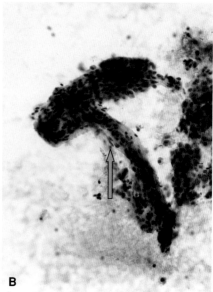

FIGURE 4.9 Comparison of benign fibrovascular stroma to a fibrovascular stalk of papillary carcinoma. The fibrovascular stroma obtained with intact fragments of benign thyroid parenchyma **(A)** is very fine with minimal surrounding fibrous tissue (***white arrow***). In contrast, the fibrovascular stroma seen in neoplasms, as typified by the denuded fibrovascular core of a papillary stalk from a papillary carcinoma **(B)**, is a heavy, thick structure noticeably larger than normal stromal vessels (***orange arrow***). Note that the papillary stalk of the papillary carcinoma comes to a blunt end where the capillaries loop upon themselves, which is again different from the sheared edges of the vessels in the benign thyroid tissue (direct smears, Papanicolaou stain).

loops can be used to separate these fibrovascular stromal elements from papillae (Fig. 4.9, e-Figs. 4.11–4.12).

Monolayered sheets are not restricted to macrofollicles. Denudation of papillae generates monolayered sheets and this is a common occurrence in the papillary variant of papillary carcinoma as a consequence of a degloving injury to papillae during the aspiration procedure (Fig. 4.10, e-Fig. 4.13). Thus, monolayered sheets are a common finding in papillary carcinoma. What distinguish the monolayered sheets of macrofollicles from those of papillary carcinoma are the nuclear alterations of papillary carcinoma. The nuclear grooves and intranuclear cytoplasmic pseudoinclusions are most obvious, but the nuclear enlargement and the resultant increased N/C ratio seen in papillary carcinoma create disorder within the monolayered sheet so that the nuclei lose their respect for one another with loss of the honeycomb arrangements and defined cell boundaries. As this disorderly conduct becomes more pronounced, epithelial fragments begin to form syncytial epithelial aggregates (Fig. 4.11, e-Fig. 4.14).

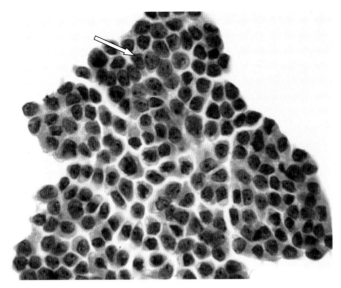

FIGURE 4.10 Monolayered sheets of papillary carcinoma. In the conventional (papillary) variant of papillary carcinoma, during the process of aspiration, the epithelium is often removed from the papillary stalks in a degloving type of injury. This epithelium presents as monolayered sheets that must be distinguished from the monolayered sheets of benign and hyperplastic thyroid. This is achieved through the recognition of the nuclear features of papillary carcinoma, such as nuclear elongation and irregular nuclear contours, altered chromatin, nuclear grooves, and intranuclear inclusions. Note the nuclear crowding and overlapping that results in distortion of the sheet architecture and loss of the cell boundaries (**white arrow**) (ThinPrep slide, Papanicolaou stain).

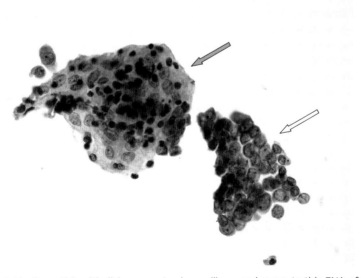

FIGURE 4.11 Syncytial epithelial aggregates in papillary carcinoma. In this FNA of a papillary carcinoma, the epithelium (**white arrow**) adjacent to the denuded papillary stalk (**orange arrow**) shows more pronounced nuclear enlargement and increased nuclear/cytoplasmic ratio. This results in a syncytial appearance of the epithelium with haphazardly distributed nuclei. In some areas, the monolayered sheetlike appearance of the epithelium may still be appreciated (ThinPrep slide, Papanicolaou stain).

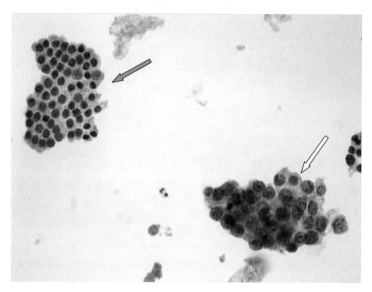

FIGURE 4.12 Comparison of monolayered sheet and syncytial aggregate. The differences between a monolayered sheet (*orange arrow*) and a syncytial aggregate or cluster (*white arrow*) become strikingly apparent when compared side by side. The monolayered sheet is flat and composed of a single cell layer in which the nuclei are arranged in an orderly manner. In contrast, the syncytial cluster is a three-dimensional mass of cells where the enlarged nuclei appear to be randomly distributed and have lost respect for each other (ThinPrep slide, Papanicolaou stain).

Syncytial aggregates are three-dimensional structures of epithelial cells in which the nuclei are disorganized and cell boundaries are difficult to discern. The nuclei in these epithelial fragments are usually enlarged and appear to overlap and crowd one another with a loss of the typical intervening cytoplasm seen in the usual monolayered sheets (Fig. 4.12, e-Fig. 4.15). This growth pattern is quite abnormal and typically seen in neoplastic conditions. However, syncytial growth patterns can be mimicked in situations where there has been substantial colloid depletion, as may occur in severe lymphocytic thyroiditis. Therefore, syncytial aggregates are not pathognomonic of neoplasia, but they should generate concern.

A form of neoplastic vascularization has been noted in Hurthle cell neoplasms. In these lesions, neovasculature can be seen in association with the clusters, sheets, and aggregates of epithelial cells. This results in an appearance appreciable on low-power magnification of capillaries amidst loosely cohesive epithelial cells [42–44] and is a good predictor of a neoplastic Hurthle cell lesion [44].

Microfollicular structures are the fourth abnormal growth pattern. Microfollicular structures are defined as acinarlike arrangements composed of 6 to 15 epithelial cells containing either a central lumen or more

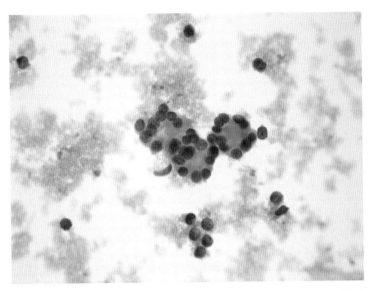

FIGURE 4.13 Microfollicular architecture. Microfollicles are three-dimensional balls of 6 to 15 follicular epithelial cells radially arranged around a small central mass of colloid or what at times may appear as a central clearing. Aspiration of intact small macrofollicles is not uncommon and finding an intact macrofollicle has little meaning. Thus, it is important to distinguish small macrofollicles from microfollicles as defined above. Similarly, the presence of a few microfollicles carries little diagnostic value. However, when microfollicles start to become a dominant architectural feature, the probability of a neoplasm increases significantly (direct smear, Papanicolaou stain).

commonly a central small mass of colloid [45] (Fig. 4.13, e-Fig. 4.16). Microfollicles occur in nonneoplastic conditions only when these conditions are seen admixed with macrofollicles. Thus, microfollicles become of diagnostic utility only when the microfollicles become a dominant form of architectural differentiation present in the sample. Any condition can generate a few microfollicles, and it would be a mistake to immediately assume that the simple identification of some microfollicles means a neoplasm is present. It should be remembered that microfollicular architecture may be seen not only in nonneoplastic conditions but also in papillary carcinoma as well as benign and malignant follicular neoplasms.

Papillary structures are the fifth epithelial architecture seen in cytologic preparations. Because of their intimate relationship to papillary carcinoma, these are discussed in Chapter 9.

COLLOID. The ratio of colloid to epithelium and the quality of the colloid identified in an aspirate has some diagnostic utility, but it is limited. In general, there is an inverse relationship between the ratio of colloid to epithelium and the likelihood of malignancy. As the colloid to epithelium ratio decreases, the possibility of a neoplasm increases. However, this relationship is imperfect and there are some neoplasms that are relatively

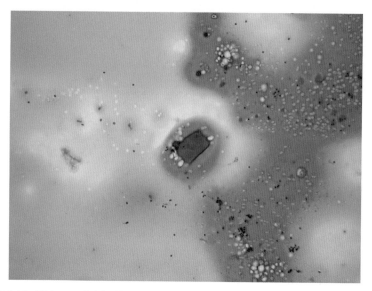

FIGURE 4.14 Watery colloid. Thin watery colloid is readily apparent on direct smears and in this example a fragment of thick, more particulate colloid is also seen. In methods of slide preparation that utilize filtration such as ThinPrep, this watery form of colloid is lost through the filter while the particulate colloid is retained, but under-represents the true colloid content of the lesion (direct smear, Papanicolaou stain).

colloid rich, such as the macrofollicular variant of papillary carcinoma that may generate substantial difficulties in interpretation on FNA in part due to its abundance of colloid [46]. Many neoplasms will be depleted of colloid, but one must be wary of the nonneoplastic conditions in which relative colloid depletion may occur.

Colloid varies substantially in its characteristics from thin watery proteinaceous material (Fig. 4.14, e-Fig. 4.17), which may be lost in processing protocols that employ filtration techniques and liquid-based preparations [18,23,47] to thick, rigid fragments of proteinaceous material that may fracture in cytologic preparations. In this form, the colloid may mimic psammoma bodies or amyloid. The absence of concentric lamination helps distinguish colloid from psammoma bodies and whereas colloid has a hyaline appearance and is angulated, sharp edged, and frequently fractured, amyloid is somewhat fuzzy or even fibrillary with round, smooth edges, and intact. Colloid when dense may also appear as strands or ropelike material that appears to be stuck on the slide and stain a dark blue on May-Grunwald-Giemsa. When seen in this form, it has been termed "chewing gum" or "bubble gum" colloid and has been associated with papillary carcinoma. However, for all of this discussion, it should be recalled that colloid provides information on the functional status of the lesion that has been aspirated and as benign lesions may be hypofunctioning

---

TABLE 4.1 Diagnostic Terminology for Thyroid FNA Proposed by the Papanicolaou Society Task Force on Standards of Practice 1996

Inadequate

Benign nonneoplastic
   Colloid nodule
   Nodular goiter
   Cystic goiter
   Thyroiditis

Cellular follicular lesion
   Favor hyperplastic (adenomatous) nodule
   Follicular neoplasm

Hurthle cell neoplasm

Malignant
   Specify

Other

Source: The Papanicolaou Society of Cytopathology Task Force on Standards of Practice. Guidelines of the Papanicolaou Society of Cytopathology for the examination of fine-needle aspiration specimens from thyroid nodules. *Diagn Cytopathol* 1996;15:84–89.

or hyperfunctioning so too may be neoplasms and colloid by itself is not sufficient to allow a classification of lesion.

NUCLEAR CHANGES. In all cytologic examinations, the recognition of neoplastic changes is dependent on identification of specific nuclear alterations. As discussed previously, most thyroid neoplasms are well differentiated and as such the nuclear changes are subtle. Although this makes the task more challenging, the recognition of neoplasia and malignancy in the thyroid is still through the detection of specific nuclear alterations. As many of the nuclear changes relate to the recognition of papillary carcinoma, these alterations will be specifically addressed in the section on papillary lesions.

FNA TERMINOLOGY AND REPORTING. Over time, there has been a variety of terminology suggested for the reporting of thyroid FNA. More recently, various recognized bodies have attempted to standardize these reporting schemes. The Papanicolaou Society task force on standards of practice produced one of the earlier standardized reporting schemes (Table 4.1) [48]. An alterative reporting system was utilized in the American Thyroid Association Guidelines Task Force for the diagnosis and management of thyroid nodules (Table 4.2) [49]. The most recent incarnation has arisen from the National Cancer Institute-sponsored Thyroid Fine Needle Aspiration State of the Science Conference (Table 4.3) [50]. All these

TABLE 4.2 Fine Needle Aspiration Terminology Used in the Management Guidelines for Patients with Thyroid Nodules and Differentiated Thyroid Cancer from the American Thyroid Association Guidelines Task Force 2006

Inadequate
Benign
Indeterminate
Suspicious for malignancy
Follicular lesion
Follicular neoplasm
Malignant

Source: Cooper DS, Doherty GM, Haugen BR, et al. Management guidelines for patients with thyroid nodules and differentiated thyroid cancer. *Thyroid* 2006;16:109–142.

terminology schemes bear significant similarities with the greatest issue arising from the "indeterminate" categories. Equally important to the FNA diagnostic category is the classification scheme of recommendations for follow-up management based on these diagnoses, which have been detailed in recent publications [51].

TABLE 4.3 Diagnostic Terminology Proposed from the National Cancer Institute Thyroid Fine Needle Aspiration State of the Science Conference 2008

Nondiagnostic (unsatisfactory)
Benign
Colloid nodule
Nodular goiter
Hyperplastic (adenomatoid) nodule
Chronic lymphocytic thyroiditis
Follicular lesion (atypia) of undetermined Significance
Neoplasm
Follicular neoplasm
Hurthle cell neoplasm
Suspicious for malignancy
Malignant
Specify

Source: Baloch ZW, LiVolsi VA, Asa SL, et al. Diagnostic terminology and morphologic criteria for cytologic diagnosis of thyroid lesions: a synopsis of the National Cancer Institute Thyroid Fine-Needle Aspiration State of the Science Conference. *Diagn Cytopathol.* 2008;36:425–437.

REFERENCES

1. Raab SS, Vrbin CM, Grzybicki DM, et al. Errors in thyroid gland fine-needle aspiration. *Am J Clin Pathol* 2006;125:873–882.
2. Berner A, Sigstad E, Pradhan M, et al. Fine-needle aspiration cytology of the thyroid gland: comparative analysis of experience at three hospitals. *Diagn Cytopathol* 2006; 34:97–100.
3. Borget I, Vielh P, Leboulleux S, et al. Assessment of the cost of fine-needle aspiration cytology as a diagnostic tool in patients with thyroid nodules. *Am J Clin Pathol* 2008;129: 763–771.
4. Santos JE, Leiman G. Nonaspiration fine needle cytology. Application of a new technique to nodular thyroid disease. *Acta Cytol* 1988;32:353–356.
5. Ciatto S, Iossa A, Cicchi P, et al. Nonaspiration fine needle cytology of thyroid tumors. *Acta Cytol* 1989;33:939.
6. Jayaram G, Gupta B. Nonaspiration fine needle cytology in diffuse and nodular thyroid lesions: a study of 220 cases. *Acta Cytol* 1991;35:789–790.
7. Rizvi SA, Husain M, Khan S, et al. A comparative study of fine needle aspiration cytology versus non-aspiration technique in thyroid lesions. *Surgeon* 2005;3:273–276.
8. Pothier DD, Narula AA. Should we apply suction during fine needle cytology of thyroid lesions? A systematic review and meta-analysis. *Ann R Coll Surg Engl* 2006;88:643–645.
9. Tublin ME, Martin JA, Rollin LJ, et al. Ultrasound-guided fine-needle aspiration versus fine-needle capillary sampling biopsy of thyroid nodules: does technique matter? *J Ultrasound Med* 2007;26:1697–1701.
10. Hamburger JI, Husain M. Semiquantitative criteria for fine-needle biopsy diagnosis: reduced false-negative diagnoses. *Diagn Cytopathol* 1988;4:14–17.
11. Hamburger JI, Husain M, Nishiyama R, et al. Increasing the accuracy of fine-needle biopsy for thyroid nodules. *Arch Pathol Lab Med* 1989;113:1035–1041.
12. Redman R, Zalaznick H, Mazzaferri EL, et al. The impact of assessing specimen adequacy and number of needle passes for fine-needle aspiration biopsy of thyroid nodules. *Thyroid* 2006;16:55–60.
13. Baloch ZW, Cibas ES, Clark DP, et al. The National Cancer Institute Thyroid fine needle aspiration state of the science conference: a summation. *Cytojournal* 2008;5:6.
14. Cai XJ, Valiyaparambath N, Nixon P, et al. Ultrasound-guided fine needle aspiration cytology in the diagnosis and management of thyroid nodules. *Cytopathology* 2006;17: 251–256.
15. Cesur M, Corapcioglu D, Bulut S, et al. Comparison of palpation-guided fine-needle aspiration biopsy to ultrasound-guided fine-needle aspiration biopsy in the evaluation of thyroid nodules. *Thyroid* 2006;16:555–561.
16. Izquierdo R, Arekat MR, Knudson PE, et al. Comparison of palpation-guided versus ultrasound-guided fine-needle aspiration biopsies of thyroid nodules in an outpatient endocrinology practice. *Endocr Pract* 2006;12:609–614.
17. Mehrotra P, Viswanathan H, Johnson SJ, et al. Ultrasound guidance improves the adequacy of our preoperative thyroid cytology but not its accuracy. *Cytopathology* 2006;17:137–144.
18. Afify AM, Liu J, Al Khafaji BM. Cytologic artifacts and pitfalls of thyroid fine-needle aspiration using ThinPrep: a comparative retrospective review. *Cancer* 2001;93:179–186.
19. Ford L, Rasgon BM, Hilsinger RL Jr., et al. Comparison of ThinPrep versus conventional smear cytopreparatory techniques for fine-needle aspiration specimens of head and neck masses. *Otolaryngol Head Neck Surg* 2002;126:554–561.
20. Cochand-Priollet B, Prat JJ, Polivka M, et al. Thyroid fine needle aspiration: the morphological features on ThinPrep slide preparations. Eighty cases with histological control. *Cytopathology* 2003;14:343–349.
21. Tulecke MA, Wang HH. ThinPrep for cytologic evaluation of follicular thyroid lesions: correlation with histologic findings. *Diagn Cytopathol* 2004;30:7–13.
22. Fadda G, Rossi ED, Raffaelli M, et al. Fine-needle aspiration biopsy of thyroid lesions processed by thin-layer cytology: one-year institutional experience with histologic correlation. *Thyroid* 2006;16:975–981.

23. Malle D, Valeri RM, Pazaitou-Panajiotou K, et al. Use of a thin-layer technique in thyroid fine needle aspiration. *Acta Cytol* 2006;50:23–27.

24. Hasteh F, Pang Y, Pu R, et al. Do we need more than one ThinPrep to obtain adequate cellularity in fine needle aspiration? *Diagn Cytopathol* 2007;35:740–743.

25. Stamataki M, Anninos D, Brountzos E, et al. The role of liquid-based cytology in the investigation of thyroid lesions. *Cytopathology* 2008;19:11–18.

26. Nassar A, Cohen C, Siddiqui MT. Utility of millipore filter and cell block in thyroid needle aspirates: which method is superior? *Diagn Cytopathol* 2007;35:34–38.

27. Sanchez N, Selvaggi SM. Utility of cell blocks in the diagnosis of thyroid aspirates. *Diagn Cytopathol* 2006;34:89–92.

28. Saleh HA, Hammoud J, Zakaria R, et al. Comparison of Thin-Prep and cell block preparation for the evaluation of Thyroid epithelial lesions on fine needle aspiration biopsy. *Cytojournal* 2008;5:3.

29. Michael CW, Pang Y, Pu RT, et al. Cellular adequacy for thyroid aspirates prepared by ThinPrep: how many cells are needed? *Diagn Cytopathol* 2007;35:792–797.

30. Prinz RA, O'Morchoe PJ, Barbato AL, et al. Fine needle aspiration biopsy of thyroid nodules. *Ann Surg* 1983;198:70–73.

31. Goellner JR, Gharib H, Grant CS, et al. Fine needle aspiration cytology of the thyroid, 1980 to 1986. *Acta Cytol* 1987;31:587–590.

32. los Santos ET, Keyhani-Rofagha S, Cunningham JJ, et al. Cystic thyroid nodules. The dilemma of malignant lesions. *Arch Intern Med* 1990;150:1422–1427.

33. Nguyen GK, Ginsberg J, Crockford PM. Fine-needle aspiration biopsy cytology of the thyroid. Its value and limitations in the diagnosis and management of solitary thyroid nodules. *Pathol Annu* 1991;26(Pt 1):63–91.

34. Baloch ZW, Tam D, Langer J, et al. Ultrasound-guided fine-needle aspiration biopsy of the thyroid: role of on-site assessment and multiple cytologic preparations. *Diagn Cytopathol* 2000;23:425–429.

35. Gupta PK, Baloch ZW. Intraoperative and on-site cytopathology consultation: utilization, limitations, and value. *Semin Diagn Pathol* 2002;19:227–236.

36. Nasuti JF, Gupta PK, Baloch ZW. Diagnostic value and cost-effectiveness of on-site evaluation of fine-needle aspiration specimens: review of 5,688 cases. *Diagn Cytopathol* 2002;27:1–4.

37. Eedes CR, Wang HH. Cost-effectiveness of immediate specimen adequacy assessment of thyroid fine-needle aspirations. *Am J Clin Pathol* 2004;121:64–69.

38. Ghofrani M, Beckman D, Rimm DL. The value of onsite adequacy assessment of thyroid fine-needle aspirations is a function of operator experience. *Cancer* 2006;108:110–113.

39. Redman R, Zalaznick H, Mazzaferri EL, et al. The impact of assessing specimen adequacy and number of needle passes for fine-needle aspiration biopsy of thyroid nodules. *Thyroid* 2006;16:55–60.

40. Zhu W, Michael CW. How important is on-site adequacy assessment for thyroid FNA? An evaluation of 883 cases. *Diagn Cytopathol* 2007;35:183–186.

41. Ghofrani M, Beckman D, Rimm DL. The value of onsite adequacy assessment of thyroid fine-needle aspirations is a function of operator experience. *Cancer* 2006;108:110–113.

42. Galera-Davidson H. Diagnostic problems in thyroid FNAs. *Diagn Cytopathol* 1997;17: 422–428.

43. Yang YJ, Khurana KK. Diagnostic utility of intracytoplasmic lumen and transgressing vessels in evaluation of Hurthle cell lesions by fine-needle aspiration. *Arch Pathol Lab Med* 2001;125:1031–1035.

44. Elliott DD, Pitman MB, Bloom L, et al. Fine-needle aspiration biopsy of Hurthle cell lesions of the thyroid gland: a cytomorphologic study of 139 cases with statistical analysis. *Cancer* 2006;108:102–109.

45. Renshaw AA, Wang E, Wilbur D, et al. Interobserver agreement on microfollicles in thyroid fine-needle aspirates. *Arch Pathol Lab Med* 2006;130:148–152.

46. Chung D, Ghossein RA, Lin O. Macrofollicular variant of papillary carcinoma: a potential thyroid FNA pitfall. *Diagn Cytopathol* 2007;35:560–564.

47. Biscotti CV, Hollow JA, Toddy SM, et al. ThinPrep versus conventional smear cytologic preparations in the analysis of thyroid fine-needle aspiration specimens. *Am J Clin Pathol* 1995;104:150–153.

48. Guidelines of the Papanicolaou Society of Cytopathology for the examination of fine-needle aspiration specimens from thyroid nodules. The Papanicolaou Society of Cytopathology Task Force on Standards of Practice. *Diagn Cytopathol* 1996;15:84–89.

49. Cooper DS, Doherty GM, Haugen BR, et al. Management guidelines for patients with thyroid nodules and differentiated thyroid cancer. *Thyroid* 2006;16:109–142.

50. Baloch ZW, LiVolsi VA, Asa SL, et al. Diagnostic terminology and morphologic criteria for cytologic diagnosis of thyroid lesions: a synopsis of the National Cancer Institute Thyroid Fine Needle Aspiration State of the Science Conference. *Diagn Cytopathol* 2008;36:425–437.

51. Layfield LJ, Abrams J, Cochand-Priollet B, et al. Post-thyroid FNA testing and treatment options: a synopsis of the National Cancer Institute Thyroid Fine Needle Aspiration State of the Science Conference. *Diagn Cytopathol* 2008;36:442–448.

5

HISTOLOGIC BIOPSY OF THYROID

Historically, the use of incisional biopsies and more recently the use of core needle biopsies had been advocated by some who felt that the preservation of tissue architecture was important in the evaluation of thyroid lesions. However, both incisional and core biopsy suffer from some significant drawbacks that lead us to recommend fine needle aspiration (FNA) in most instances with histologic sampling reserved for limited applications.

Currently, incisional biopsy is infrequently employed and for obvious reasons. Incisional biopsy is an open procedure with greater consumption of health-care resources. Incisional biopsy also requires entry into the same compartment that may have to be reentered for later surgery, potentially complicating the later procedure. Needless to say that the patient is left with a scar in addition to the loss of the time required for the procedure.

Needle core biopsy overcomes some of these limitations. Core biopsy is done as an outpatient, thereby reducing health-care resource consumption and is less invasive into the anterior compartment of neck than an incisional biopsy. However, needle core biopsy carries substantially greater risks than FNA and in particular the risk of hemorrhage and significant hematoma [1–4].

Both incisional biopsy and needle core biopsy are traumatic to a lesion that has been sampled and may disrupt, scar, or even infarct the lesion. This may also occur with FNA, but as FNA typically employs a smaller gauge needle, the frequency and severity of lesional injury is reduced. In most cases, lesional injury is not of major significance, but if a follicular lesion is diagnosed and requires careful evaluation of the capsule to determine malignancy, previous sampling procedures can compromise the correct interpretation of the histologic diagnosis on a subsequent surgical specimen.

Some tout the potential need for ancillary studies as necessitating a histologic sample. It should be remembered that any ancillary technique applicable to a histologic specimen can be applied to FNA specimens. For example, if immunoperoxidase staining is required, a formalin-fixed cell block preparation from a good FNA needle rinse can provide numerous fragments for interpretation.

With regards to diagnostic accuracy, studies to date have not been able to document any consistent superiority of either FNA or core needle biopsy [2,3,5]. Admittedly, the attempts to study this question have been flawed and because of inherent pathologist biases favoring certain specimen types for interpretation, it will be difficult to establish that one technique is truly superior to the other. At best, the studies suggest that both FNA and core biopsy results achieve similar diagnostic accuracy in the majority of cases. In a small minority of patients, one sampling technique will establish a diagnosis where the other will fail (FNA success while core biopsy nondiagnostic, or alternatively core biopsy diagnostic with a non-diagnostic FNA); however, this cannot be prospectively predicted in a given patient. It should be pointed out that the studies have suggested a reduction in inadequate samples when needle core biopsy is engaged [2,5,6]. It also goes without saying that the greatest diagnostic accuracy is achieved when an expert histopathologist interprets the histology and similarly the best results are achieved when the FNA is interpreted by an expert cytopathologist. Thus, the choice of core needle biopsy or FNA is occasionally determined by the preference of the individual collecting the sample, but more frequently is determined by the preference of the pathologist who interprets the sample either explicitly or implicitly.

CORE NEEDLE BIOPSY TECHNIQUE

Because of the critical anatomic structures located in the region, core needle biopsy of the thyroid is typically performed with the use of ultrasound guidance to confirm needle position and ensure that the needle throw will not cause injury to other structures and thus avoid disastrous complications. In most situations, a spring-loaded coring device is used for sample collection. As many of these devices employ a large gauge needle (anywhere from 12 to 20 gauge), local anesthesia is required for the procedure. Once anesthesia is obtained, using sterile technique a scalpel is used to introduce a small incision in the skin to allow needle penetration, followed by positioning of the needle into the lesion. Once the needle position is confirmed, the spring is triggered. In double action devices, the needle is advanced through the target lesion, thereby collecting a small core of tissue within a hollowed portion of the needle (the biopsy notch). Then an outer cutting cannula is activated, sliding over the needle to capture a core of tissue within the biopsy notch [7]. In single action devices, the needle is motionless and placed into position in the lesion and when the spring is activated, the outer cannula slides over the tissue trapped within the biopsy notch of the needle [1,8–10]. The single action device is more controlled as the needle does not moved beyond its original position and therefore somewhat safer to use in the confined anatomic compartment in which the thyroid is located. The needle is then withdrawn from the lesion and the core sample expose by retracting a protective needle sheath. The tissue is recovered from the needle either by teasing it away using a fine gauge hypodermic needle or by gently swirling the needle with the sample in a liquid collection fluid such as sterile saline or fixative. Care must be taken to minimize trauma to the core, as crush artifact is easily introduced and the cores may be disrupted or fractured into tiny pieces. Typically, the procedure yields one to three cores, which usually are of approximately 1 to 2 cm in length depending on the sampling device employed. As the procedure is more traumatic than FNA, hemostasis is essential with a period of postprocedural observation required to ensure that no significant hemorrhagic complications arise.

How to Prepare a Thyroid Biopsy for Histology

The ideal handling of a thyroid core or incisional biopsy involves careful gross examination to ensure that the small pieces are not disrupted. Core biopsies should be carefully placed on small pieces of sponge or lens paper to maintain their integrity during processing. Fixation should be in neutral buffered formalin at room temperature or, if overnight, at 4°C. Prolonged fixation is not required for small tissue cores or pieces, and they can be processed through dehydration and embedded in wax within a few hours of excision. Manipulation during embedding should be minimized, again aiming to maintain intact small cores.

Sections of paraffin-embedded tissue should be cut at 4 μm or less and mounted on glass slides. The usual routine stain is the conventional hematoxylin and eosin stain. Some pathologists prefer the use of hematoxylin–phloxine–saffron, but this is a matter of choice and habit. Additional sections can be used for special stains and immunohistochemistry; the use of charged slides is recommended for the latter. Details of the various applications are provided in further chapters.

If the clinical diagnosis requires the application of molecular tools, flow cytometry, or culture for microbial organisms, samples should be obtained prior to fixation for these studies. Paraffin-embedded tissue can be used for some molecular testing, and for the identification of infectious organisms by polymerase chain reaction (PCR) but this is suboptimal and should be used only if the diagnosis was not expected prior to histologic examination.

How to Evaluate a Histological Thyroid Biopsy

The initial evaluation of a histological biopsy of thyroid should determine the adequacy of the sample. The report should document whether thyroid tissue is included, as well as other tissues that are often sampled, such as skeletal muscle and fat.

Unlike cytologic preparations, there is no definition of adequacy for these biopsies. There are no requirements for number or length of cores or number of follicular structures to allow interpretation. Obviously, interpretation requires identification of sufficient appropriate material to render a diagnosis.

If adequate, tissue cores and incisional biopsies allow complete evaluation of lesional architecture and cytology, as discussed in the chapters that follow. However, the determination of invasion through capsules and into vascular spaces is not possible and therefore requires thorough examination of the entire lesion. For this reason, the complete evaluation of follicular lesions of thyroid requires resection of the entire lesion, usually entailing at least a lobectomy or hemithyroidectomy. Staging of thyroid cancers usually requires these definitive resections as well.

REFERENCES

1. Screaton NJ, Berman LH, Grant JW. US-guided core-needle biopsy of the thyroid gland. *Radiology* 2003;226:827–832.
2. Khoo TK, Baker CH, Hallanger-Johnson J, et al. Comparison of ultrasound-guided fine-needle aspiration biopsy with core-needle biopsy in the evaluation of thyroid nodules. *Endocr Pract* 2008;14:426–431.
3. Liu Q, Castelli M, Gattuso P, et al. Simultaneous fine-needle aspiration and core-needle biopsy of thyroid nodules. *Am Surg* 1995;61:628–632.
4. Munn JS, Castelli M, Prinz RA, et al. Needle biopsy of nodular thyroid disease. *Am Surg* 1988;54:438–443.
5. Renshaw AA, Pinnar N. Comparison of thyroid fine-needle aspiration and core needle biopsy. *Am J Clin Pathol* 2007;128:370–374.
6. Mehrotra P, Hubbard JG, Johnson SJ, et al. Ultrasound scan-guided core sampling for diagnosis versus freehand FNAC of the thyroid gland. *Surgeon* 2005;3:1–5.
7. Taki S, Kakuda K, Kakuma K, et al. Thyroid nodules: evaluation with US-guided core biopsy with an automated biopsy gun. *Radiology* 1997;202:874–877.
8. Harvey JN, Parker D, De P, et al. Sonographically guided core biopsy in the assessment of thyroid nodules. *J Clin Ultrasound* 2005;33:57–62.
9. Lieu D. Cytopathologist-performed ultrasound-guided fine-needle aspiration and core-needle biopsy: a prospective study of 500 consecutive cases. *Diagn Cytopathol* 2008;36:317–324.
10. Strauss EB, Iovino A, Upender S. Simultaneous fine-needle aspiration and core biopsy of thyroid nodules and other superficial head and neck masses using sonographic guidance. *AJR Am J Roentgenol* 2008;190:1697–1699.

6

ANCILLARY TOOLS IN THYROID DIAGNOSIS

Most thyroid tumors can be readily diagnosed using cytologic and histopathologic criteria, which allow the pathologist to distinguish benign from malignant lesions, and guarantee accurate classification of the majority of malignant tumors. However, in several situations, the pathologist is confronted with thyroid lesions in which the distinction between benign and malignant can be quite subtle, or the exact classification of malignancy is not evident on routine examination. The accuracy of diagnosis has clinical consequences and implies different modalities of treatment. On the one hand, there is the need to avoid excessive treatment and psychological discomfort to the patient. On the other hand, patients with potentially aggressive disease need to be guaranteed effective management at the initial stages of disease when it is still curable. For this reason, the approach to these challenging situations should include the application of ancillary techniques, such as immunohistochemistry, immunophenotyping, and molecular profiling, that can improve the standard morphologic assessment both in surgical specimens [1] and in cytology samples obtained by fine needle aspiration (FNA) [2].

Genetic studies have identified a process of cumulative molecular events involved in thyroid tumor initiation and progression, resulting in genomic instability and the capacity for independent cellular growth, invasion, and metastasis [3]. It seems unrealistic to expect a single tool, in the form of a magic biomarker, to be able to effectively resolve the diagnostic dilemmas in thyroid pathology. Each marker differentially expressed in tumorous and nontumorous tissues represents a snapshot of the molecular events succeeding in the tissue environment. The amount of information a single marker offers is often insufficient to understand tumor biology or to render accurate diagnosis. The use of combined immunohistochemical markers as a panel seems to be an alternative to aid some of the diagnostic challenges in surgical pathology and cytopathology of thyroid specimens [1,4–6]. Most importantly, genomic and proteomic technological approaches are being developed to introduce molecular signatures capable of separating benign from malignant thyroid tumors, and in the last group, to distinguish tumors with indolent and aggressive behavior [7–11].

The availability and application of these ancillary tools varies from laboratory to laboratory. In this section, we briefly review the technologies available. The application of individual tests is discussed in the sections that follow, where the significance of their results will clarify differential diagnosis.

IMMUNOHISTOCHEMISTRY

The application of immunohistochemistry is valuable to distinguish lesions of differing histogenesis [1]. This tool can readily determine if a lesion is epithelial or represents a lymphoma or sarcoma. Specific antibodies can identify the profile of a metastatic carcinoma, or distinguish a medullary from a follicular carcinoma. There are several antibodies that have been proposed as markers of malignancy, especially for thyroid follicular lesions of an indeterminate nature. These are discussed in detail in the sections that follow.

Immunoperoxidase staining has been optimized for most antibodies for their use on formalin-fixed, paraffin-embedded tissue with or without epitope retrieval techniques. Therefore, when working with FNA samples, any immunoperoxidase staining should be performed on material that has been collected fresh and then undergone formalin fixation with paraffin embedding as a cell block. Occasionally, this may not be possible. For example, an FNA sample may have been deposited into a commercial liquid fixative for liquid-based preparation. In the absence of alternatives, it may be possible to use this material for immunoperoxidase staining. However, if this will be employed, it is important to ensure that validation studies have shown that the results of immunoperoxidase studies performed on material handled in the manner proposed are comparable to standard formalin-fixed tissue.

CELL SURFACE IMMUNOPHENOTYPING AND PLOIDY

The pathologic evaluation of lymphoid populations is a greatly facilitated by the use of cell surface immunophenotyping by either flow cytometry or laser scanning cytometry [12]. With the use of these techniques, surface light chain restriction is demonstrable in many B-cell malignancies and a number of antigens are detectable that are difficult or impossible to detect in formalin-fixed, paraffin-embedded tissue. One limitation of cell surface immunophenotyping is the requirement for a fresh cell suspension. In this arena, FNA excels at providing superb cell suspensions and if the FNA has been performed adequately, yields tremendous cellularity. A cell suspension may also be obtained from a needle core biopsy following maceration and vigorous agitation, but the cellularity typically is far lower than that obtainable from an FNA.

Ploidy and cell cycle determinations are also possible with the use of either flow or laser scanning cytometry. Ploidy analysis was popular during the 1980s when it was thought that this gross method of DNA analysis would be both diagnostic and predictive [13–15]. However, it became apparent that benign thyroid lesions could exhibit aneuploidy [14], so the diagnostic value was not proven. Nonetheless, there are data supporting the predictive value of aneuploidy as a marker of more aggressive behavior in documented malignancies of follicular epithelial derivation [16].

MOLECULAR ANALYSIS

The progress in molecular biology of cancer has resulted in highly specific and sensitive tests that can identify cancers, provide more accurate subtyping of malignancies, and determine the appropriate use of targeted therapies. While some of these alterations result in proteomic changes that can be identified by immunohistochemistry, some require identification of changes in RNA or DNA of tumor cells. DNA is quite stable and often can be extracted from formalin-fixed, paraffin-embedded tissue. While RNA can also be obtained from these sources, it is highly dependent on careful handling and the quality is often poor. It is therefore recommended that tissue be prepared specially for these ancillary techniques.

Most commercial cytology fixatives are alcohol based and provide a suitable yield of DNA and RNA for molecular studies [6,17–19]. It is therefore recommended that thyroid aspirates be prepared with either collection of fresh sample in a sterile balanced salt solution of culture medium or have at least some material fixed in this way for ancillary studies, even if smears are used for primary diagnosis.

DNA extraction of even small sequence lengths can be performed to identify specific mutations that play a role in thyroid cancers, specifically BRAF mutations in papillary thyroid carcinomas, ras mutations in follicular lesions, and ret mutations in medullary carcinomas. Other mutations, such as β-catenin mutations in poorly differentiated carcinomas, have surrogate markers in immunohistochemical changes (e.g., nuclear translocation of this cell surface-related protein).

RNA-based evaluation using RT-PCR has been the gold standard for documentation of the ret/PTC gene rearrangements [20]. This approach has been used because of the inconsistent breakpoints within large introns that make DNA analysis unreliable. In early studies, immunohistochemical identification of ectopic ret protein in follicular epithelial cells was used as a surrogate marker of this molecular event, but the antisera and antibodies against ret have not proven to be reliable for this purpose [1].

CYTOGENETICS

Cytogenetic analysis and *in situ* hybridization are powerful tools to analyze major genetic changes such as rearrangements and chromosomal losses. The thyroid is the site of several major translocations, including the family of ret/PTC rearrangements [21] and the Pax8-PPARγ fusion [22].

These changes can be identified by PCR and sequencing, but this is a cumbersome approach. RT-PCR can be used to document expression of these fusions, but this has proven difficult due to variable expression levels. FISH-based approaches have been reported and seem to offer a reasonable alternative for morphologists [22,23].

CULTURE

In the case of potentially infective lesions, culture may be required to reach a definitive diagnosis. This is readily performed if either a portion of an FNA needle rinse into sterile balanced salt solution or a portion of the core from a needle core biopsy is used for microbiological studies.

REFERENCES

1. Fischer S, Asa SL. Application of immunohistochemistry to thyroid neoplasms. *Arch Pathol Lab Med* 2008;132:359–372.
2. Filie AC, Asa SL, Geisinger KR, et al. Utilization of ancillary studies in thyroid fine needle aspirates: a synopsis of the National Cancer Institute Thyroid Fine Needle Aspiration State of the Science Conference. *Diagn Cytopathol* 2008;36:438–441.
3. Kondo T, Ezzat S, Asa SL. Pathogenetic mechanisms in thyroid follicular-cell neoplasia. *Nat Rev Cancer* 2006;6:292–306.
4. Erickson LA, Lloyd RV. Practical markers used in the diagnosis of endocrine tumors. *Adv Anat Pathol* 2004;11:175–189.
5. Bartolazzi A, Gasbarri A, Papotti M, et al. Application of an immunodiagnostic method for improving preoperative diagnosis of nodular thyroid lesions. *Lancet* 2001;357: 1644–1650.
6. Saggiorato E, De PR, Volante M, et al. Characterization of thyroid "follicular neoplasms" in fine-needle aspiration cytological specimens using a panel of immunohistochemical markers: a proposal for clinical application. *Endocr Relat Cancer* 2005;12:305–317.
7. Barden CB, Shister KW, Zhu B, et al. Classification of follicular thyroid tumors by molecular signature: results of gene profiling. *Clin Cancer Res* 2003;9:1792–1800.
8. Finley DJ, Zhu B, Barden CB, et al. Discrimination of benign and malignant thyroid nodules by molecular profiling. *Ann Surg* 2004;240:425–436.
9. Giordano TJ, Kuick R, Thomas DG, et al. Molecular classification of papillary thyroid carcinoma: distinct BRAF, RAS, and RET/PTC mutation-specific gene expression profiles discovered by DNA microarray analysis. *Oncogene* 2005;24:6646–6656.
10. Al Brahim N, Asa SL. Papillary thyroid carcinoma: an overview. *Arch Pathol Lab Med* 2006;130:1057–1062.
11. Serra S, Asa SL. Controversies in thyroid pathology: the diagnosis of follicular neoplasms. *Endocr Pathol* 2008;19:156–165.
12. Al Za'abi AM, Geddie WB, Boerner SL. Equivalence of laser scanning cytometric and flow cytometric immunophenotyping of lymphoid lesions in cytologic samples. *Am J Clin Pathol* 2008;129:780–785.
13. Bronner MP, Clevenger CV, Edmonds PR, et al. Flow cytometric analysis of DNA content in Hurthle cell adenomas and carcinomas of the thyroid. *Am J Clin Pathol* 1988;89:764–769.
14. Joensuu H, Klemi PJ. DNA aneuploidy in adenomas of endocrine organs. *Am J Pathol* 1988;132:145–151.
15. Klemi PJ, Joensuu H, Eerola E. DNA aneuploidy in anaplastic carcinoma of the thyroid gland. *Am J Clin Pathol* 1988;89:154–159.
16. Baloch ZW, LiVolsi VA. Prognostic factors in well-differentiated follicular-derived carcinoma and medullary thyroid carcinoma. *Thyroid* 2001;11:637–645.

17. Rezk S, Khan A. Role of immunohistochemistry in the diagnosis and progression of follicular epithelium-derived thyroid carcinoma. *Appl Immunohistochem Mol Morphol* 2005;13:256–264.

18. Cheung CC, Carydis B, Ezzat S, et al. Analysis of ret/PTC gene rearrangements refines the fine needle aspiration diagnosis of thyroid cancer. *J Clin Endocrinol Metab* 2001;86: 2187–2190.

19. Salvatore G, Giannini R, Faviana P, et al. Analysis of BRAF point mutation and RET/PTC rearrangement refines the fine-needle aspiration diagnosis of papillary thyroid carcinoma. *J Clin Endocrinol Metab* 2004;89:5175–5180.

20. Sugg SL, Ezzat S, Rosen IB, et al. Distinct multiple *ret*/PTC gene rearrangements in multifocal papillary thyroid neoplasia. *J Clin Endocrinol Metab* 1998;83:4116–4122.

21. Tallini G, Asa SL. RET oncogene activation in papillary thyroid carcinoma. *Adv Anat Pathol* 2001;8:345–354.

22. Kroll TG, Sarraf P, Pecciarini L, et al. PAX8-PPARgamma1 fusion oncogene in human thyroid carcinoma. *Science* 2000;289:1357–1360.

23. Rhoden KJ, Unger K, Salvatore G, et al. RET/papillary thyroid cancer rearrangement in nonneoplastic thyrocytes: follicular cells of Hashimoto's thyroiditis share low-level recombination events with a subset of papillary carcinoma. *J Clin Endocrinol Metab* 2006;91:2414–2423.

7

CYSTIC LESIONS

SIMPLE COLLOID CYSTS AND HEMORRHAGIC CYSTS

Cystic change within nodules of the thyroid gland is easily identified on ultrasound. Large cysts become the target for fine needle aspiration (FNA) as core biopsy is not suited for sampling of these lesions. Some cysts will not have any solid component, and are typically of low clinical suspicion. However, many are ultrasonographically "complex cysts" with both cystic and solid components [1]. The cyst contents are often not of particular diagnostic value and sampling of the solid component is mandated either through evacuation of the cyst contents followed by repeat aspiration of any residual solid mass or under ultrasound guidance [2,3].

Simple colloid cysts of the thyroid are common due to excess colloid accumulation within inactive follicles. Aspiration of these cysts yields abundant colloid that is often watery in consistency and frequently lost in ThinPrep preparations, but readily apparent on direct smears (Fig. 7.1, e-Figs. 7.1–7.2). Although epithelium may be completely absent in these samples, usually some simple, bland, monolayered sheets of follicular epithelial are present and readily lead to a benign diagnosis. In the absence of follicular epithelium, but a tremendous abundance of colloid, it is accepted that a benign diagnosis can still be rendered.

Hemorrhagic cysts, sometimes referred to as "degenerate cysts" or "degenerative changes," are exceedingly common, much to the annoyance of both aspirators and pathologists alike. The majority of these hemorrhagic cysts presumably arise from ischemic involution of hyperplastic nodules due to overtaxing a tenuous vascular supply. Infarction generates a cystic cavity containing blood that undergoes lysis, leaving hemosiderin-laden macrophages and foamy macrophages with altered "old" erythrocytes that are characteristically resilient to common erythrolytic processes that readily lyze "young" circulating erythrocytes (Fig. 7.2, e-Fig. 7.3) [4]. Follicular epithelium may be identified in the aspirate of some of these lesions, but these lesions are the genesis of one of the major controversies in the realm of FNA adequacy, as follicular epithelium is frequently absent.

It should be remembered that hemorrhagic cysts may have an iatrogenic origin due to hematoma formation resulting from previous

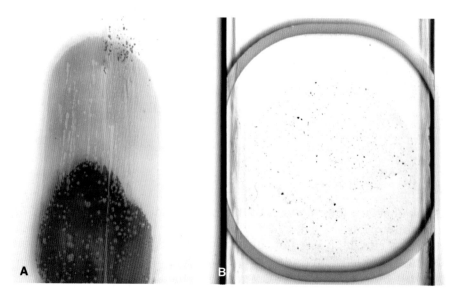

FIGURE 7.1   This photograph of a direct smear **(A)** and of a ThinPrep slide **(B)** of a colloid cyst demonstrates the abundance of colloid evident in the direct smear that is frequently depleted in the ThinPrep slide as the colloid is able to pass through the pores of the TransCyt filter (direct smear and ThinPrep, Papanicolaou stain).

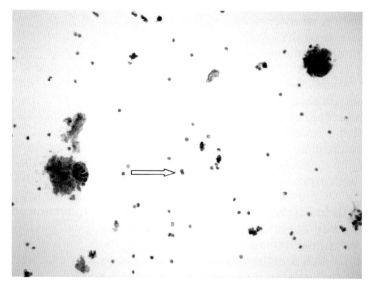

FIGURE 7.2   Fine needle aspiration of a hemorrhagic cyst of the thyroid. The aspirate usually reveals a background of proteinaceous material admixed with old erythrocytes (*white arrow*) and macrophages (both hemosiderin-laden and foamy). Erythrocytes from the blood obtained during the FNA procedure are readily lysed by the agents in most commercially available preservative/fixative solutions. However, old erythrocytes, indicative of remote hemorrhage, are resistant to most of the usual mediators of erythrolysis (ThinPrep, Papanicolaou stain).

FNA or core biopsy and can be rapidly enlarging due to the rapid expansion of a hematoma and thereby can frighten both the patient and clinician. However, the major differential diagnosis of concern with benign hemorrhagic cysts is that of a cystic papillary carcinoma [1]. Herein is the explanation of the need for follicular epithelium to evaluate the nature of the underlying lesion and the reason for the mandate to sample any solid components. Statistically, a hemorrhagic cyst is far more likely to be a benign lesion than a cystic papillary carcinoma, but to establish the diagnosis pathologically one must carefully evaluate the epithelium for the presence or absence of diagnostic features of papillary carcinoma [5] (see Chapter 9).

Hemorrhagic cysts also generate dilemmas due to the cytologic "atypia" that can be seen in the degenerative or regenerative epithelial cells [6]. Typically, these cells are large with preserved or even lowered nuclear/cytoplasmic ratio, but with large, rounded nuclei and often large nucleoli. The cells may resemble enlarged oncocytes. These cells typically form small simple flat sheets or are seen individually. It should be remembered that most thyroid carcinomas are well differentiated and these suspect cells do not fit the description of the typical culprits. Thus a degree of tolerance should be exercised when dealing with rare individual cells or small groups of these large "atypical" cells in a hemorrhagic cystic lesion.

THYROGLOSSAL DUCT CYSTS

These congenital lesions occur anywhere along the midline developmental tract of the thyroid from the base of the tongue to the mediastinum, but are frequently in the region of the hyoid bone [7]. They are identified clinically as mass lesions and are biopsied to exclude malignancy [8,9].

By FNA, these lesions are typically devoid of colloid or contain watery colloid appearing as a thin proteinaceous fluid. Cyst contents in the form of vacuolated macrophages are almost universal. In most aspirates of thyroglossal duct cysts, epithelial elements are completely lacking and no specific diagnosis can be rendered. Follicular epithelial cells are usually absent, but when present, they are in the form of simple monolayered sheets with bland nuclear morphology and when this occurs, it becomes impossible to determine, cytologically, if the thyroid gland (particularly the pyramidal lobe) or an extrathyroidal mass has been sampled. The most common epithelial elements found in FNA of thyroglossal duct cysts are squamous cells or ciliated respiratory epithelial cells. From the foregoing discussion, it is self-evident that a definitive diagnosis of thyroglossal duct cyst is not possible by cytologic features alone and it is actually a clinicopathological correlation that suggests the diagnosis.

Histologically, thyroglossal duct cysts are usually colloid-rich cysts that resemble simple cysts within thyroid parenchyma. They often arise

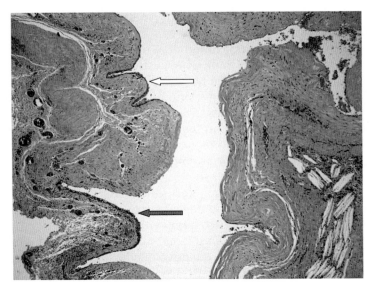

FIGURE 7.3 Thyroglossal duct cysts are typically found in the soft tissue adjacent to and occasionally involving the hyoid bone. The cyst lining is frequently denuded, but when preserved, it is composed of respiratory epithelium (*orange arrow*) (Fig. 7.4A) or squamous epithelium (*white arrow*) (Fig. 7.4B). Thyroid tissue may occasionally be identified in the wall of the cyst (Fig. 7.5). Various stigmata of degenerative changes are typically seen including cholesterol clefts with associated inflammatory reactions as is apparent in the lower right corner of this figure (hematoxylin & eosin).

within soft tissue and have only a small amount of associated thyroid parenchyma (Figs. 7.3–7.5, e-Figs. 7.4–7.8).

It is important to exclude the presence of thyroid carcinoma (most often papillary carcinoma) that can arise within a thyroglossal duct cyst [10] even as high as base of tongue [11]. To achieve this, the epithelium must be scrutinized for the diagnostic nuclear changes of papillary carcinoma whether in FNA or histology. If papillary carcinoma is confirmed in the biopsy, one may attempt to distinguish a papillary carcinoma arising within the thyroid gland from one within the thyroglossal duct or the third possibility of metastatic papillary carcinoma to a midline lymph node adjacent to the thyroid gland. Histologically, it may be impossible to determine on a needle core biopsy if the tumor is either within the thyroid gland or within thyroglossal duct cyst. However, a metastasis may be diagnosed on a core biopsy if a portion of the lymph node and, critically, its capsule are identified in the sample. If the lymph node capsule is not evident in the core biopsy and one is left with only tumor and lymphoid tissue, then the situation is identical to FNA in that the findings may be explained by a nodal metastasis, but the alternative of a lymphoid infiltrate adjacent to the tumor still in its place of origin cannot be excluded.

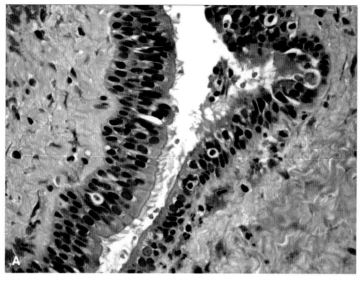

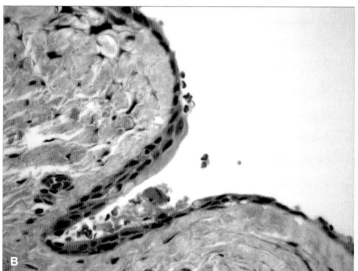

FIGURE 7.4 Epithelial lining of thyroglossal duct cysts. Ciliated respiratory epithelium **(A)** is frequently found to line thyroglossal duct cysts. Presumably, through a metaplastic process, squamous epithelium **(B)** is also common (hematoxylin & eosin stain).

BRANCHIAL CLEFTLIKE CYSTS

Lymphoepithelial cysts with histological features characteristic of branchial cleft cysts occur in the thyroid gland [12]. These cysts have a squamous epithelial lining with abundant underlying lymphoid tissue, including lymphoid aggregates with large reactive germinal centers (Figs. 7.6–7.8, e-Figs. 7.9–7.12). They are usually associated with chronic lymphocytic thyroiditis.

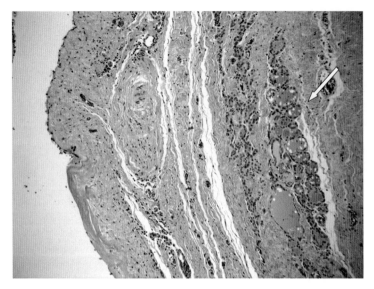

FIGURE 7.5 Thyroid tissue in a thyroglossal duct cyst. Thyroid tissue (*white arrow*) is not always identifiable in thyroglossal duct cysts and when present, the tissue is typically seen within the wall of the cyst (hematoxylin & eosin stain).

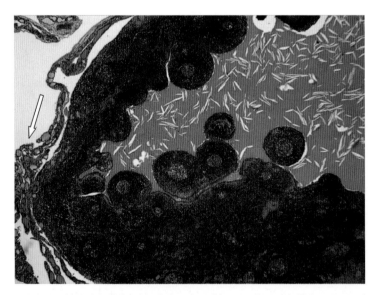

FIGURE 7.6 Lymphoepithelial cyst of the thyroid. Lymphoepithelial cysts (or branchial cleftlike cysts) occur within the thyroid gland and have the features typical of branchial cleft cysts that arise elsewhere in the neck. They are thought to originate from either the ultimobranchial body or branchial cleft derivatives and are frequently associated with autoimmune thyroiditis. In this illustration, a small amount of thyroid tissue is evident on one side (*white arrow*) (hematoxylin & eosin stain).

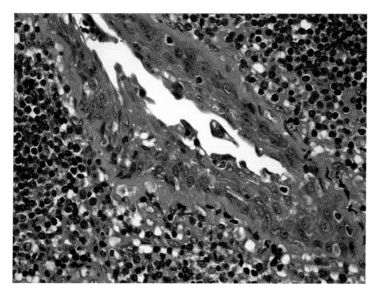

FIGURE 7.7   Lymphoepithelial cyst of the thyroid gland is lined by squamous epithelium that overlies lymphoid tissue with numerous primary and secondary follicles (hematoxylin & eosin stain).

Aspiration may yield bland squamous epithelium, but often only lymphocytes are identified [13].

Because of the histological resemblance to branchial cleft cysts, it is postulated that these lymphoepithelial cysts are branchial in origin. The

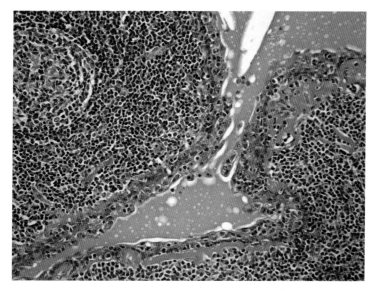

FIGURE 7.8   The epithelium of the lymphoepithelial cysts is typically infiltrated by lymphoid cells and may show foci of denudation, but a careful search will usually reveal the areas of squamous differentiation (hematoxylin & eosin stain).

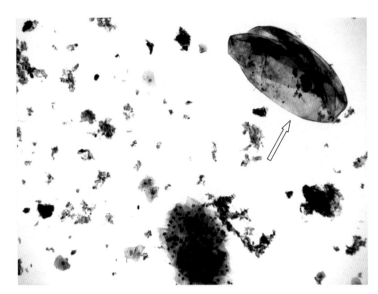

FIGURE 7.9 Paraesophageal diverticulum. Occasionally, paraesophageal diverticulum (Zenker's diverticulum) may present as a left-sided thyroid mass. Due to inflammatory reactions leading to fibrosis, these diverticula may be adherent to, and indistinguishable from, the thyroid gland on ultrasound examination. These diverticula appear as cystic lesions with mature keratinizing squamous cells on FNA and may be identified by the additional presence of bacteria and food such as vegetable matter (*white arrow*) and meat (skeletal muscle) (ThinPrep, Papanicolaou stain).

histogenesis of branchial cleft cysts is thought to be from the ultimo-branchial body, originating from branchial pouches four and/or five, which also contribute to the embryological development of the thyroid. These branchial cleftlike cysts may also arise from branchial cleft derivatives, and their enlargement may be related to the immunological mechanisms associated with autoimmune thyroiditis.

PHARYNGEAL OR ESOPHAGEAL DIVERTICULUM

Although ultrasound may be able to identify a pharyngeal or esophageal diverticulum that presents as a "thyroid" mass, occasionally the anatomic origin of these lesions is inapparent and thus becomes the subject of FNA or core biopsy [14]. In aspiration, they typically present with mature squamous cells, macrophages, variable inflammatory cells, bacteria, and food including meat and vegetable material revealing their true nature (Fig. 7.9, e-Figs. 7.13–7.14).

REFERENCES

1. Abbas G, Heller KS, Khoynezhad A, et al. The incidence of carcinoma in cytologically benign thyroid cysts. *Surgery* 2001;130:1035–1038.

2. Kini SR. *Thyroid*. New York: Igaku-Shoin Ltd., 1996.

3. Baloch ZW, LiVolsi VA, Asa SL, et al. Diagnostic terminology and morphologic criteria for cytologic diagnosis of thyroid lesions: a synopsis of the National Cancer Institute Thyroid Fine-Needle Aspiration State of the Science Conference. *Diagn Cytopathol* 2008;36:425–437.

4. Nassar A, Gupta P, LiVolsi VA, et al. Histiocytic aggregates in benign nodular goiters mimicking cytologic features of papillary thyroid carcinoma (PTC). *Diagn Cytopathol* 2003;29:243–245.

5. Bellantone R, Lombardi CP, Raffaelli M, et al. Management of cystic or predominantly cystic thyroid nodules: the role of ultrasound-guided fine-needle aspiration biopsy. *Thyroid* 2004;14:43–47.

6. Faquin WC, Cibas ES, Renshaw AA. "Atypical" cells in fine-needle aspiration biopsy specimens of benign thyroid cysts. *Cancer* 2005;105:71–79.

7. Sprinzl GM, Koebke J, Wimmers-Klick J, et al. Morphology of the human thyroglossal tract: a histologic and macroscopic study in infants and children. *Ann Otol Rhinol Laryngol* 2000;109:1135–1139.

8. Shahin A, Burroughs FH, Kirby JP, et al. Thyroglossal duct cyst: a cytopathologic study of 26 cases. *Diagn Cytopathol* 2005;33:365–369.

9. Katz AD, Hachigian M. Thyroglossal duct cysts. A thirty year experience with emphasis on occurrence in older patients. *Am J Surg* 1988;155:741–744.

10. Yang YJ, Haghir S, Wanamaker JR, et al. Diagnosis of papillary carcinoma in a thyroglossal duct cyst by fine-needle aspiration biopsy. *Arch Pathol Lab Med* 2000;124:139–142.

11. Seoane JM, Cameselle-Teijeiro J, Romero MA. Poorly differentiated oxyphilic (Hurthle cell) carcinoma arising in lingual thyroid: a case report and review of the literature. *Endocr Pathol* 2002;13:353–360.

12. Apel RL, Asa SL, Chalvardjian A, et al. Intrathyroidal lymphoepithelial cysts of probable branchial origin. *Hum Pathol* 1994;25:1238–1242.

13. Asanuma K, Nishio A, Itoh N, et al. Multiple branchial cleft-like cysts in a female patient with Hashimoto's thyroiditis. *Endocr J* 2000;47:303–307.

14. Walts AE, Braunstein G. Fine-needle aspiration of a paraesophageal diverticulum masquerading as a thyroid nodule. *Diagn Cytopathol* 2006;34:843–845.

8

INFLAMMATORY AND LYMPHOID LESIONS

ACUTE INFLAMMATION

Acute inflammation of the thyroid occurs in the setting of infection and/or trauma, after radiation, or in association with tumor necrosis. Infection is rare in economically advantaged countries, and when it does occur it is often associated with structural abnormalities including fistulas [1–4]. It is more commonly seen in impoverished areas of the world [5,6] or in immunocompromised hosts [7]. Acute inflammation often is attributed to direct extension from adjacent oropharyngeal structures, but there may also be hematogenous dissemination of systemic infection or there may be local infection associated with severe trauma. Fine needle aspiration (FNA) frequently shows acute inflammatory cells, macrophages, necrotic debris, granulation tissue vascular fragments, and rarely an identifiable infectious agent (Figs. 8.1–8.4, e-Figs. 8.1–8.8). Histologic biopsy will identify acute inflammatory cells, often with microabscess formation, necrotic debris, and evidence of vascular damage. The degree of inflammation may vary, particularly in immunocompromised hosts. The material should be stained to identify infectious organisms that may be bacterial, fungal, or viral. Cultures for microbes can be helpful and may provide important information about sensitivity to specific antibacterial or antifungal therapies.

The important differential diagnosis is anaplastic thyroid carcinoma that can have large areas of tumor necrosis that can resemble acute inflammation but is generally sterile, yielding no organisms on culture.

GRANULOMATOUS (SUBACUTE) INFLAMMATION

Granulomatous inflammation of the thyroid may occur as a result of a variety of disorders:

1. De Quervain's thyroiditis [7,8]
2. Palpation thyroiditis [9]
3. Sarcoidosis [10,11]
4. Infectious processes (mycoses, mycobacterial infection, etc.) [1]

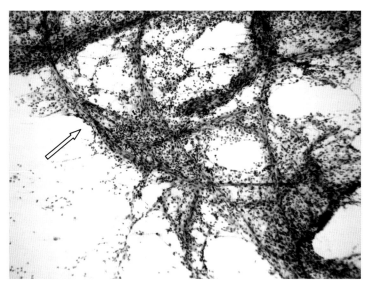

FIGURE 8.1 Fine needle aspiration of acute inflammatory lesions of the thyroid show neutrophils, macrophages, and capillary structures resembling granulation tissue (*white arrow*). Necrotic material may or may not be evident. A specific etiology is typically not apparent (direct smear, Papanicolaou stain).

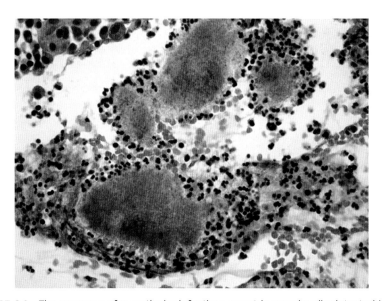

FIGURE 8.2 The presence of a particular infectious agent is occasionally detected in fine needle aspiration of acute inflammatory lesions of the thyroid such as in this case in which the "sulfur granules" characteristic of Actinomyces are evident (cell block, hematoxylin & eosin stain).

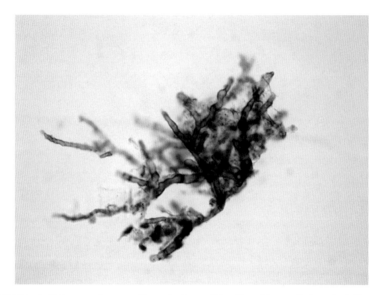

FIGURE 8.3 In this case, fine needle aspiration of the thyroid revealed acute inflammation in addition to a fungus with dichotomously branching, thick walled hyphae of a uniform diameter and regular septation, consistent with *Aspergillus* sp (ThinPrep, Papanicolaou stain).

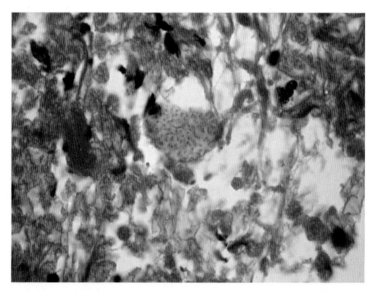

FIGURE 8.4 *Toxoplasma gondii* cysts identified in this thyroid fine needle aspiration from an immunosuppressed male, in which the background reveals acute inflammation with extensive necrosis (cell block, hematoxylin & eosin stain).

De Quervain's thyroiditis is an idiopathic, possibly autoimmune or viral, disorder also known as subacute thyroiditis or granulomatous thyroiditis. This distinct clinicopathologic entity rarely results in thyroid biopsy because of its characteristic clinical manifestations. Patients usually develop painful thyroid enlargement, typically close to 10 days following a viral infection of upper respiratory tract. There may be associated transient hyperthyroidism and associated biochemical disturbances that are attributed to rupture of thyroid follicles and release of stored thyroid hormone. This may be followed by a transient phase of hypothyroidism due to tissue damage. The disease is self-limited and resolves spontaneously.

Other forms of subacute and granulomatous inflammation include "painless" subacute thyroiditis and the focal type of granulomatous inflammation that results from palpation of the thyroid during clinical examination ("palpation thyroiditis").

Sarcoidosis may involve the thyroid gland and infections may occur that are granulomatous in nature. Fungal infections are more common in immunocompromised patients while tuberculosis is rare.

FNA reveals granulomatous inflammation admixed with follicular epithelium and a variable amount of colloid (Figs. 8.5 and 8.6, e-Figs. 8.9–8.18). Multinucleated giant cells may be seen engulfing colloid in cases of de Quervain's and palpation thyroiditis, both of which lack necrosis as does sarcoidosis. When necrosis is appreciated, the possibility of an infectious etiology should be considered and a careful search for organisms should be initiated. Unless an infectious agent is identified on routine or special staining, FNA is often not able to establish a specific definitive diagnosis and one is left with the rather generic diagnosis of "granulomatous thyroiditis."

Histologic examination may provide a more specific diagnosis by revealing the folliculocentric nature of de Quervain's thyroiditis with widespread granulomas that are centered on ruptured follicles. This contrasts with the more focal and haphazard arrangement of granulomas in infections and the interstitial positioning of granulomas in sarcoidosis. In contrast, palpation thyroiditis is also folliculocentric, but focal and usually limited to single follicles with infiltration of the colloid by macrophages (Fig. 8.7, e-Figs. 8.19–8.21).

CHRONIC INFLAMMATION

Chronic lymphocytic thyroiditis is a very common disorder. The inflammation may be diffuse or focal. It may be primary, due to autoimmune disease, or it may be secondary to infection, medication, or radiation. It should be remembered that the mere presence of lymphoid tissue does not indicate an inflammatory lesion as lymphoid tissue may be found in association with branchial cleftlike cysts, ultimobranchial body remnants, papillary carcinomas, and other malignancies that have undergone degeneration or

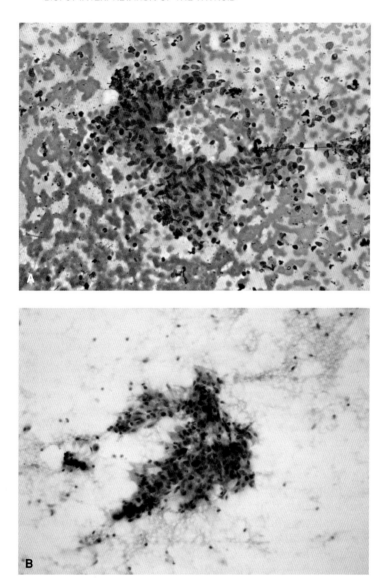

FIGURE 8.5 Granulomatous thyroiditis shows a background of mixed lymphoid cells, colloid, and fragments of bland follicular epithelium. Although numerous multinucleated giant cells are typically identified, their presence is not diagnostic of granulomatous thyroiditis. It should be recalled that papillary carcinoma may contain a plethora of multinucleated giant cells. It is the granuloma itself that identifies the process of granulomatous inflammation. Granulomas are weakly cohesive and typically fragment during aspiration and smear production. Their appearance is similar in air-dried Diff Quik-stained direct smears **(A)** and alcohol fixed, Papanicolaou-stained slides **(B)** where epithelioid histiocytes mass into a clusters of large cells with relatively abundant cytoplasm and elongate, often "carrot-shaped" nuclei (**A:** air-dried direct smear, Diff Quik stain; **B:** alcohol-fixed direct smear, Papanicolaou stain).

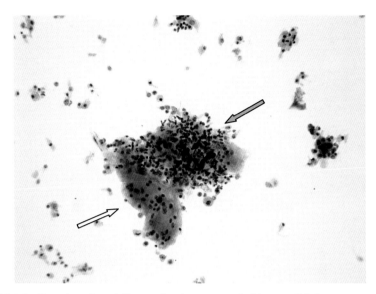

FIGURE 8.6 Granulomatous inflammation is as recognizable on a ThinPrep preparation as on direct smears, although the granulomas tend to be more ball-like and compacted. In this example, a multinucleated giant cell (*white arrow*) is seen adjacent to the granuloma (*orange arrow*) (ThinPrep, Papanicolaou stain).

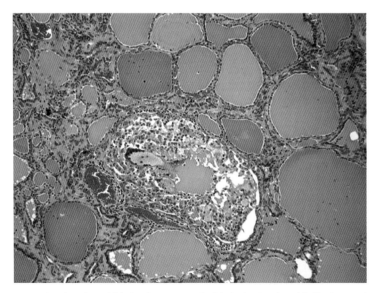

FIGURE 8.7 Palpation thyroiditis is often recognizable by its focal and folliculocentric nature. In this example, the surrounding follicles are unaffected by the granulomatous process which appears to be directed toward the colloid of the follicle (hematoxylin & eosin stain).

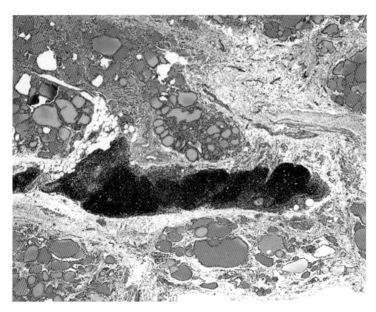

FIGURE 8.8 The presence of intrathyroidal thymic tissue may be confused with chronic inflammation of the thyroid gland. It may be encounter near solid cell nests and its thymic nature may be recognized by the presence of a lobular architecture and Hassle's corpuscles (hematoxylin & eosin stain).

necrosis. Thymic tissue within or around thyroid is a common source of difficulty, but it is usually distinguished by the presence of Hassle's corpuscles and/or other epithelioid elements (Figs. 8.8 and 8.9, e-Figs. 8.22–8.23). Therefore, the identification of chronic inflammation in a thyroid biopsy creates a complex diagnostic dilemma. The thyroid biopsy that contains chronic inflammatory cells represents one of the most difficult areas and must be carefully evaluated for the presence of associated pathologies. More importantly, the presence of inflammation in the thyroid results in reactive atypia of adjacent follicular epithelium that can result in the erroneous diagnosis of papillary thyroid carcinoma.

Autoimmune thyroiditis has been classified by many authors in various ways [9]. The commonest form is Hashimoto's thyroiditis, a well-defined clinicopathologic syndrome consisting of goiter, hypothyroidism, and lymphocytic thyroiditis that is widely accepted to be of autoimmune etiology [12,13]. Patients have antibodies to thyroglobulin and to thyroid peroxidase (formerly known as the "microsomal antigen") [14]. Some patients also have antibodies to a colloid component other than thyroglobulin ("second colloid antigen") and occasionally to thyroid hormones. Patients with this disorder are most often women with a female to male ratio of 10:1 and onset between 30 and 50 years of age. The thyroid typically becomes a diffuse, lobulated, asymmetrical, nontender goiter. Most patients with long-standing disease are hypothyroid. Occasionally,

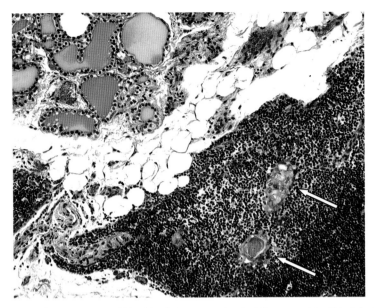

FIGURE 8.9 The presence of the Hassle's corpuscles (*white arrows*) in this intrathyroid lymphoid tissue confirms that it is ectopic thymic tissue (hematoxylin & eosin stain).

there is a transient episode of hyperthyroidism known as "Hashitoxicosis" early in the course of the disease. This has been attributed to the release of stored hormones during tissue destruction or due to stimulation by antibodies directed against the TSH receptor [14].

Other forms of autoimmune chronic lymphocytic thyroiditis include a nongoitrous variant that may be associated with variable degrees of atrophy, the juvenile variant that has a tendency to be associated with hyperplasia, painless thyroiditis with hyperthyroidism, and postpartum thyroiditis. The distinction of these different forms of chronic thyroiditis is largely based on clinical and biochemical features. There are subtle morphological differences in some of the variants, but the main differences involve the presence and degree of oncocytic change, and the presence and degree of fibrosis. In contrast to these autoimmune disorders, diffuse toxic goiter of autoimmune etiology, known as "Graves' disease," is usually associated with only mild focal inflammation, and is, therefore, not discussed in this differential diagnosis and the reader is referred to Chapter 9 (Papillary lesions) for a review of this subject.

Biopsy of the thyroid in patients with chronic lymphocytic thyroiditis usually results from the identification of a nodule. The presence of thyroid growth-stimulating immunoglobulins (TGI) in these patients and/or compensatory TSH excess due to tissue destruction and hypothyroidism have been implicated in the development of hyperplastic nodules that present as discrete masses. A nodular appearance on ultrasound of cases of lymphocytic thyroiditis may be accentuated by the difference in echotexture between portions of the gland densely infiltrated with lymphoid cells and the often fibrotic stroma, alternating with those portions of the gland that are relatively spared from inflammation and are epithelial rich.

FNA of Lymphocytic Thyroiditis

In FNA samples, the hallmark of lymphocytic thyroiditis is the presence of a significant lymphoid population. Lymphoid cells may represent one of the following four conditions:

1. Aspiration of a chronic inflammatory infiltrate in the thyroid.
2. Hemodilution of the sample with peripheral blood.
3. Aspiration of a perithyroid lymph node.
4. Aspiration of a lymphoma.

In many cases, it is a simple task to recognize the lymphocytic infiltrate as a component of lymphocytic thyroiditis. However, when the lymphoid population is more scant, it may be difficult to determine if the lymphoid cells represent an inflammatory cell population or simply lymphocytes carried into a hemodiluted sample. This can be made more difficult in samples processed by liquid-based methods such as ThinPrep that employ erythrolysis, removing the red blood cells and leaving behind the leukocytes to generate a pseudo-inflammatory infiltrate. Lymphoid cells that normally circulate in the blood are essentially small lymphocytes; therefore, to confirm a true inflammatory infiltrate, one should look for centroblasts, plasma cells, tingible body macrophages, and germinal center fragments. The finding of mast cells or a significant number of eosinophils also suggests a true inflammatory infiltrate rather than contaminating blood.

Lymphoid infiltrates are composed of very specific cells. The three lymphoid cells that are the foundation of most of inflammatory infiltrates are small lymphocytes, centrocytes, and centroblasts. The morphology of the lymphoid cells is often best appreciated on air-dried samples.

Small lymphocytes are smaller than a neutrophil and have scant cytoplasm with round, regular nuclei, dark chromatin, and lack nucleoli. Centrocytes, or small cleaved cells, are slightly larger than small lymphocytes and are characterized by cleaved nuclei containing clumped chromatin and inconspicuous nucleoli. Visualization of nuclear clefting is dependent on the orientation of the nucleus and will not be evident in all cells. Nuclear clefts are exaggerated by some degree in direct smears that are wet-fixed, as the alcohol-induced shrinkage artifact tends to accentuate the nuclear irregularities. Centroblasts, or large noncleaved cells, are large lymphoid cells with a small quantity of cytoplasm and round nuclei with a fine chromatin pattern and one to three nucleoli that are often marginalized against the nuclear membrane (Figs. 8.10–8.12, e-Figs. 8.24–8.28).

The ratio of these lymphoid cells to one another is variable and in some cases small lymphocytes may dominate, but when secondary follicular structures develop, the proportion of centrocytes and centroblasts is increased and germinal center fragments may be appreciated in the

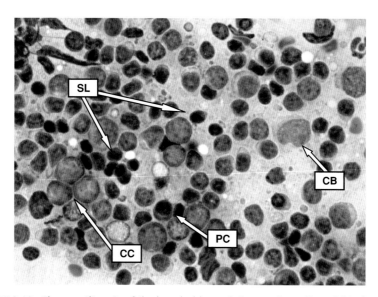

FIGURE 8.10   The constituents of the lymphoid population can be quite variable, but when the lymphoid infiltrate is well developed with follicular differentiation, four distinct lymphoid cells are apparent. These include small lymphocytes (SL), centrocytes (CC), notable due to the nuclear clefting seen as a pale line crossing the nucleus, and small indistinct nucleoli, centroblast (CB), identified as larger cells with one to three nucleoli and plasma cells (PC). The presence of mast cells as well as numerous eosinophils may be encounter in lymphocytic thyroiditis (direct smear, Diff Quik stain).

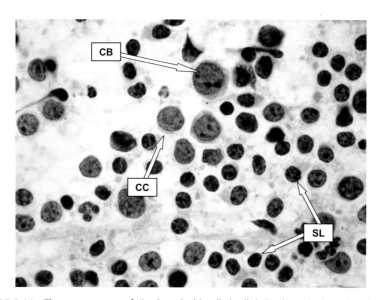

FIGURE 8.11   The appearance of the lymphoid cells is slightly altered when direct smears are wet fixed in alcohol, but the components of the lymphoid follicles are still readily apparent including small lymphocytes (SL), centrocytes (CC), and centroblast (CB) (direct smear, Papanicolaou stain).

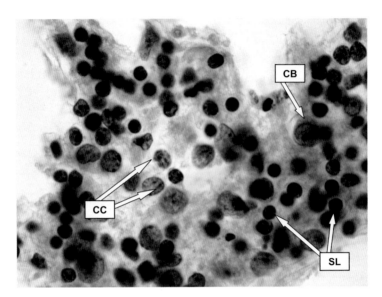

FIGURE 8.12 ThinPrep appearance of lymphoid cells in lymphocytic thyroiditis. The liquid preparation of ThinPrep without smearing causes the lymphoid cells to round up and appear smaller with less cytoplasm. In addition, there tends to be increased cell dissociation as a result of the resuspension of the sample during slide preparation. In this example, a germinal center fragment is present in which small lymphocytes (SL), centrocytes (CC), and centroblast (CB) may be seen (ThinPrep, Papanicolaou stain).

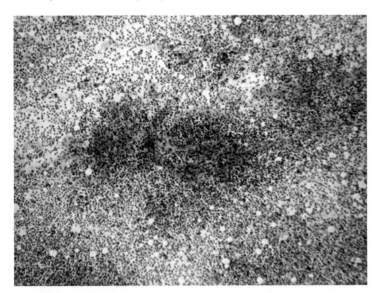

FIGURE 8.13 When the lymphoid population shows florid follicular differentiation, numerous germinal center fragments may be found. Their cohesive nature makes them apparent at low power examination, but can also lead to confusion with epithelial fragments, particularly when there is an abundance of centroblastic cells that may resemble Hürthle cells. The clues to the correct diagnosis are the identification of the other lymphoid cells (small lymphocytes and centrocytes) in addition to finding of follicular dendritic cells and tingible body macrophages (Fig. 8.14) (direct smear, Papanicolaou stain).

aspirate (Fig. 8.13, e-Fig. 8.29). The recognition of germinal center fragments is added by the identification of tingible body macrophages (Fig. 8.14A, e-Fig. 8.30) and follicular dendritic cells (Fig. 8.14B, e-Fig. 8.31), with enmeshed centroblasts and centrocytes. Plasma cells will be present in many cases and other lymphoid cells such as immunoblasts may be seen.

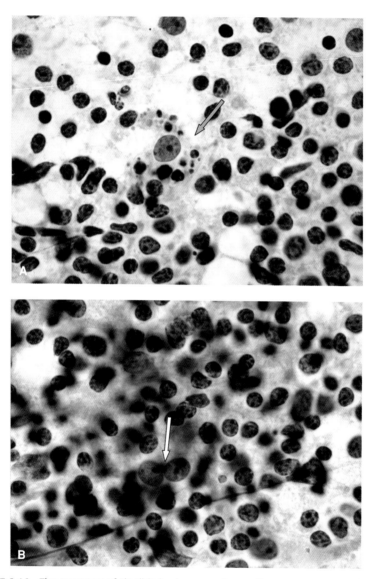

FIGURE 8.14 The presence of tingible body macrophages (**A:** *orange arrow*) and follicular dendritic cells (**B:** *white arrow*) confirm that a cohesive mass of cells is a germinal center fragment and not an epithelial cell cluster. The tingible body macrophage is identified by the presence of ingested hematophilic material (tingible bodies), whereas the follicular dendritic cells are binucleate, with each nucleus containing a well-defined central nucleolus (direct smear, Papanicolaou stain).

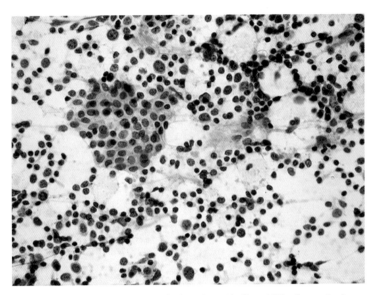

FIGURE 8.15 Bland follicular epithelium in lymphocytic thyroiditis. It may be impossible to distinguish lymphocytic thyroiditis from aspiration of a periglandular lymph node. Thus to establish the diagnosis of lymphocytic thyroiditis, thyroid epithelium or colloid (Fig. 8.17) must be identified (direct smear, Papanicolaou stain).

It can be very difficult or impossible to distinguish lymphoid tissue of a chronic inflammatory infiltrate from lymphoid tissue of a lymph node, as the component cells are the same in each. In histology, this is not a concern as the lymphoid infiltrate can be seen to be within the thyroid gland, or alternatively the architecture of the nodal tissue (cortex, medulla, sinuses, and capsule) can be identified. However, in FNA samples, these anatomic findings are lacking and, therefore, an alternative approach must be applied to distinguish an inflammatory infiltrate within the thyroid gland from aspiration of a periglandular lymph node. In fact, the primary indicator is the presence of thyroid epithelium. Thus, to diagnose lymphocytic thyroiditis, the inflammatory infiltrate must be combined with follicular epithelium (Fig. 8.15, e-Fig. 8.32). Care must be taken to ensure that germinal center fragments are not mistaken for epithelial groups (Fig. 8.16, e-Figs. 8.33–8.37). Rarely, colloid may be present in the absence of follicular epithelium and this too can serve as evidence of the needle entering the thyroid gland (Fig. 8.17, e-Fig. 8.38). However, colloid depletion is common in lymphocytic thyroiditis and it is uncommon in a FNA of lymphocytic thyroiditis to identify colloid without any epithelial cells.

The follicular epithelium seen in lymphocytic thyroiditis is often bland; however, Hashimoto's thyroiditis is one of the more commonly aspirated forms of lymphocytic thyroiditis and oncocytic cells (also known as Hürthle cells) are frequently found. It is important to note that while Hürthle cells are common in Hashimoto's thyroiditis, the presence of

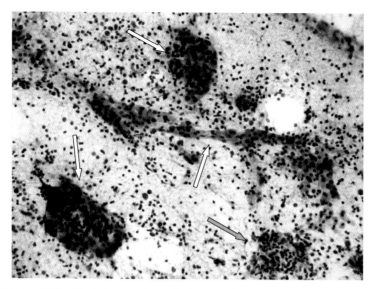

FIGURE 8.16 Epithelial clusters and germinal center fragment in lymphocytic thyroiditis. Because of their cohesiveness, germinal center fragments can be misidentified as epithelial cell clusters. This is particularly true in cases where epithelium is scarce and has not undergone Hürthle cell change. In this example, the Hürthle cell changes in the epithelium (*white arrows*) make the appearance of the epithelial cells so distinct so as to render the germinal center fragment (*orange arrow*) obvious (direct smear, Papanicolaou stain).

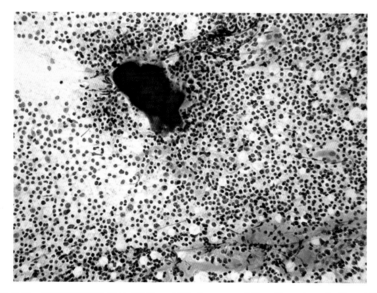

FIGURE 8.17 Colloid in lymphocytic thyroiditis. In cases of florid lymphocytic thyroiditis, the abundance of the lymphoid population may be such that finding follicular epithelium is almost impossible. In such cases, the identification of colloid acts as surrogate evidence of the inflammation occurring within the thyroid gland and not representing inadvertent aspiration of a lymph node adjacent to the thyroid gland (direct smear, Papanicolaou stain).

Hürthle cells in an FNA does not indicate Hashimoto's thyroiditis. Onco-cytes are follicular epithelial cells that have undergone a metaplastic change characterized by an increase in cytoplasm that appears more vac-uolated and granular with the granularity being a result of an increase in mitochondrial content. These mitochondria, due to their high protein con-tent, take up more eosin and, therefore, not only is the cytoplasm granular but also the granules are eosinophilic, a feature readily apparent on Pap stain material (Fig. 8.18, e-Fig. 8.39). Hürthle cells may also show signifi-cant cytoplasmic vacuolation and may begin to resemble macrophages (Fig. 8.19, e-Fig. 8.40). The nuclei of oncocytes are significantly enlarged, round, and regular with a prominent, central eosinophilic nucleolus.

The epithelium may be relatively unscathed in thyroiditis and appear as simple monolayered sheets. However, with colloid depletion, the ep-ithelium may begin to take on the architecture of syncytial aggregates. Mi-crofollicles should not be present in significant numbers and transgressing vessels should be absent. Nuclear changes can occur in both the regular follicular epithelial cells and oncocytic cells of lymphocytic thyroiditis. There is often an irregular alteration of the chromatin that appears more pale and granular. Nuclear membrane irregularities up to and including nuclear grooving is a common finding. Nucleoli increase in prominence in regular follicular epithelium and are extremely prominent in oncocytic cells (Fig. 8.20, e-Fig. 8.41). Clearly, these changes mimic to some degree

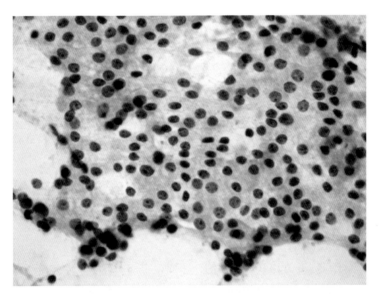

FIGURE 8.18 Hürthle cell change is very common in lymphocytic thyroiditis, but also oc-curs in hyperplasia and neoplasia. Hürthle cells are characterized by more voluminous cyto-plasm that often appears granular and vacuolated. Due to an increase in protein-rich mito-chondria, Papanicolaou staining makes the cytoplasmic "granules" appear eosinophilic and imparts an eosinophilic blush to the cytoplasm that contrasts with the typical cyanophilia of the follicular epithelial cell cytoplasm (direct smear, Papanicolaou stain).

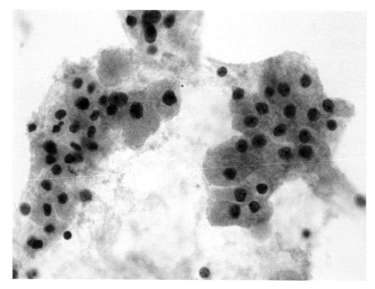

FIGURE 8.19 The cytoplasmic vacuolation that occurs in Hürthle cells may be to such a degree that the epithelial cells begin to mimic macrophages. Notice the persistence of the eosinophilic cytoplasmic granules (ThinPrep, Papanicolaou stain).

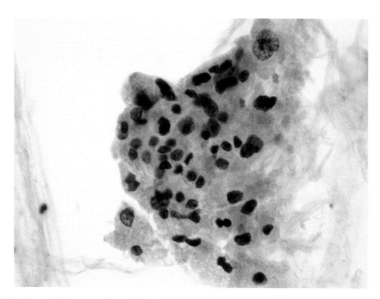

FIGURE 8.20 In typical Hürthle cell change, the nuclei are enlarged with more granular chromatin and a central, prominent, eosinophilic nucleolus. Hürthle cells often develop atypical nuclear changes as illustrated in this case where there is significant nuclear pleomorphism, more irregular angulated nuclear contours, and increased hyperchromasia (ThinPrep, Papanicolaou stain).

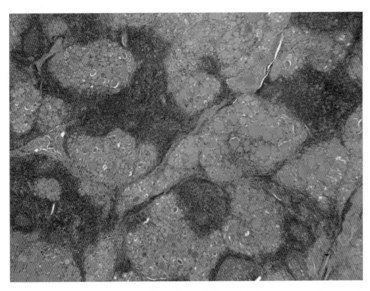

FIGURE 8.21   This low-power image of lymphocytic thyroiditis shows the demarcation of the lymphoid tissue that has infiltrated the fibrous stroma from residual epithelial islands. On a larger scale, these different tissues have differing echogenicity that may generate an ultrasound appearance suggests of nodules within the thyroid gland (hematoxylin & eosin stain).

the changes of papillary carcinoma, and in the presence of lymphocytic thyroiditis an extra degree of caution is warranted with a demand for all features of papillary carcinoma to be present before issuing a definitive diagnosis. Well-formed intranuclear inclusions are not a feature of lymphocytic thyroiditis and can be used to distinguish papillary carcinoma from thyroiditis.

Histologic Biopsy of Lymphocytic Thyroiditis

Similar to the FNA appearance of lymphocytic thyroiditis, in histologic sections, the tissue is diffusely infiltrated by a lymphoid population, including small lymphocytes, centrocytes, centroblasts, plasma cells, and occasionally immunoblasts. Lymphoid follicles may form and develop germinal centers (Figs. 8.21 and 8.22, e-Figs. 8.42–8.45).

The glandular epithelium exhibits variable degrees of damage. Residual thyroid follicles are either atrophic, with sparse colloid and flattened epithelium, or exhibit oxyphilic metaplasia [15] (Figs. 8.23 and 8.24, e-Figs. 8.46–8.48). As in FNA specimens, the follicular epithelial cells may also exhibit marked cytologic atypia that can be characterized by irregular nuclear membranes, grooves, and even clearing of nucleoplasm (Fig. 8.25, e-Figs. 8.49–8.50). These features, which in the face of inflammation are considered reactive, mimic papillary carcinoma [9,16]. Areas of squamous metaplasia may be found [17].

As the disease evolves, fibrosis becomes more conspicuous and in some patients, there is progression to the "fibrous variant" with less

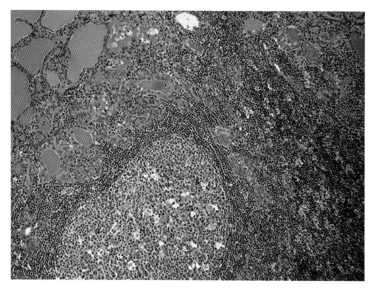

FIGURE 8.22 The histology of lymphocytic thyroid will reveal the same cellular constituents of the lymphoid population as seen in fine needle aspiration and when well-developed, lymphoid follicles will be present (hematoxylin & eosin stain).

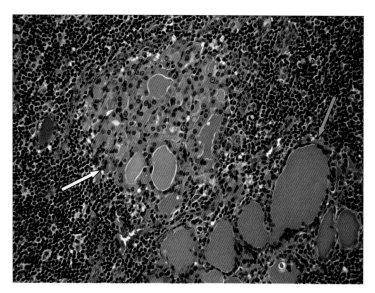

FIGURE 8.23 The epithelium undergoes a number of changes in lymphocytic thyroiditis. Epithelial atrophy (*orange arrow*) is common with flattened and attenuated epithelium and may progress to develop colloid depletion. Oncocytic (Hürthle cell) change is also common (*white arrow*). As seen in this illustration, it is frequent to have adjacent epithelium showing different alterations (hematoxylin & eosin stain).

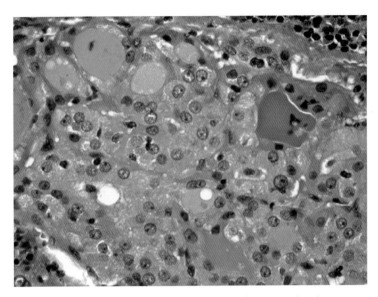

FIGURE 8.24   Oncocytic (Hürthle cell) change may be extensive in some cases of Hashimoto's thyroiditis. As in cytologic preparations, the oncocytic cells have abundant granular, eosinophilic cytoplasm as a result of increased mitochondrial content. The cytoplasmic vacuolation seen in the cytologic preparations is evident in the histology, but not commonly noted by most authors. The Hürthle cells are characterized by nuclear enlargement with prominent eosinophilic nucleoli (hematoxylin & eosin stain).

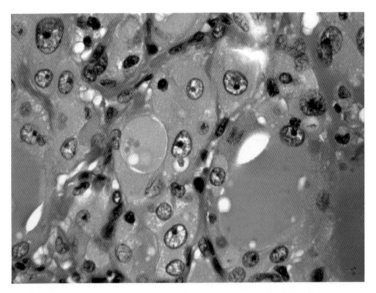

FIGURE 8.25   Nuclear abnormalities are frequent in benign Hürthle cells in Hashimoto's thyroiditis. These include nuclear pleomorphism along with alterations of the chromatin structure (particularly increased chromatin coarseness and parachromatin clearing) and increased nucleolar prominence. Nuclear membrane irregularity is frequent and it is fairly common to find nuclear grooves (hematoxylin & eosin stain).

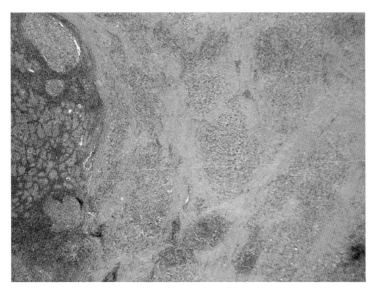

FIGURE 8.26   Pronounced fibrosis may develop in some cases of lymphocytic thyroiditis. In this low-power image, it is evident that much of the thyroid parenchyma has been replaced by fibrous tissue. There are only a few residual islands of thyroid follicles present with foci of lymphoid tissue (hematoxylin & eosin stain).

prominent lymphocytic infiltration, more prominent squamous metaplasia, and intense fibrosis that almost totally replaces thyroid tissue (Figs. 8.26 and 8.27, e-Figs. 8.51–8.54) [18]. Fine needle biopsy of these fibrotic glands is usually not undertaken but when attempted, usually yields a hypocellular specimen.

Ancillary Tests

The nodules that usually precipitate tissue evaluation are cellular areas composed of follicles with variable colloid storage. It is not uncommon for them to be composed predominantly of oncocytes. The cytologic atypia that resembles that of papillary carcinoma and the fibrosis that can trap follicular epithelium create difficult diagnostic problems. The distinction of papillary carcinoma from a reactive process, hyperplasia or adenoma can be extremely difficult. Application of special techniques is particularly important in this setting. The reader is referred to the sections on papillary carcinoma (Chapter 9) to understand the roles of immunohistochemical stains for HBME-1, CK19, and galectin-3 in this regard. Patients with chronic lymphocytic thyroiditis have intense diffuse positivity for CK19 that precludes any value of this marker in limited biopsies; therefore, it is not recommended in this setting.

Molecular studies were thought to provide valuable ancillary information that could assist in the diagnosis of borderline lesions of thyroid. As discussed in Chapter 9, the identification of BRAF mutations and ret/PTC

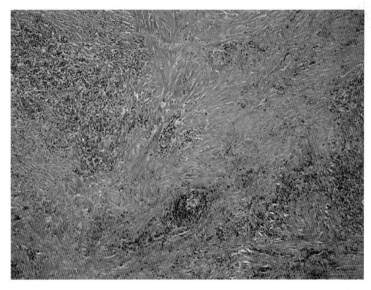

FIGURE 8.27 Little of the thyroid parenchyma can be identified in fibrosing lymphocytic thyroiditis. Residual lymphoid follicles are seen, but much of the remainder of the tissue is simply fibrous tissue. Where preserved, the thyroid epithelium may undergo Hürthle cell change and frequently shows squamous metaplasia (e-Figs. 98–99) (hematoxylin & eosin stain).

rearrangements in papillary thyroid carcinoma can assist in the diagnosis of this malignancy. In the setting of chronic lymphocytic thyroiditis, the identification of a classical papillary carcinoma can be confirmed by the identification of one of these more common molecular alterations. Recent data indicate that glands with Hashimoto's disease express ret/PTC gene rearrangements and other molecular alterations associated with papillary carcinoma [19–22]. In some cases, this may be attributed to nodules of oncocytes or micropapillary carcinomas in the tissue submitted for examination, and some authors have shown that these studies are negative if these lesions are carefully excluded from the inflamed tissue examined [23]. In general, ret/PTC expression in oncocytic nodules in this setting identifies gene rearrangements that correlate with other features of papillary carcinoma.

RIEDEL'S THYROIDITIS

Riedel's thyroiditis is an uncommon fibroinflammatory lesion that is characterized clinically by a hard goiter and tracheal compression [24]. It is most common in middle age (average age 47.8 years, range 23 to 77 years) and is more frequent in women, with a female to male ratio of about 5:1. Most patients are euthyroid but those with significant tissue destruction manifest hypothyroidism. It is frequently associated with other fibrosing lesions involving the retroperitoneum, mediastinum, gallbladder, eyes, and parotid glands. Because of these associations, the disorder is considered to be a manifestation

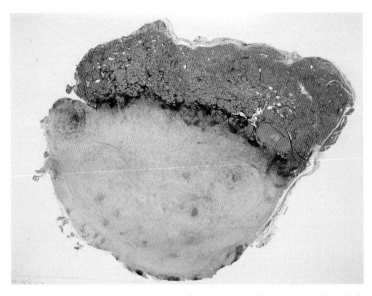

FIGURE 8.28 In Riedel's thyroiditis, the thyroid parenchyma is replaced by dense fibrous tissue. In this low-power image, the fibrotic portion of the thyroid glands appears like a nodule demarcated by an external band of uninvolved thyroid tissue (hematoxylin & eosin stain).

of a systemic fibrosing lesion. Suggestions of a relationship with Hashimoto's disease or other autoimmune endocrinopathies have not been upheld.

This lesion is characterized histologically by a chronic inflammatory infiltrate that involves some or occasionally all of the thyroid, and extends into surrounding soft tissue and skeletal muscle (Figs. 8.28–8.30, e-Figs. 8.55–8.60). This is an important distinction from chronic lymphocytic thyroiditis and other autoimmune disorders that affect all thyroid tissue but are limited to that tissue. The identification of uninvolved thyroid tissue is a key feature of this disorder. The inflammatory infiltrate is composed of lymphocytes, monocytes, granulocytes, and eosinophils but is devoid of giant cells and granulomas, does not form lymphoid follicles, and is not associated with oncocytic change of the follicular epithelium; in fact, the latter is usually completely destroyed by the process. A characteristic feature is vasculitis that may be infiltrative, occlusive, or sclerosing. The degree of inflammation and extent of fibrosis are not consistent but vary from case to case and from area to area within a given specimen.

The role of FNA biopsy is limited by the fibrotic nature of the lesion that usually results in acellular or paucicellular aspirates. The identification of atypia can be misleading [25].

The differential diagnosis includes chronic lymphocytic thyroiditis, solitary fibrous tumor, sclerosing papillary carcinoma, paucicellular variant of anaplastic thyroid carcinoma, and lymphomas. The distinction from chronic lymphocytic thyroiditis is discussed above. The features of the

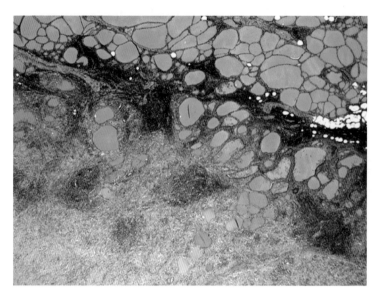

FIGURE 8.29 The interface between the normal tissue and the fibrotic nodule of Riedel's thyroiditis shows the presence of the lymphoid infiltrate. Note the lack of lymphoid follicles, which are typically absent in cases of Riedel's thyroiditis (hematoxylin & eosin stain).

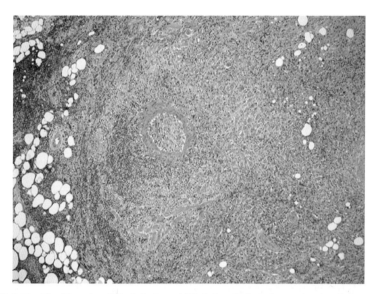

FIGURE 8.30 The fibrosis of Riedel's thyroiditis is locally invasive and extends beyond the thyroid gland to involve adjacent structures of the neck. It is this extrathyroidal extension that characterizes Riedel's thyroiditis and distinguishes it from the other forms of fibrosing thyroiditis. In this image, note the entrapment of the adjacent adipose tissue by the fibrosis and the vascular occlusion (hematoxylin & eosin stain).

sclerosing tumors are discussed in other chapters and lymphoma is the subject of the next section.

LYMPHOMA

Primary thyroid lymphoma is rare and accounts for less than 5% of thyroid malignancies [26]. The classical clinical presentation of a primary non-Hodgkin lymphoma of the thyroid is that of an elderly, female patient with a rapidly enlarging thyroid mass, often with compressive symptoms. These tumors almost always arise in a thyroid gland affected by chronic lymphocytic thyroiditis that represents a significant risk factor for the development of primary thyroid lymphoma [27–30].

The majority of primary non-Hodgkin lymphomas of the thyroid gland are diffuse large B-cell lymphomas (DLBCL) [31–35]. In a relatively large retrospective study of primary thyroid lymphomas, Derringer et al. [31] found that approximately one half of the large cell lymphomas appear as DLBCL alone, while the other half appeared combined with an extranodal marginal zone lymphoma of mucosa-associated lymphoid tissue (MALT) type. Even in those cases of DLBCL alone, some traits of marginal zone lymphoma were evident, prompting the suggestion that most primary thyroid lymphomas are of the MALT type [31]. Extranodal margin zone lymphoma of MALT type is the next most common lymphoma [31,34,35] with a variety of other morphologic subtypes being reported at low frequencies including follicular lymphoma [31,36–39], Burkitt lymphoma [34,39], small lymphocytic lymphoma [39], and peripheral T-cell lymphoma [36]. Hodgkin lymphoma has also rarely been reported to involve the thyroid gland [39].

In cases where there is a known history of Hashimoto's thyroiditis with the onset of a rapidly enlarging thyroid nodule, a primary thyroid lymphoma is usually suspected. However, the differential diagnosis is that of anaplastic carcinoma and as such biopsy is often required. The method of biopsy for the diagnosis is a matter of debate, but in our opinion it is often achievable through FNA.

The approach to the FNA diagnosis of non-Hodgkin lymphoma of the thyroid is not different from the approach to diagnosis at other anatomic sites. The method requires excellent cytomorphology combined with appropriate ancillary studies and in particular immunophenotyping, which is achieved through the use of either flow cytometry or laser scanning cytometry combined with immunoperoxidase studies as required. Thus, in cases with sufficient clinical suspicion for lymphoma or when an abnormal lymphoid population is present on cytomorphology, a portion of the needle rinse is collected into sterile balanced salt solution or cell culture media and maintained in a fresh state until cell surface immunophenotyping is undertaken.

In the situation of diffuse large B-cell lymphoma, the cytomorphology is usually grossly abnormal. The aspirate is composed of a relatively

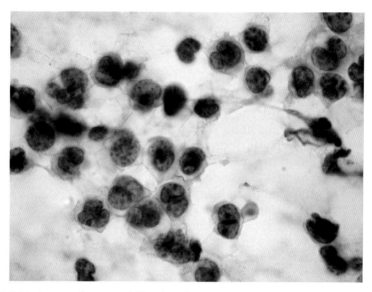

FIGURE 8.31 Large cell non-Hodgkin's lymphoma may be cytomorphologically apparent due to the pronounced abnormalities evident in a monotonous population of large centroblast or immunoblastlike lymphoid cells (direct smear, Papanicolaou stain).

monotonous population of large centroblastlike cells, typically with obvious cytologic atypia (Fig. 8.31, e-Figs. 8.61–8.62). A small number of small lymphocytes may be seen in the background, representing reactive T cells. As these cases typically arise in a background of lymphocytic thyroiditis, it is not uncommon for the aspirate to have a more complex background, and it is possible to find follicular structures and germinal center fragments with a mixed lymphoid population in the background, reflective of the benign thyroiditis. Necrosis is not usually appreciated and mitoses may be seen, but are not typically present in large numbers.

Cell surface immunophenotyping demonstrates a light chain restricted B-cell population (CD19+, CD20+) (Fig. 8.32, e-Fig. 8.63). It is important to note that aberrant kappa/lambda ratios that would exceed some definitions of monoclonality have been detected by flow cytometry in cases of Hashimoto's thyroiditis without evidence of lymphoma and wherein polymerase reaction studies do not demonstrate heavy chain gene rearrangement [40]. Thus, caution should be exercised when interpreting light chain restriction and one must ensure that a morphologically abnormal population is evident in the cytology. There are few reports detailing the complete cell surface immunophenotype of diffuse large B-cell lymphoma of the thyroid. By immunoperoxidase staining, the tumors have been found to be negative for CD5 [30], usually negative for CD10 [31], but occasional positive cases have been noted [30].

Extranodal margin zone lymphoma can have a subtle cytomorphology and be overlooked, in part, because of a complex and "mixed"

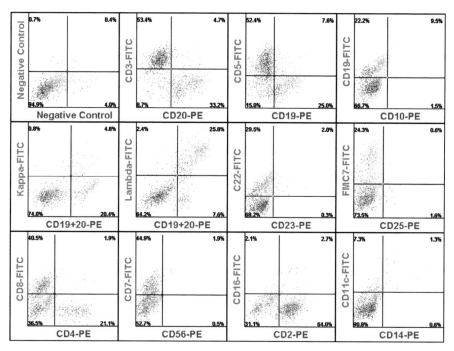

FIGURE 8.32   Cell surface immunophenotype of a large cell lymphoma of the thyroid. This immunophenotype obtained by laser scanning cytometry demonstrate a reactive background population of T cells (blue) with normal pan T-cell antigen expression. Two different B-cell populations are evident. There is a small population of polyclonal B cells (red) with a larger population of lambda light-chain-restricted B cells that are negative for CD5 and CD10 (green). The cytomorphology shows a population of abnormal, large, centroblastlike cells, consistent with a large, B-cell non-Hodgkin lymphoma.

background of lymphoid cells. Here the key is the identification of an abnormal population of monocytoid or plasmacytoid cells lymphoid cells combined with an aberrant immunophenotype. Monocytoid cells have noticeably more abundant pale-staining cytoplasm with round to oval or slightly irregular nuclei containing open chromatin and a small nucleolus. Typically present individually, monocytoid cells will occasionally cluster together and appear more epithelioid. Plasmacytoid cells are well named and resemble plasma cells with an eccentrically placed nucleus and chromatin clumping. Large centroblastlike cells may be seen and the background population is often composed of a variety of cell types including plasma cells wherein Dutcher bodies may become prominent. Benign follicular structures may be present, representing the concomitant thyroiditis. Lymphoepithelial lesions cannot be reliably identified in cytologic preparations. Immunophenotyping will demonstrate a light chain restricted B-cell population that is typically negative for CD5 and CD10 that is often, but not invariably, positive for CD43 on immunoperoxidase staining.

The findings on core and open biopsy are similar to those in the fine needle aspiration and are well described by Derringer et al. [31] in their report on the largest current series of primary thyroid lymphoma. In diffuse large B-cell lymphoma, sheetlike arrangements of abnormal centroblast or immunoblastlike lymphoid cells efface the normal thyroid parenchyma (Figs. 8.33 and 8.34, e-Figs. 8.64–8.66). This infiltrate often shows both vascular invasion and extension into the periglandular tissue with a variable degree of associated fibrosis. The rare follicular lymphoma involving the thyroid gland demonstrates neoplastic follicles composed of varying ratios of centrocytic and centroblast cells deposited throughout the thyroid tissue (Fig. 8.35, e-Figs. 8.67–8.68). In extranodal marginal zone lymphoma involving the thyroid gland, sheetlike arrangements of plasmacytoid or monocytoid cells infiltrate and efface the normal thyroid (Figs. 8.36 and 8.37, e-Figs. 8.69–8.72). Lymphoid follicles may be preserved. Lymphoepithelial lesions are identified in two forms. In the first form, the lymphoma cells invade the thyroid follicular epithelium, but not the colloid (Figs. 8.38 and 8.39, e-Figs. 8.73–8.74). In the second form, the lymphoepithelial islands consist of follicles filled with and distended by lymphoma cells (Figs. 8.40 and 8.41, e-Figs. 8.75–8.76).

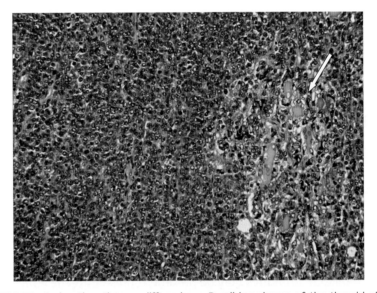

FIGURE 8.33 As in other tissues, diffuse large B-cell lymphoma of the thyroid gland is evident as a sheetlike growth of abnormal centroblastlike lymphoid cells. Immunoperoxidase staining of this case showed that the abnormal cells were CD20+, CD10+, Bcl-6+, Bcl-2+, MUM1−, CD23−, and CD5−. In this illustration, much of the normal architecture of the thyroid gland has been obliterated, but a few residual thyroid follicles are still evident (*white arrow*) (hematoxylin & eosin stain).

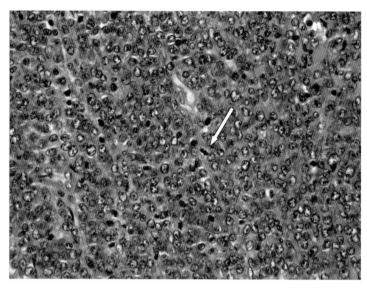

FIGURE 8.34 Diffuse large B-cell lymphoma of the thyroid has a rather monotonous appearance of abnormal centroblastlike cells. Occasional mitoses may be evident (*arrow*) (hematoxylin & eosin stain).

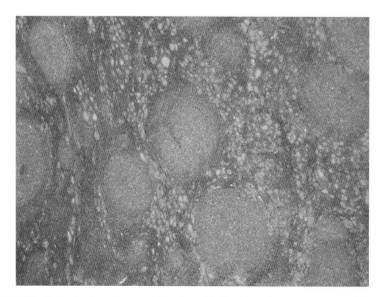

FIGURE 8.35 Follicular lymphoma of the thyroid gland is not as common as diffuse large B-cell lymphoma, but is recognized by the presence of neoplastic follicles scattered throughout the thyroid parenchyma (hematoxylin & eosin stain).

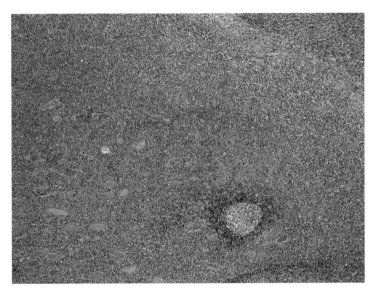

FIGURE 8.36 This case of extranodal margin zone lymphoma of the thyroid shows dense infiltration of the thyroid parenchyma by sheets of abnormal plasmacytoid lymphoid cells. Note that a single lymphoid follicle is still evident as are scattered thyroid follicles. At this magnification, lymphoepithelial lesions cannot be seen (hematoxylin & eosin stain).

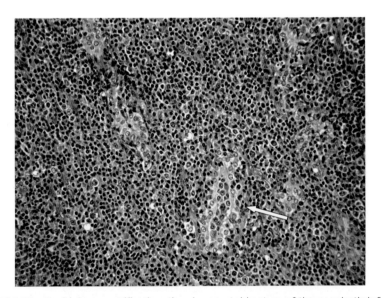

FIGURE 8.37 At a higher magnification, the plasmacytoid nature of the neoplastic infiltrate of extranodal marginal zone lymphoma can be appreciated in addition to lymphoepithelial lesions (*white arrow*) (hematoxylin & eosin stain).

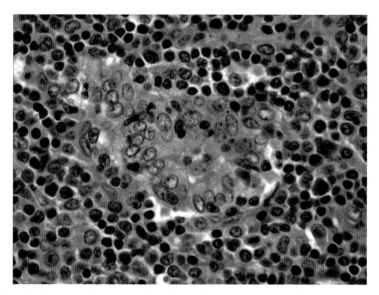

FIGURE 8.38 Two varieties of lymphoepithelial lesion may be identified when extranodal marginal zone lymphoma involves the thyroid gland. In the first form, neoplastic lymphoid cells invade follicular epithelial cells (hematoxylin & eosin stain).

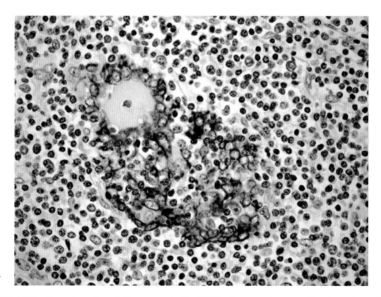

FIGURE 8.39 The density of the neoplastic infiltrate my obscure the lymphoepithelial lesions in extranodal marginal zone lymphoma. In this situation, a pan-keratin immunoperoxidase stain may aid in identification of the epithelial elements that may be otherwise indistinguishable (AE1:AE3 and hematoxylin stain).

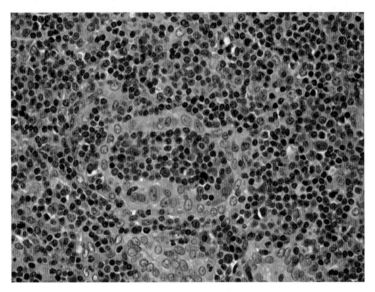

FIGURE 8.40 Colloid variant of a lymphoepithelial lesion. When extranodal marginal zone lymphoma involves the thyroid gland, a variant of lymphoepithelial lesion may be found in which the neoplastic lymphoid cells invade into the colloid portion of the follicle, often leaving the epithelium relatively well preserved (hematoxylin & eosin stain).

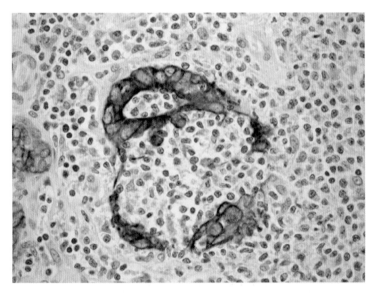

FIGURE 8.41 Keratin staining in the colloid variant of a lymphoepithelial lesion. Once again, immunoperoxidase staining for mixed keratins (AE1:AE3) may help illuminate lymphoepithelial lesions of the colloid variant in extranodal marginal zone lymphoma of the thyroid (AE1:AE3 and hematoxylin stain).

PLASMACYTOMA

Extramedullary plasmacytoma of the thyroid gland is rare with isolated cases reports and a few small series appearing in the literature [41–46]. These typically arise in the setting of Hashimoto's thyroiditis with a morphologic appearance identical to plasmacytoma seen in other organ sites. The major differential diagnostic considerations include lymphomas with a plasmacytoid appearance, in particular plasmacytoid extranodal marginal zone lymphoma, as well as plasmacytoma arising in thyroid cartilage and secondarily involving the thyroid gland or as a component of multiple myeloma. Other considerations include benign inflammatory processes with an excess of plasma cells and plasma cell granuloma [47,48]. The distinction of reactive from neoplastic processes relies on demonstration of clonality. Rarely, plasmacytoma may cause diagnostic problems with other primary thyroid tumors that have a prominent plasmacytoid appearance such as medullary carcinoma [44], whose similarities in morphology are compounded by the potential for amyloid to be detected in both lesions.

THYMOMA

Thymomas occurring within the thyroid gland or in the immediate vicinity of the thyroid gland and thereby mimicking a thyroid nodule have been described in a number of case reports [49–59]. These lesions are thought to arise from entrapped thymic remnants and represent one of four clinicopathologic entities as described by Chan and Rosai [54] of which three occur in the thyroid gland. These four entities include the benign ectopic hamartomatous thymoma (which does not occur within the thyroid gland), ectopic cervical thymomas that like their mediastinal kindred may be benign, locally invasive or metastasize, and the malignant spindle epithelial tumor with thymuslike differentiation (SETTLE) and carcinoma showing thymuslike differentiation (CASTLE).

Ectopic thymomas show a strong female predominance. The tumors frequently present as a painless thyroid mass that is "cold" on thyroid scanning. Local mass effect or compressive symptomology may be present, but most are otherwise asymptomatic with the exception of one case report that described myasthenialike symptoms [56].

The cytologic and histologic appearance of ectopic thymomas mirrors that seen in their mediastinal counterparts with variable combinations of lymphoid cells admixed with either epithelioid or spindle epithelial cells. When epithelial rich, these lesions must be distinguished from other epithelial and spindle cell tumors of the thyroid; for this reason, CASTLE and SETTLE are discussed in Chapters 11 and 12, respectively. On the other hand, lymphocyte rich thymomas wherein the epithelial component is not appreciated may masquerade as lymphocytic thyroiditis or even lymphoma [55–59]. The diagnosis of a lymphocyte rich ectopic thymoma may be discovered through the recognition of the characteristic immature T-cell phenotype of thymic lymphocytes by immunophenotyping of cell surface antigens with flow [58] or laser scanning cytometry. However, it is clear from the reports in the literature that most of these cases have not been discovered until the lesion was excised.

LANGERHANS CELL HISTIOCYTOSIS

Langerhans cell histiocytosis (LCH) rarely involves the thyroid gland [60–69]. LCH of the thyroid gland shows a slight female predominance and the disease most often occurs in the setting of systemic disease in children and young adults [64]. The clinical presentation is typically that of a variably sized "cold" nodule involving the thyroid gland or thyromegaly due to diffuse infiltration.

The diagnosis has been achieved on FNA, which usually reveals minimal colloid with a background of eosinophils, neutrophils, lymphocytes, and numerous Langerhans cells, seen individually and in sheetlike groupings. Langerhans cells are large histiocytoid cells that often appear epithelioid, stellate, or somewhat spindled with a moderate amount of vacuolated cytoplasm and characterized by elongated nuclei with significant nuclear membrane irregularities reaching a pinnacle in the form of a prominent, longitudinal nuclear groove or deep clefts (Figs. 8.42 and

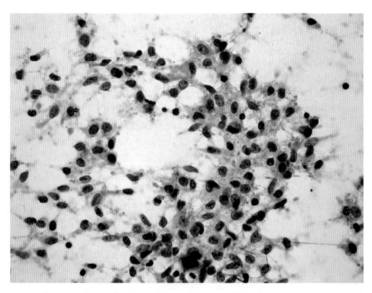

FIGURE 8.42 Fine needle aspiration of Langerhans cell histiocytosis often reveals little to no thyroid elements. Instead, one finds a population of epithelioid, stellate, or spindle histiocytoid cells with moderately abundant vacuolated cytoplasm. The background may show eosinophils and mixed lymphoid cells. Necrosis may be present and mitoses occasionally encountered. Even at this magnification, nuclear grooving is apparent (direct smear, Papanicolaou stain).

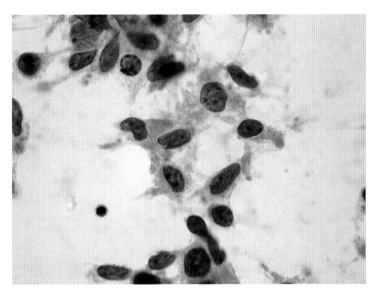

FIGURE 8.43   Nuclear grooves are marked in Langerhans cells of Langerhans cell histiocytosis and may appear as a thin line to a marked cleft to a deep chasm that apparently partitions the nucleus. Rare intranuclear inclusions may also be found (direct smear, Papanicolaou stain).

8.43, e-Figs. 8.77–8.81). The chromatin pattern is fine with inconspicuous nucleoli and intranuclear inclusions may be seen. Although there is nuclear atypia, frankly malignant cells are absent. Mitoses are usually present. On FNA, LCH has a reputation for misdiagnosis as subacute thyroiditis, follicular neoplasms, as well as undifferentiated carcinoma and papillary carcinoma [61,64]. Likely LCH, due to its rarity, was not considered in the differential diagnoses in these cases and the Langerhans cells were unrecognized.

Histologically, LCH may show focal involvement with a septal distribution, a defined nodular mass, or a diffuse infiltrate that replaces the normal thyroid parenchyma by sheets of Langerhans cells (Fig. 8.44, e-Figs. 8.82–8.84). The Langerhans cells may infiltrate among the thyroid follicles where the two may blend together almost imperceptibly. In this situation, identification of the follicular epithelium may be aided by application of a keratin immunoperoxidase stain (Fig. 8.45, e-Fig. 8.85). Eosinophils are frequently present and may collect around and within microscopic foci of necrosis forming eosinophilic microabscesses (Fig. 8.46, e-Fig. 8.86). Mitoses are typically identified, but should not lead to a consideration of Langerhans cell sarcoma, as this diagnosis is dependent on the finding of Langerhans cells that are cytologically frankly and grossly malignant. A background of lymphocytic thyroiditis may be appreciated in some cases [64,65,67].

Langerhans cells have a characteristic immunoprofile with expression of S-100 protein and CD1a (Fig. 8.47, e-Fig. 8.87) and are variably

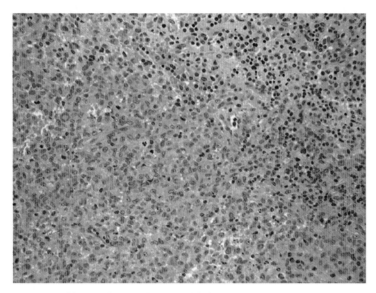

FIGURE 8.44 Core biopsy of Langerhans cell histiocytosis. In this case, the Langerhans cell histiocytosis has diffusely infiltrated and replaced the thyroid parenchyma. Eosinophils and mixed lymphoid cells are evident in the background (hematoxylin & eosin stain).

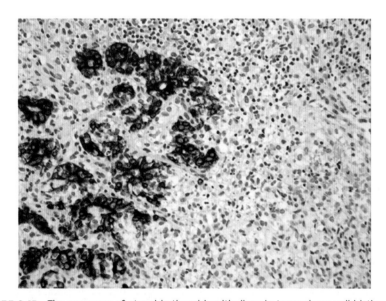

FIGURE 8.45 The presence of atrophic thyroid epithelium in Langerhans cell histiocytosis may be revealed by immunoperoxidase staining for keratin, which also helps to demonstrate that the abnormal cell infiltrate is not of epithelial origin (CAM 5.2 & hematoxylin stain).

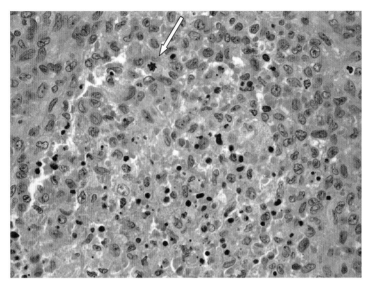

FIGURE 8.46   Necrosis is frequently identified in Langerhans cell histocytosis and may be associated with an eosinophilic microabscesses. Mitoses are also commonly identified (*white arrow*). The possibility of Langerhans cell sarcoma should be entertained when the Langerhans cells are cytologically malignant (hematoxylin & eosin stain).

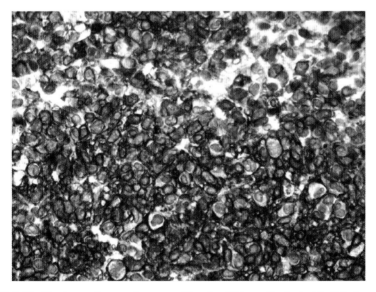

FIGURE 8.47   The Langerhans cells are positive for CD1a as illustrated in this figure. The cells are also frequently positive for S-100 protein, but are typically negative or very weakly positive for CD45, CD68, and lysozyme (CD1a & hematoxylin stain).

and weakly positive for CD45, CD68, and lysozyme. The characteristic ultrastructure feature within the cytoplasm of the Langerhans cells is the Birbeck granule, a pentalaminar "tennis racketlike" structure measuring approximately 200 to 400 nm in length with a width of 33 nm. The differential diagnosis of LCH involving the thyroid gland is broad and includes inflammatory and neoplastic conditions. The key to the correct diagnosis is the recognition of the Langerhans cells. The inflammatory background may lead to consideration of acute, chronic, or subacute thyroiditis. Here, the presence of the eosinophils is a rather unique and helpful feature pointing to LCH as a consideration. The neoplasms that may be considered include poorly differentiated primary or metastatic carcinoma, lymphoma, or even melanoma. The low nuclear/cytoplasmic ratio of the Langerhans cells and the absence of frank malignant features should mitigate against these diagnoses. It is the awareness of Langerhans cell histiocytosis that should elicit a careful examination of unusual lesions for Langerhans cells. Confirmation of the diagnosis can be obtained through immunoperoxidase and ultrastructural studies.

REFERENCES

1. Moinuddin S, Barazi H, Moinuddin M. Acute blastomycosis thyroiditis. *Thyroid* 2008;18:659–661.
2. Gopan T, Strome M, Hoschar A, et al. Recurrent acute suppurative thyroiditis attributable to a piriform sinus fistula in an adult. *Endocr Pract* 2007;13:662–666.
3. Herndon MD, Christie DB, Ayoub MM, et al. Thyroid abscess: case report and review of the literature. *Am Surg* 2007;73:725–728.
4. Sai Prasad TR, Chong CL, Mani A, et al. Acute suppurative thyroiditis in children secondary to pyriform sinus fistula. *Pediatr Surg Int* 2007;23:779–783.
5. Sivakumar S. Role of fine needle aspiration cytology in detection of microfilariae: report of 2 cases. *Acta Cytol* 2007;51:803–806.
6. Indumathi VA, Shivakumar NS. Disseminated nocardiosis in an elderly patient presenting with prolonged pyrexia: diagnosis by thyroid abscess culture. *Indian J Med Microbiol* 2007;25:294–296.
7. Zavascki AP, Maia AL, Goldani LZ. Pneumocystis jiroveci thyroiditis: report of 15 cases in the literature. *Mycoses* 2007;50:443–446.
8. Volpé R. Subacute (de Quervain's) thyroiditis. *Clin Endocrinol Metab* 1979;8:81–95.
9. LiVolsi VA. *Surgical pathology of the thyroid*. Philadelphia: WB Saunders, 1990.
10. Orlandi F, Mussa A, Gonzatto I, et al. Two cases of sarcoidosis of the thyroid. *Sarcoidosis Vasc Diffuse Lung Dis* 2000;17:88–89.
11. Weiss IA, Limaye A, Tchertkoff V, et al. Sarcoidosis of the thyroid clinically mimicking malignancy. *N Y State J Med* 1989;89:578–580.
12. Volpé R. Lymphocytic (Hashimoto's) thyroiditis. In: Werner SC, Ingbar SC, eds. *The thyroid*. New York: Harper and Row, 1978:996–1008.
13. Jansson R, Karlsson A, Forsum U. Intrathyroidal HLA-DR expression and T lymphocyte phenotypes in Graves' thyrotoxicosis, Hashimoto's thyroiditis and nodular colloid goitre. *Clin Exp Immunol* 1984;58:264–272.
14. Asa SL. The pathology of autoimmune endocrine disorders. In: Kovacs K, Asa SL, eds. *Functional endocrine pathology*. Boston: Blackwell Scientific Publications, 1991:961–978.
15. Friedman NB. Cellular involution in thyroid gland: significance of Hürthle cells in myxedema, exhaustion atrophy, Hashimoto's disease and reaction in irradiation, thiouracil therapy and subtotal resection. *J Clin Endocrinol* 1949;9:874–882.

16. Rosai J, Carcangiu ML, DeLellis RA. Tumors of the thyroid gland. In: *Atlas of tumor pathology*. 3rd series, fascicle 5. Washington, DC: Armed Forces Institute of Pathology, 1992.

17. Dube VE, Joyce GT. Extreme squamous metaplasia in Hashimoto's thyroiditis. *Cancer* 1971;27:434–437.

18. Katzmann JA, Vickery AL. The fibrosing variant of Hashimoto's thyroiditis. *Hum Pathol* 1974;5:161–170.

19. Wirtschafter A, Schmidt R, Rosen D, et al. Expression of the RET/PTC fusion gene as a marker for papillary carcinoma in Hashimoto's thyroiditis. *Laryngoscope* 1997;107:95–100.

20. Rhoden KJ, Unger K, Salvatore G, et al. RET/papillary thyroid cancer rearrangement in nonneoplastic thyrocytes: follicular cells of Hashimoto's thyroiditis share low-level recombination events with a subset of papillary carcinoma. *J Clin Endocrinol Metab* 2006;91:2414–2423.

21. Kang DY, Kim KH, Kim JM, et al. High prevalence of RET, RAS, and ERK expression in Hashimoto's thyroiditis and in papillary thyroid carcinoma in the Korean population. *Thyroid* 2007;17:1031–1036.

22. Sheils OM, O'eary JJ, Uhlmann V, et al. Ret/PTC-1 activation in Hashimoto thyroiditis. *Int J Surg Pathol* 2000;8:185–189.

23. Sugg SL, Ezzat S, Rosen IB, et al. Distinct multiple *ret*/PTC gene rearrangements in multifocal papillary thyroid neoplasia. *J Clin Endocrinol Metab* 1998;83:4116–4122.

24. Papi G, LiVolsi VA. Current concepts on Riedel thyroiditis. *Am J Clin Pathol* 2004; 121(suppl):S50–S63.

25. Blumenfeld W. Correlation of cytologic and histologic findings in fibrosing thyroiditis. A case report. *Acta Cytol* 1997;41:1337–1340.

26. Ansell SM, Grant CS, Habermann TM. Primary thyroid lymphoma. *Semin Oncol* 1999;26:316–323.

27. Holm LE, Blomgren H, Lowhagen T. Cancer risks in patients with chronic lymphocytic thyroiditis. *N Engl J Med* 1985;312:601–604.

28. Kato I, Tajima K, Suchi T, et al. Chronic thyroiditis as a risk factor of B-cell lymphoma in the thyroid gland. *Jpn J Cancer Res* 1985;76:1085–1090.

29. Pedersen RK, Pedersen NT. Primary non-Hodgkin's lymphoma of the thyroid gland: a population based study. *Histopathology* 1996;28:25–32.

30. Niitsu N, Okamoto M, Nakamura N, et al. Clinicopathologic correlations of stage IE/IIE primary thyroid diffuse large B-cell lymphoma. *Ann Oncol* 2007;18:1203–1208.

31. Derringer GA, Thompson LD, Frommelt RA, et al. Malignant lymphoma of the thyroid gland: a clinicopathologic study of 108 cases. *Am J Surg Pathol* 2000;24:623–639.

32. Ruggiero FP, Frauenhoffer E, Stack BC Jr. Thyroid lymphoma: a single institution's experience. *Otolaryngol Head Neck Surg* 2005;133:888–896.

33. Kossev P, LiVolsi V. Lymphoid lesions of the thyroid: review in light of the revised European-American lymphoma classification and upcoming World Health Organization classification. *Thyroid* 1999;9:1273–1280.

34. Lam KY, Lo CY, Kwong DL, et al. Malignant lymphoma of the thyroid. A 30-year clinicopathologic experience and an evaluation of the presence of Epstein–Barr virus. *Am J Clin Pathol* 1999;112:263–270.

35. Cho JH, Park YH, Kim WS, et al. High incidence of mucosa-associated lymphoid tissue in primary thyroid lymphoma: a clinicopathologic study of 18 cases in the Korean population. *Leuk Lymphoma* 2006;47:2128–2131.

36. Colovic M, Matic S, Kryeziu E, et al. Outcomes of primary thyroid non-Hodgkin's lymphoma: a series of nine consecutive cases. *Med Oncol* 2007;24:203–208.

37. Satge D, Ott G, Sasco AJ, et al. A low-grade follicular thyroid carcinoma in a woman with Down syndrome. *Tumori* 2004;90:333–336.

38. Goodlad JR, MacPherson S, Jackson R, et al. Extranodal follicular lymphoma: a clinicopathological and genetic analysis of 15 cases arising at non-cutaneous extranodal sites. *Histopathology* 2004;44:268–276.

39. Thieblemont C, Mayer A, Dumontet C, et al. Primary thyroid lymphoma is a heterogeneous disease. *J Clin Endocrinol Metab* 2002;87:105–111.

40. Chen HI, Akpolat I, Mody DR, et al. Restricted kappa/lambda light chain ratio by flow cytometry in germinal center B cells in Hashimoto thyroiditis. *Am J Clin Pathol* 2006;125:42–48.
41. Macpherson TA, Dekker A, Kapadia SB. Thyroid-gland plasma cell neoplasm (plasmacytoma). *Arch Pathol Lab Med* 1981;105:570–572.
42. Aozasa K, Inoue A, Yoshimura H, et al. Plasmacytoma of the thyroid gland. *Cancer* 1986;58:105–110.
43. Kovacs CS, Mant MJ, Nguyen GK, wt al. Plasma cell lesions of the thyroid: report of a case of solitary plasmacytoma and a review of the literature. *Thyroid* 1994;4:65–71.
44. Bourtsos EP, Bedrossian CW, De Frias DV, et al. Thyroid plasmacytoma mimicking medullary carcinoma: a potential pitfall in aspiration cytology. *Diagn Cytopathol* 2000;23:354–358.
45. Kuo SF, Chang HY, Hsueh C, et al. Extramedullary plasmacytoma of the thyroid. *N Z Med J* 2006;119:U2005.
46. De Schrijver I, Smeets P. Thyroid enlargement due to extramedullary plasmacytoma. *JBR-BTR* 2004;87:73–75.
47. Martinez F, Filipowicz E, Hudnall SD. Plasma cell granuloma of the thyroid. *Arch Pathol Lab Med* 2002;126:595–598.
48. Deniz K, Patiroglu TE, Okten T. Plasma cell granuloma of the thyroid. *APMIS* 2008;116:167–172.
49. Yamashita H, Murakami N, Noguchi S, et al. Cervical thymoma and incidence of cervical thymus. *Acta Pathol Jpn* 1983;33:189–194.
50. Miyauchi A, Kuma K, Matsuzuka F, et al. Intrathyroidal epithelial thymoma: an entity distinct from squamous cell carcinoma of the thyroid. *World J Surg* 1985;9:128–135.
51. Harach HR, Saravia DE, Franssila KO. Thyroid spindle-cell tumor with mucous cysts. An intrathyroid thymoma? *Am J Surg Pathol* 1985;9:525–530.
52. Asa SL, Dardick I, Van Nostrand AWP, et al. Primary thyroid thymoma: a distinct clinicopathologic entity. *Hum Pathol* 1988;19:1463–1467.
53. Weigensberg C, Daisley H, Asa SL, et al. Thyroid thymoma in childhood. *Endocr Pathol* 1990;1:123–127.
54. Chan JK, Rosai J. Tumors of the neck showing thymic or related branchial pouch differentiation: a unifying concept. *Hum Pathol* 1991;22:349–367.
55. Vengrove MA, Schimmel M, Atkinson BF, et al. Invasive cervical thymoma masquerading as a solitary thyroid nodule. Report of a case studied by fine needle aspiration. *Acta Cytol* 1991;35:431–433.
56. Oh YL, Ko YH, Ree HJ. Aspiration cytology of ectopic cervical thymoma mimicking a thyroid mass. A case report. *Acta Cytol* 1998;42:1167–1171.
57. Milde P, Sidawy MK. Thymoma presenting as a palpable thyroid nodule: a pitfall in fine needle aspiration (FNA) of the neck. *Cytopathology* 1999;10:415–419.
58. Ponder TB, Collins BT, Bee CS, et al. Diagnosis of cervical thymoma by fine needle aspiration biopsy with flow cytometry. A case report. *Acta Cytol* 2002;46:1129–1132.
59. Cohen JB, Troxell M, Kong CS, et al. Ectopic intrathyroidal thymoma: a case report and review. *Thyroid* 2003;13:305–308.
60. Sahoo M, Karak AK, Bhatnagar D, et al. Fine-needle aspiration cytology in a case of isolated involvement of thyroid with Langerhans cell histiocytosis. *Diagn Cytopathol* 1998;19:33–37.
61. Saiz E, Bakotic BW. Isolated Langerhans cell histiocytosis of the thyroid: a report of two cases with nuclear imaging–pathologic correlation. *Ann Diagn Pathol* 2000;4:23–28.
62. Sampathkumar S, Younger C, Cramer H, et al. Langerhans' cell histiocytosis involving the pituitary, thyroid, lung, and liver. *Endocr Pract* 2002;8:217–221.
63. Zhu H, Hu DX. Langerhans cell histiocytosis of the thyroid diagnosed by fine needle aspiration cytology. A case report. *Acta Cytol* 2004;48:278–280.
64. Elliott DD, Sellin R, Egger JF, et al. Langerhans cell histiocytosis presenting as a thyroid gland mass. *Ann Diagn Pathol* 2005;9:267–274.

65. Deepak DS, Woodcock BE, Macfarlane IA. A thyroid mass composed of Langerhans' cell histiocytosis and auto-immune thyroiditis associated with progressive hypothalamic-pituitary failure. *Int J Clin Pract* 2007;61:2130–2131.

66. Yagci B, Kandemir N, Yazici N, et al. Thyroid involvement in Langerhans cell histiocytosis: a report of two cases and review of the literature. *Eur J Pediatr* 2007;166:901–904.

67. Lassalle S, Hofman V, Santini J, et al. Isolated Langerhans cell histiocytosis of the thyroid and Graves' disease: an unreported association. *Pathology* 2008;40:525–527.

68. Ramadas PT, Kattoor J, Mathews A, et al. Fine needle aspiration cytology of Langerhans cell thyroid histiocytosis and its draining lymph nodes. *Acta Cytol* 2008;52:396–398.

69. Lollar K, Farrag TY, Cao D, et al. Langerhans cell histiocytosis of the thyroid gland. *Am J Otolaryngol* 2008;29:201–204.

9

PAPILLARY LESIONS

GRAVES' DISEASE

It is rare that a patient with Graves' disease will undergo biopsy of the thyroid except in the event of a cold nodule developing within the hyperplastic gland. However, in that setting, it is possible that nonnodular tissue is included in the specimen and it is important to distinguish the papillary hyperplasia from the pathology of the nodule in question. The pathology of Graves' disease varies with the clinical status and therapy. In its florid form, the gland develops a diffuse increase in cellularity with epithelial hyperplasia forming papillary invaginations into the lumen of follicles that are devoid of colloid or contain only scant colloid with peripheral scalloping (Figs. 9.1 and 9.2, e-Figs. 9.1–9.3). The papillae have fibrovascular cores, but usually are lined by tall columnar cells with basally oriented nuclei that are crowded but round and regular (Fig. 9.3, e-Figs. 9.4–9.5), without the irregularity of contour or the clearing with peripheral margination of chromatin, which are the hallmarks of papillary carcinoma. Inflammatory cells are scarce and usually are not found in biopsies, but rather are only found scattered in foci of the gland at surgical resection (Fig. 9.4, e-Fig. 9.6). The features of this disorder resemble papillary carcinoma superficially, since there is complex papillary architecture that in biopsies can mimic malignancy. In larger specimens, it is evident that the papillae in Graves' disease are organized within follicles rather than having the haphazard pattern of papillary carcinoma. More critically, the cytologic features are not as those of papillary carcinoma; the nuclei are crowded but usually retain their basal orientation. They do not have the convoluted membrane with grooves and inclusions that characterize papillary carcinoma and they are usually evenly dark and basophilic rather than clear. The differential diagnosis based on these features is the hyperplastic or adenomatous nodule with papillary architecture discussed in the next section. In fine needle aspiration (FNA) specimens, marginal vacuoles or fireflare appearance in May–Grünwald–Giemsa stained smears was initially described as a distinctive feature of thyrotoxic goiter in hyperthyroidism. These vacuoles are thought to represent dilated endoplasmic reticulum, a manifestation of active pinocytosis containing colloid, or diffusion of thyroid hormone [1]. However, marginal vacuoles are found in

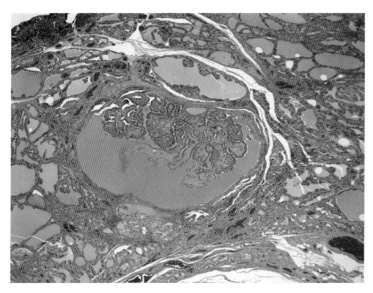

FIGURE 9.1 The appearance of Graves' disease is tremendously variable due to the severity of disease and the effects of prior therapy. In more florid cases, the thyroid follicles contain intrafollicular papillary projections of hyperplastic epithelium (hematoxylin & eosin stain).

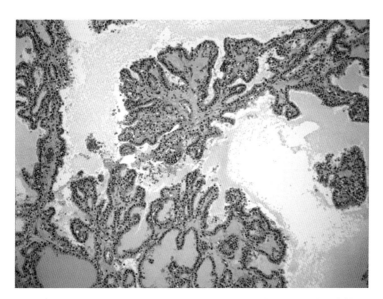

FIGURE 9.2 The papillae of Graves' disease have fibrovascular cores of variable thickness, but often are delicate with the papillae showing a branching pattern. These papillary structures must be distinguished from the papillae of papillary carcinoma. Note the reduced colloid content of the follicle (hematoxylin & eosin stain).

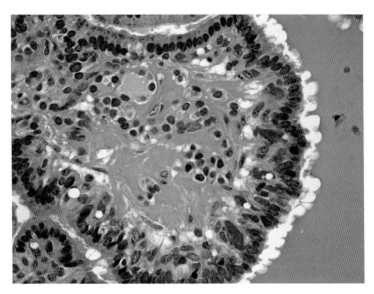

FIGURE 9.3   The epithelium in Graves' disease is composed of tall columnar cells with basally oriented nuclei that are crowded, but round to elongated and regular. These nuclei lack the nuclear features of papillary carcinoma, namely nuclear membrane irregularities, grooves, optically clear nuclei, and intranuclear inclusions. Note that the colloid shows prominent scalloping (hematoxylin & eosin stain).

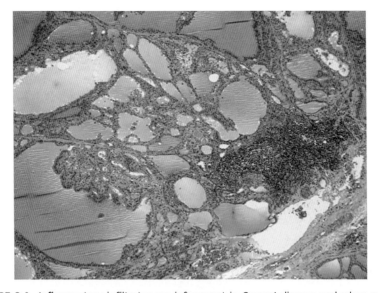

FIGURE 9.4   Inflammatory infiltrates are infrequent in Graves' disease and when present tend to be widely separated. Therefore, biopsy specimens from Graves' disease usually do not show significant lymphoid tissue (hematoxylin & eosin stain).

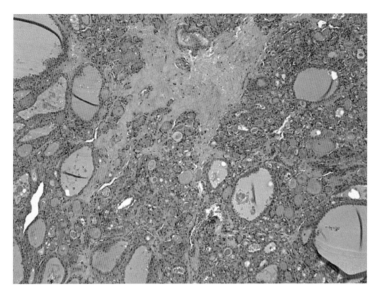

FIGURE 9.5 Administration of antithyroid mediations (Tapazole, propylthiouracil) to pa-tients with Graves' disease results in regression of the hyperplasia. The follicles tend to re-plenish their stores of colloid and focal fibrosis may develop (hematoxylin & eosin stain).

various nontoxic thyroid lesions [2], including papillary carcinoma, and are therefore of little diagnostic assistance.

With the administration of antithyroid mediations (Tapazole, propy-lthiouracil), the hyperplasia recedes, follicles resume their more typical ap-pearance, and colloid accumulates within their lumens (Fig. 9.5, e-Figs. 9.7 and 9.8). Radioactive iodine administration results in additional changes, including fibrosis, moderate focal chronic inflammation and the presence of conspicuous "smudged" nuclei, and nuclei that are large, hy-perchromatic, and cytologically atypical (Fig. 9.6, e-Figs. 9.9 and 9.10).

HYPERPLASTIC NODULES AND ADENOMAS WITH PAPILLARY ARCHITECTURE

The "papillary hyperplastic nodule" of the thyroid is usually identified in girls, often in teenagers in and around the age of menarche. These lesions present as solitary nodules and they may be associated with clinical or subclinical hyperfunction; they are usually hot on radioiodine scan. These lesions are characterized by a unique architecture that is best recognized at low magnification. Although they do have true papillae with fibrovas-cular cores, the papillae are usually organized and have a centripetal pat-tern within enlarged, distorted follicles. These nodules are distinguished from papillary carcinoma in that they are totally encapsulated or at least very well delineated without evidence of invasion, they often have central

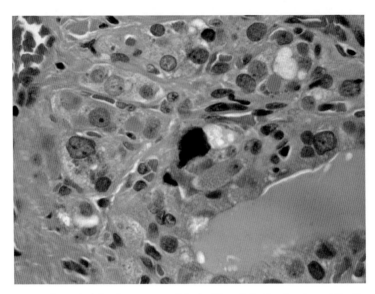

FIGURE 9.6 A characteristic change associated with radioiodine treatment for Graves' disease is pronounced nuclear atypia with cells containing hyperchromatic and "smudged" nuclei (hematoxylin & eosin stain).

cystic change, they usually have at least focal subfollicle formation in the centers of broad edematous papillae, and most importantly, they do not have the nuclear features of papillary carcinoma (Figs. 9.7–9.11, e-Figs. 9.11–9.15). Although one analysis of clonality has suggested that these are

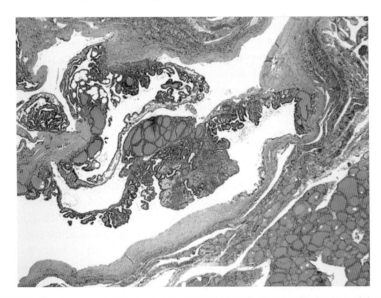

FIGURE 9.7 The low power histologic appearance of a papillary hyperplastic nodule reveals a delineating fibrous capsule with central cystic change and subfollicle formation in the center of a broad edematous papilla (hematoxylin & eosin stain).

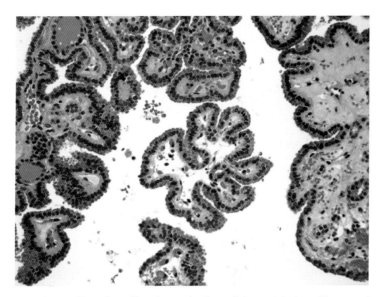

FIGURE 9.8   The papillae of papillary hyperplastic nodule contain true fibrovascular stalks that are apparent histologically and cytologically (Fig. 9.10) (hematoxylin & eosin stain).

polyclonal hyperplasias [3], the detection of Gsα or TSH receptor activating mutations in such nodules suggests that they are neoplasms [4–8]. These specific mutations that activate TSH signaling account for their functional hyperactivity as well as their structural morphology that resembles

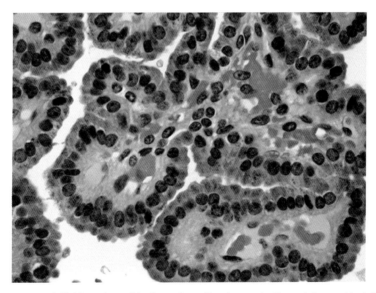

FIGURE 9.9   By definition, the epithelium of papillary hyperplastic nodule must lack the nuclear features of papillary carcinoma. Thus, there must be an absence of nuclear irregularities, grooves, optical clarity, and intranuclear inclusions (hematoxylin & eosin stain).

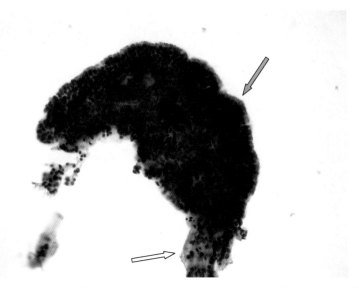

FIGURE 9.10   Aspiration of a papillary hyperplastic nodule may yield an intact papilla, as in this illustration, where the fibrovascular stalk (*white arrow*) is visible and seen protruding from the still largely intact epithelial covering (*orange arrow*). These papillary stalks may generate a suspicion of papillary carcinoma, but it is critical to note that the epithelium lacks the nuclear features of papillary carcinoma (Fig. 9.11) (ThinPrep, Papanicolaou stain).

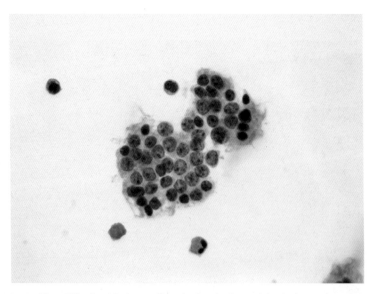

FIGURE 9.11   The epithelium from papillary hyperplastic nodules lacks nuclear grooves and intranuclear inclusions. However, given the presence of the papillae and the potential for minor nuclear atypia, papillary hyperplastic nodules are notorious for generating cytologic diagnoses of "suspicious for papillary carcinoma" or even "papillary carcinoma" (ThinPrep, Papanicolaou stain).

localized Graves' disease. Their behavior is almost always benign. Some have advocated the name "papillary adenoma" for these tumors; while scientifically appropriate, this term carries historical connotations that some feel are unacceptable [9].

In adults, one can have a similar histologic appearance in a "hot" nodule, that is, a thyroid nodule that is associated with clinical toxicity or subclinical hyperthyroidism and iodine uptake on scan. These lesions may be solitary but in adults they are more often seen in the setting of sporadic nodular goiter.

On FNA and on histologic evaluation, particularly at frozen section, papillary hyperplastic nodules or adenomas can be very alarming and lead to a false-positive diagnosis of papillary carcinoma. Indeed, these entities give rise to well-formed papillae but on higher magnification, they lack the cytologic criteria for the diagnosis of papillary carcinoma, including powdery nuclear chromatin, multiple micro- and/or macronucleoli, intranuclear cytoplasmic inclusions, and linear chromatin grooves [10]. Immunohistochemical studies have shown that HBME-1 can be useful to distinguish these lesions in histologic samples, since papillary carcinoma is frequently positive (see below), but benign lesions are negative for this marker [11].

PAPILLARY CARCINOMA: CLASSICAL TYPE

Papillary carcinoma represents the most common thyroid epithelial malignancy diagnosed in regions of the world where goiters are not endemic. Although malignant, these lesions are usually indolent and most have an excellent prognosis with a 20-year survival rate of 90% or better [12,13]. When these lesions do metastasize, they most often do so initially via lymphatics with initial regional lymph node metastases. Metastases beyond the neck are unusual in common papillary carcinoma.

Papillary carcinomas may be multifocal. This has been interpreted as reflective of intraglandular lymphatic dissemination. However, the identification of such microcarcinomas in up to 24% of the population [14] and the detection of different clonal rearrangements [15] or X chromosome inactivation patterns [16] in the different lesions from a single patient support the interpretation of multifocal primary lesions in most patients.

The terminology is misleading. Papillary carcinomas can exhibit papillary architecture (e-Fig. 9.16) but they may also have follicular (e-Fig. 9.17) or mixed papillary and follicular patterns [9,17–23]. It is now recognized that the diagnosis of papillary carcinoma is based on what the WHO has described as "a distinctive set of nuclear characteristics" [24]. As such, the histologic diagnosis of papillary carcinoma of the thyroid has become a cytologic diagnosis based on nuclear features; this explains the utility of FNA in the diagnosis of thyroid nodules. Although papillary structures (Figs. 9.12–9.16, e-Figs. 9.18–9.23) are not required for a diagnosis of papillary

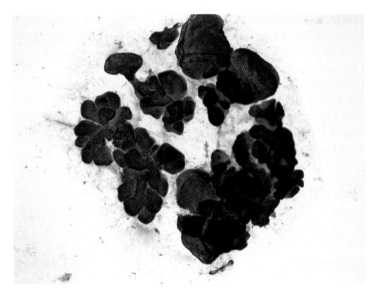

FIGURE 9.12 Papillae from a conventional papillary carcinoma may present as complex three-dimensional structures when aspirated intact (direct smear, Papanicolaou stain).

carcinoma and the presence of papillary structures is not pathognomic of papillary carcinoma, the identification of a lesion with a papillary architecture should prompt a careful search for the nuclear features of papillary carcinoma.

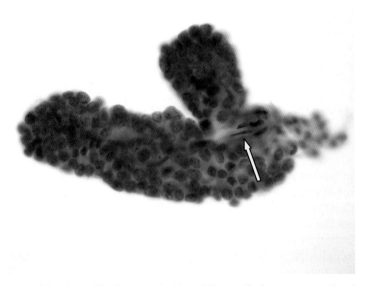

FIGURE 9.13 Higher magnification examination of the papilla from a conventional papillary carcinoma reveals the central fibrovascular core (*white arrow*) (ThinPrep, Papanicolaou stain).

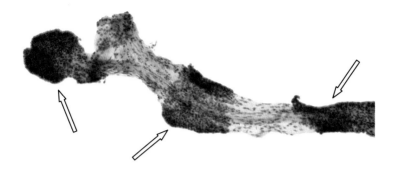

FIGURE 9.14   Denudation of the epithelium from papillae (degloving injury to the papillae) is a frequent occurrence and can be accentuated during resuspension in ThinPrep slide production. This image shows partial denudation of a fibrovascular stalk of a papillary carcinoma where a few fragments of epithelium are preserved (*arrows*). The degloving injury generates separate epithelial fragments and naked fibrovascular stalks (Figs. 9.15 and 9.16) (ThinPrep, Papanicolaou stain).

NUCLEAR FEATURES OF PAPILLARY CARCINOMA

Some of the changes seen in papillary carcinoma are part of the neoplastic process and less specific to papillary carcinoma itself. Common to most

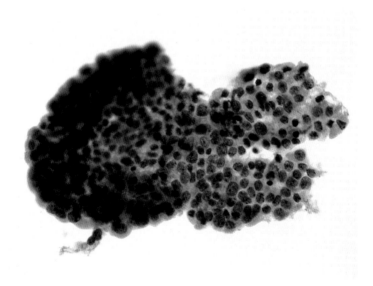

FIGURE 9.15   The de-gloved epithelium from papillae generated by aspiration and resuspension in ThinPrep slide production may present as monolayered sheets. Occasionally, the epithelium from the tip of the papillae will retain a rounded tiplike architecture, but lacks the fibrovascular cores (ThinPrep, Papanicolaou stain).

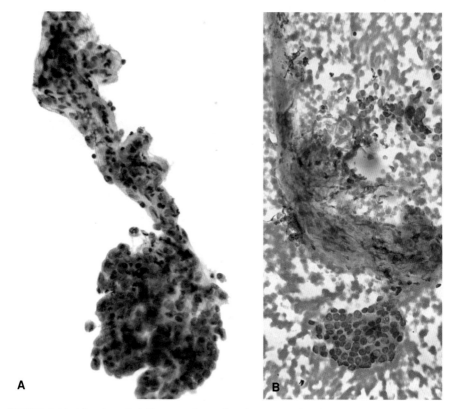

A

B

FIGURE 9.16 The denuded fibrovascular stalks of a conventional papillary carcinoma seen in FNA may be overlooked as "fibrous tissue," as often the lumen of the capillaries is not easily identified in either alcohol-fixed, Papanicolaou-stained slides **(A)** or air-dried, Diff Quik-stained material **(B)**. A clue to their significance may be found when the epithelium is still adherent to the vascular structures as seen in the lower portion of these two examples (**A**: ThinPrep, Papanicolaou stain; **B**: direct smear, Diff Quik stain).

thyroid neoplasia is the presence of nuclear enlargement, loss of nuclear roundness, increased chromatin granularity, and increased prominence of the nucleolus.

NUCLEAR ENLARGEMENT AND ELONGATION. The nuclei in thyroid neoplasia enlarge and do so out of proportion to any increase in cytoplasm, resulting in an increased nuclear/cytoplasmic (N/C) ratio. This nuclear enlargement may also be recognized by any of the following three manifestations of increased N/C ratio (Figs. 9.17 and 9.18, e-Figs. 9.24 and 9.25):

1. Loss of the apparent basal polarization of the nuclei (seen histologically).
2. Nuclear crowding and overlapping in the epithelial fragments (seen cytologically and histologically).

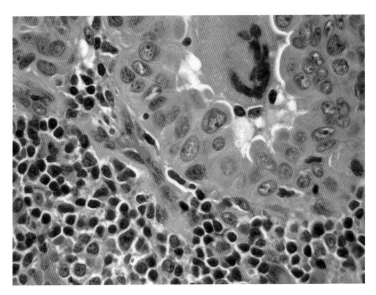

FIGURE 9.17   Neoplastic change in papillary carcinoma manifests as a number of nuclear changes including nuclear enlargement, loss of nuclear roundness, increased chromatin granularity, and increased prominence of the nucleolus. The increase in nuclear size distorts the architecture of the epithelium causing nuclear crowding, overlapping, and loss of basal polarization of the nuclei (hematoxylin & eosin stain).

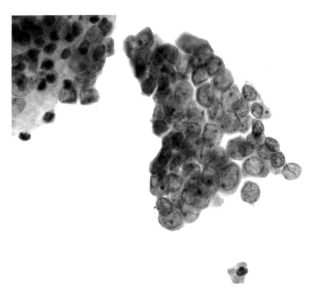

FIGURE 9.18   In FNA samples, the nuclear enlargement of papillary carcinoma generates nuclear crowding and overlapping and the epithelial fragments develop a syncytial architecture. The increase in nuclear size is accentuated in ThinPrep slides as the wet fixation cause the epithelial cells to "round up" with an apparent reduction in cytoplasm, thereby exaggerating the shift in nuclear/cytoplasmic ratio (ThinPrep, Papanicolaou stain).

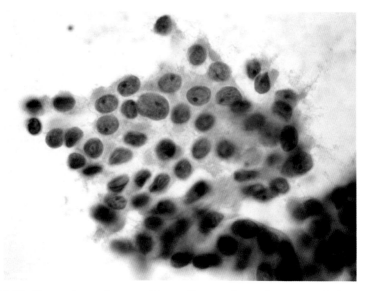

FIGURE 9.19 The nuclear enlargement in papillary carcinoma is asymmetrical so that the nuclei lose their spherical shape and become more elongated and ovoid. Variation in the degree of nuclear enlargement results in nuclear pleomorphism (direct smear, Papanicolaou stain).

3. Transition from monolayered sheets to syncytial aggregates (seen in cytological preparations).

The nuclear enlargement is usually inconsistent from cell to cell, generating a mild degree of pleomorphism and the nuclear enlargement is asymmetrical, resulting in a nucleus that has lost its typical spherical shape and becomes ovoid (Fig. 9.19, e-Fig. 9.26). Hypothetically, this reflects the disordered nuclear scaffolding that occurs as a result of the oncogenesis of papillary carcinoma and manifests a number of other profound alterations in nuclear structure that take on diagnostic importance.

NUCLEAR MEMBRANE IRREGULARITY, NUCLEAR GROOVES, AND INTRANUCLEAR INCLUSIONS. The nuclear membranes of papillary carcinoma show irregularities of varying degrees. Most nuclei are oval with smooth, regular margins. However, in papillary carcinoma nuclei may have markedly irregular nuclear membranes, resulting in a "crumpled paper" or "raisin-like" appearance (Fig. 9.20, e-Fig. 9.27). One manifestation of this nuclear membrane irregularity is the nuclear groove. The nuclear grooves seen in papillary carcinoma have been given a variety of names, including linear chromatin ridge, chromatin band, nuclear folds, nuclear crease, or more accurately invaginations. Nuclear grooves actually reflect an invagination of the nuclear membrane that runs parallel to the long axis of the elongated nucleus [9, 25–26] (Figs. 9.21–9.24, e-Figs. 9.28–9.34). Many grooves are fine and difficult to resolve by light microscopy. When well oriented and

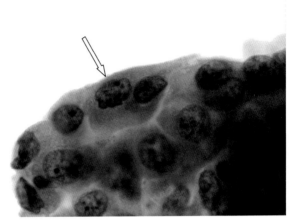

FIGURE 9.20 Nuclear membrane irregularities are common in papillary carcinoma. The majority of nuclei will be round with minimal nuclear membrane irregularities, but in some cases the nuclear membranes can become significantly irregular in contour (*arrow*) (ThinPrep, Papanicolaou stain).

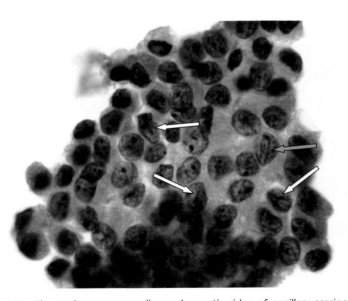

FIGURE 9.21 The nuclear groove or linear chromatin ridge of papillary carcinoma is seen as a thin line that runs along the long axis of the nucleus (*white arrows*). If see from above and well resolved, it is possible to determine that the groove is actually two parallel lines (*orange arrow*), representing the edges of the invagination, much like viewing a valley or canyon from above (ThinPrep, Papanicolaou stain).

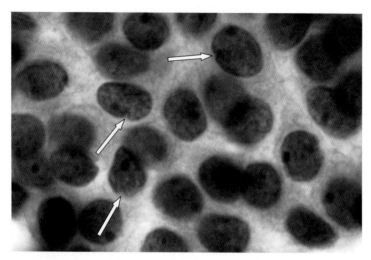

FIGURE 9.22 When nuclear grooves are viewed from the side, the profile of the invagination becomes apparent as a valley or "notch" (*arrows*) (ThinPrep, Papanicolaou stain).

well resolved, one can appreciate that the groove is composed of two parallel lines representing the edges of the nuclear groove where the membrane has invaginated (Figs. 9.21 and 9.24, e-Figs. 9.28, 9.29, 9.32–9.34). If the orientation of the nucleus is such as to view the groove on edge, the invagination may be appreciated as a "notch" (Fig. 9.22, e-Figs. 9.30, 9.32–9.34).

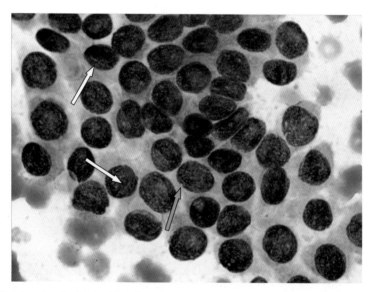

FIGURE 9.23 On air-dried, Diff Quik-stained direct smears, the nuclear grooves appear as thin pale lines crossing the nuclear surface (*white arrows*). A nuclear notch is apparent in one nucleus (*orange arrow*) (direct smear, Diff Quik stain).

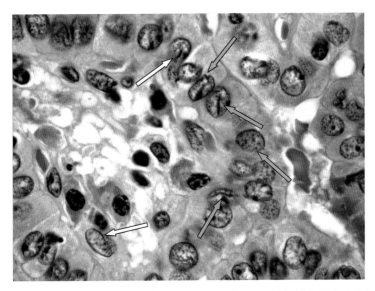

FIGURE 9.24 The appearance of nuclear grooves (*white arrows*) in histological slides is the same as in cytologic preparations. When viewed from above, the valleylike nature of the invagination that forms the nuclear groove is apparent (*orange arrows*) and nuclear notches may be identified (*green arrows*) (hematoxylin & eosin stain).

It must be noted that nuclear grooves in follicular epithelial cells are also seen in a variety of settings, most notably in lymphocytic thyroiditis and are not specific for papillary carcinoma. Quantification studies have shown that papillary carcinoma tends to have more grooves than other lesions [27–33], but have not shown that a specific number of grooves establishes a definitive diagnosis. One further caveat is that nuclear grooves are of diagnostic help only when identified within a follicular epithelial cell. Macrophages (histiocytes) are characterized by elongated oval nuclei with nuclear grooves that can mimic papillary carcinoma [34] and clearly the identification of grooves in histiocytes is of no diagnostic value with regards to papillary carcinoma.

When carried to an extreme and reflecting profound nuclear skeletal derangement, invagination of the nuclear membrane produces intranuclear cytoplasmic pseudoinclusions [25,27,33,35], shortened to "intranuclear inclusions." Intranuclear inclusions have a high specificity for papillary carcinoma, although not 100%. However, to have this degree of specificity, the object in question must be an intranuclear inclusion and not a mimic such as an area of chromatin pallor. Thus, to be considered an intranuclear inclusion, the object must fulfill four criteria. These criteria have been derived to achieve highly specific cytologic diagnoses, but are equally applicable to histologic preparations (Figs. 9.25–9.29, e-Figs. 9.35–9.43):

1. Size criterion: the diameter of an intranuclear inclusion must be at least one quarter the diameter of the nucleus (Fig. 9.26).

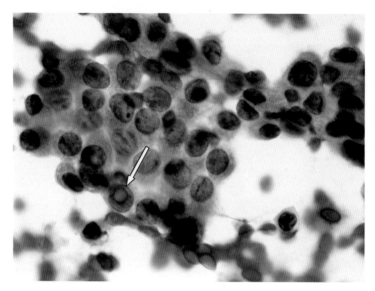

FIGURE 9.25 Cytoplasmic intranuclear pseudoinclusions (*white arrow*) are the pinnacle of deformations of the nuclear structure in papillary carcinoma. These represent invaginations of the cytoplasm into the nucleus and although not pathognomic of papillary carcinoma, nor identifiable in every case of papillary carcinoma, intranuclear inclusions are very important in establishing the cytologic diagnosis (direct smear, Papanicolaou stain).

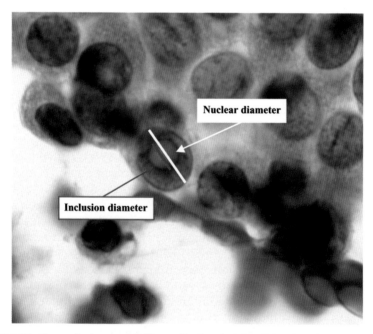

FIGURE 9.26 Four criteria are useful in confirming that the object is a true intranuclear inclusion. Firstly, the cell must be an epithelial cell. Secondly, the diameter of an intranuclear inclusion should be at least one quarter the diameter of the nucleus in which it is found. This criterion is overly strict as many intranuclear inclusions will be smaller than this criterion allows. However, the mimics of intranuclear inclusions also tend to be of small size and this criterion helps eliminate those mimics (direct smear, Papanicolaou stain).

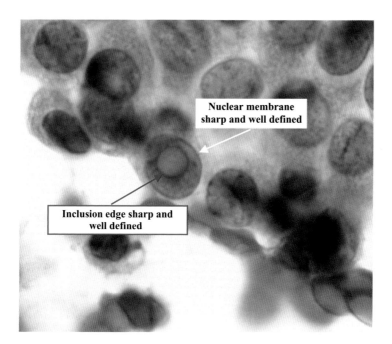

Nuclear membrane
sharp and well defined

Inclusion edge sharp and
well defined

FIGURE 9.27   The edge of the intranuclear inclusion is actually the nuclear membrane as it invaginates into the nucleus. Therefore, the edge of the intranuclear inclusion should be as sharply defined as that of the nuclear membrane elsewhere. Similarly, the intranuclear inclusion should be round and regular (direct smear, Papanicolaou stain).

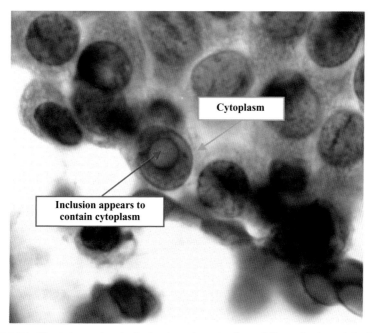

Cytoplasm

Inclusion appears to
contain cytoplasm

FIGURE 9.28   The intranuclear inclusion is an invagination of the cytoplasm into the nucleus and therefore the inclusion itself must appear similar to the cytoplasm and different from the nucleoplasm (direct smear, Papanicolaou stain).

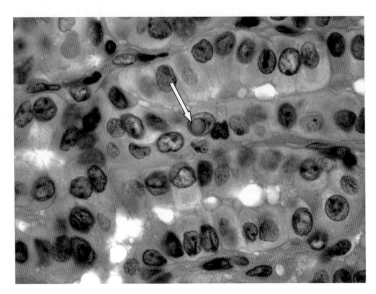

FIGURE 9.29   The same criteria used in the cytologic identification of intranuclear inclusions can be used in histologic examination. The inclusion (*white arrow*) should have a diameter at least one quarter of the diameter of the nucleus and should be round, regular, and demarcated by a sharp edge, while its contents should appear similar to the cytoplasm of the epithelial cell in which it is found. Note the numerous nuclear grooves and notches in this case (hematoxylin & eosin stain).

2. Edge criterion: the inclusion must have sharply defined borders and should be round and regular (Fig. 9.27).
3. Contents criterion: the inclusion should contain material that appears similar to the cytoplasm of the cell (Fig. 9.28).
4. Epithelial cell criterion: the cell housing the inclusion must be an identifiable follicular epithelial cell.

The most overly rigid criterion is the size requirement. There are certainly many intranuclear inclusions that are smaller than this criterion allows. However, artifacts that mimic intranuclear inclusion tend to be small and this size criterion helps eliminate the possibility of misinterpreting these mimics.

The edge of the intranuclear inclusion is generated by the invaginated nuclear membrane, and as such must be as sharply defined as the other portions of the nuclear membrane and the inclusion itself should appear round and regular. This criterion is also overly rigid, for it requires the nucleus to have an ideal orientation to the observer. Thus, a perfectly orientated intranuclear inclusion will have a very sharp, crisp edge. When the inclusion is off angle in cytologic preparations, the intranuclear inclusion is viewed through some of the nucleoplasm and the edges may not be as clear and defined. In histologic preparations, tangential sectioning may rarely produce a similar problem. Relaxation of requirement for sharp-edged inclusions results in a risk of considering areas of chromatin clearing as inclusions and these regions of chromatin clearing do not convey the same diagnostic significance as the inclusion.

The third criterion for an intranuclear inclusion requires the identification of cytoplasm within the inclusion and this is most often apparent in the tinctorial characteristics of the inclusion compared to the cytoplasm outside the nucleus. In Papanicolaou-stained cytologic preparations, the inclusion should be cyanophilic to faintly eosinophilic; in Romanowsky-stained preparations, the inclusion is pale blue; and in material stained with hematoxylin and eosin, the inclusion is pink. In histologic preparations, this criterion is absolute. However, in cytologic preparations, this criterion may again be considered somewhat harsh, as an inclusion oriented so there is nucleoplasm between the observer and the inclusion will appear more basophilic due to the overlying chromatin.

The final criterion is not overly harsh and must be met. For an intranuclear inclusion to be accepted, it must be seen within a follicular epithelial cell. Intranuclear inclusions have no specificity for papillary carcinoma if they are not within follicular epithelial cells.

The presence of intranuclear inclusions is not pathognomonic of papillary carcinoma even when the four criteria above are satisfied. Intranuclear inclusions are known to occur in other lesions such as medullary carcinoma and this diagnosis requires accurate distinction of C cells from follicular epithelial cells. They have also been reported in histologic sections of follicular epithelial cells in Hashimoto's thyroiditis [36], however the authors of this book feel that true intranuclear inclusions as define above represent a neoplastic change. Some investigators have proposed that a specific number of inclusions can predict papillary carcinoma [27,30,37]; however, the frequency of intranuclear inclusions varies among the subtypes of papillary carcinoma. For example, intranuclear inclusions are more frequent and florid in the tall cell variant of papillary carcinoma, while the follicular variant of papillary carcinoma is notorious for having fewer intranuclear inclusions that often do not appear to be as well developed as in conventional papillary carcinomas. For this reason, intranuclear inclusions are not a prerequisite for the diagnosis of papillary carcinoma, although in cytologic practice, the potential for misdiagnosis increases when intranuclear inclusions are lacking.

OPTICALLY CLEAR NUCLEI. The chromatin of neoplastic thyroid cells is altered and frequently becomes more pale and granular (powdery) in comparison to resting thyroid cells. Whereas chromatin changes are seen in many different thyroid neoplasms and are relatively nonspecific, the chromatin structure in papillary carcinoma is predisposed to the development of peripheral margination. As a result, the center of the nucleus develops a "ground glass" appearance [38] or when pronounced, appears to be optically clear. The chromatin is pushed to the edge of the nucleus and the central clearing with thickened outline of the nucleus yield an appearance that

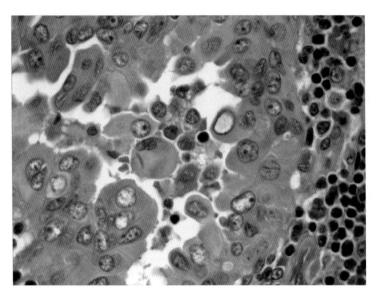

FIGURE 9.30   Formalin fixation may result in artifactual margination and clearing of the chromatin within nuclei of papillary carcinoma generating optically clear or "Orphan Annie eye" nuclei. Although classically associated with papillary carcinoma, this artifact has been noted to occur in other lesions and is not seen with other fixatives (hematoxylin & eosin stain).

resembles the large oval eyes of the cartoon character Orphan Annie, hence the term "Orphan Annie eye nuclei" (Fig. 9.30, e-Figs. 9.44 and 9.45). This is a fixation artifact [39] seen in formalin-fixed tissue and is not typically evident in frozen sections. It should be noted that the occurrence of optically clear nuclei is variable and influenced by the fixation conditions and has been reported in lesions other than papillary carcinoma [39]. Optically clear nuclei are not described in routinely processed FNA of papillary carcinoma. However, it has been reported that optically clear nuclei can be induced in direct smears of the FNA specimens if the smears are first air dried and then rehydrated followed by staining with a modified Pap stain [40–42].

NUCLEOLI. The nucleoli of thyroid neoplasms are increased in prominence in comparison to resting follicular epithelium. The nucleoli do not take on the size and intensity of those seen in adenocarcinomas that arise elsewhere in the body, but are instead seen as one to three micronucleoli, positioned toward the nuclear membrane. A usual nucleolar feature is the development of "bare nucleoli" in which the chromatin surrounding the nucleolus is cleared, giving the appearance of the nucleolus residing within a hole (e-Fig. 9.46).

OTHER FEATURES SEEN WITH PAPILLARY CARCINOMA

PSAMMOMA BODIES. Psammoma bodies are calcified, hematoxyphilic, concentrically laminated, spherical bodies (Figs. 9.31 and 9.32, e-Figs.

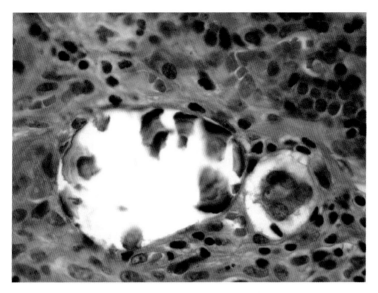

FIGURE 9.31 Psammoma bodies are calcified, concentrically laminated, spherical bodies that are typically basophilic. Because of their rigid nature, fracture is common during histologic sectioning, but even in the remaining fragments, the laminated nature of the structure is apparent (hematoxylin & eosin stain).

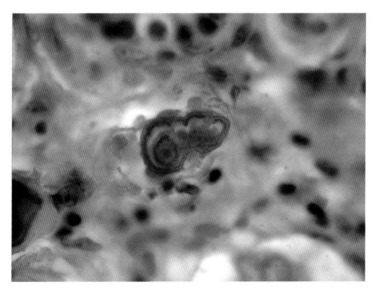

FIGURE 9.32 Fusion of psammoma bodies into a single mass may result in concretions that lose their spheric outline. Note that the individual psammoma bodies retain their internal concentric laminations (hematoxylin & eosin stain).

9.47–9.51). It is common for psammoma bodies to fuse together, making larger concretions, and thereby lose their spherical form. Psammoma bodies are found in 40% to 50% of classical papillary carcinomas, either in the tumor or in the surrounding nontumorous thyroid. In contrast, they are distinctively uncommon in other variants of papillary carcinoma. Psammoma bodies alone are not diagnostic of papillary carcinoma. However, the presence of true psammoma bodies should be considered suspicious and prompt a careful search for a neoplasm with the nuclear changes of papillary carcinoma. Dense colloid, amyloid, collagenous structures, foreign bodies, and dystrophic calcification may mimic the appearance of psammoma bodies. These mimics are usually distinguished by their lack of concentric laminations that characterize psammoma bodies.

The pathogenesis of psammoma bodies is a matter of debate. Historically, it was felt that psammoma bodies resulted from either thickening of the papilla's basal lamina followed by vascular thrombosis, calcification and tumor cell necrosis, or necrosis and calcification of intralymphatic tumor thrombi [43]. However, these theories do not account for the formation of psammoma bodies in nonpapillary tumors (such as meningioma) nor for the observations of intracytoplasmic psammoma bodies (Figs. 9.33–9.35, e-Figs. 9.49–9.51). Thus, alterative theories have suggested calcification of hyaline stromal structures [44] or mechanisms similar to

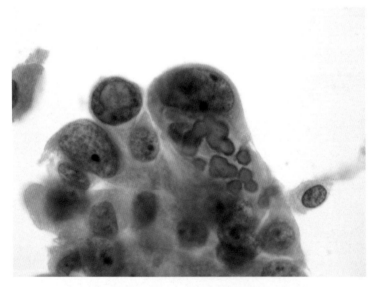

FIGURE 9.33 The pathogenesis of psammoma bodies is somewhat debated. In this example and the following figures (Figs. 9.34 and 9.35), it is apparent that psammoma bodies may have an intracytoplasmic origin that does not support the hypothesis of cellular necrosis leading to psammoma body development. In this image, epithelial cells of a papillary carcinoma are seen to contain intracytoplasmic psammoma bodies in which a central pinpoint nidus is evident with the first few layers of lamination (ThinPrep, Papanicolaou stain).

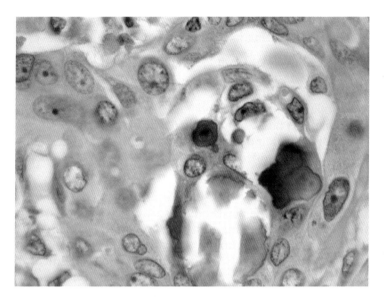

FIGURE 9.34   This is a histologic section of the tumor illustrated in Figure 9.33 in which a typical "mature" psammoma body is evident at the low portion of the image and smaller psammoma bodies are seen adjacent to it. Note the intracytoplasmic location of the psammoma bodies (hematoxylin & eosin stain).

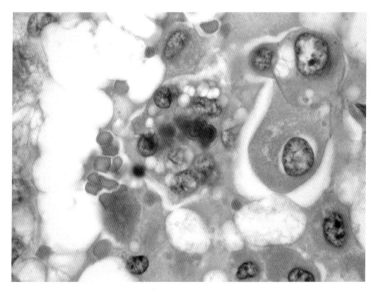

FIGURE 9.35   These psammoma bodies are clearly intracytoplasmic, but have all the features expected for a psammoma body, namely spherical, concentrically laminated, basophilic masses (hematoxylin & eosin stain).

those proposed for serous tumors involving nanobacteria acting as a nidus for psammoma body formation [45,46].

COLLOID. Colloid depletion is relatively common in papillary carcinoma. When present, the colloid of papillary carcinoma has some notable features. Histologically, the colloid is often darker staining than in the normal thyroid and often there is peripheral scalloping of the colloid in follicles of irregular shape (e-Fig. 9.52). Cytologically, the so-called "chewing gum colloid" of papillary carcinoma appears more dense and "sticky" than usual (e-Figs. 9.53 and 9.54). In either case, these changes are not diagnostically specific.

MULTINUCLEATED GIANT CELLS. Multinucleated giant cells of macrophage derivation are occasionally seen in association with papillary carcinoma, often scattered amongst the papillae (Figs 9.36–9.38, e-Figs. 9.55–9.60) [47]. Aspiration of papillary carcinoma may reveal these multinucleated giant cells [48–53], whose appearance is identical to multinucleated giant cells found in other conditions such as granulomatous thyroiditis. The presence of multinucleated giant cells is thus not specifically diagnostic of papillary carcinoma, but should raise the possibility of this diagnosis.

EPITHELIAL CELLS VARIANTS SEEN IN FNA OF PAPILLARY CARCINOMA. In FNA samples from papillary carcinoma, one occasionally encounters epithelial cells that have an appearance similar to squamous metaplastic cells

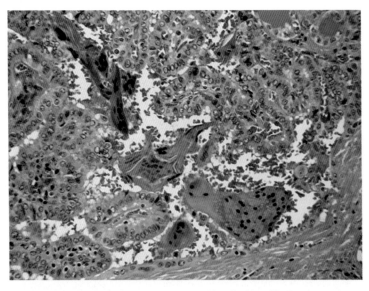

FIGURE 9.36 Multinucleated giant cells are occasionally identified among the papillae of papillary carcinoma (hematoxylin & eosin stain).

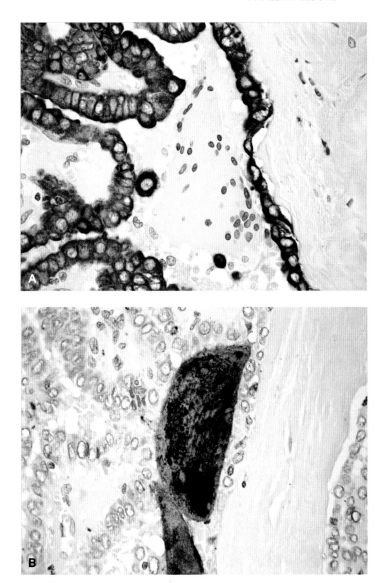

FIGURE 9.37 The multinucleated giant cells seen in papillary carcinoma are of macrophage/monocyte derivation as indicated by their lack of expression of the pan-keratins AE1:AE3 **(A)** and expression of the macrophage marker KP-1 (CD68) **(B)**.

as seen in gynecologic cytology. These metaplasticlike cells represent follicular epithelial cells with a relative abundance of glassy cytoplasm with squared-off cytoplasmic edges imparting a cobblestone appearance to the epithelial groups (Fig. 9.39, e-Figs. 9.61–9.62). These are not true squamous metaplastic cells, but a variant follicular epithelial cell. Very rarely, keratinizing squamous cells may be seen in FNA of papillary

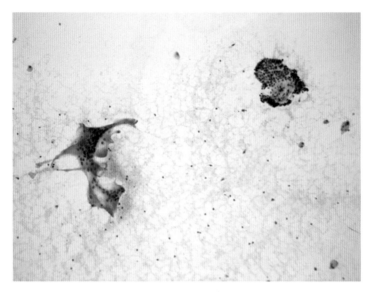

FIGURE 9.38 Multinucleated giant cells are occasionally seen in FNA from conventional papillary carcinoma. Although the finding of multinucleated giant cells should prompt a careful examination of the epithelial fragments for the nuclear features of papillary carcinoma, the presence of multinucleated giant cells is not diagnostic of papillary carcinoma (direct smear, Papanicolaou stain).

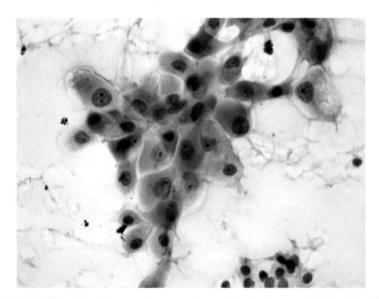

FIGURE 9.39 FNA of papillary carcinomas will occasionally show epithelial cells with features similar to squamous metaplastic cells as seen in gynecologic cytology. The term "metaplasticlike cells" is somewhat of a misnomer as these cells are not truly squamous in differentiation, although true keratinizing squamous cells may rarely be encountered in papillary carcinoma with foci of squamous differentiation (Papanicolaou stain).

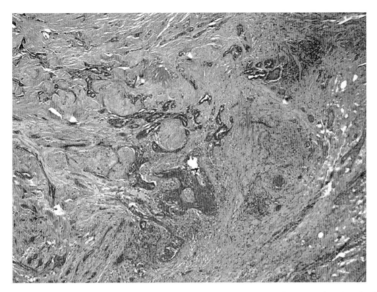

FIGURE 9.40   Foci of squamous differentiation are occasionally identified in histologic samples of papillary carcinoma. In this case, the focus of squamous differentiation is seen within the desmoplastic stroma of an invasive tumor (hematoxylin & eosin stain).

carcinoma if foci of squamous differentiation have developed. However, this is uncommon in cytologic preparations and more frequently encountered in histologic samples (Figs. 9.40 and 9.41, e-Figs. 9.63 and 9.64).

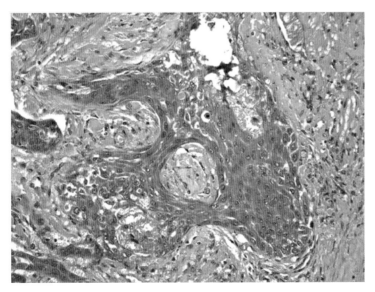

FIGURE 9.41   The regions of squamous differentiation in papillary carcinoma have all the characteristic features of squamous epithelium including intercellular bridging and dyskeratotic cells (hematoxylin & eosin stain).

Epithelial cells with septate vacuoles are also seen in FNA of papillary carcinoma and represent epithelial cells with pronounced dilation of their endoplasmic reticulum [54] (Fig. 9.42, e-Figs. 9.65–9.67). Often the epithelial cells with septate vacuoles also have a metaplasticlike appearance and are more common when cystic change is present within the tumor.

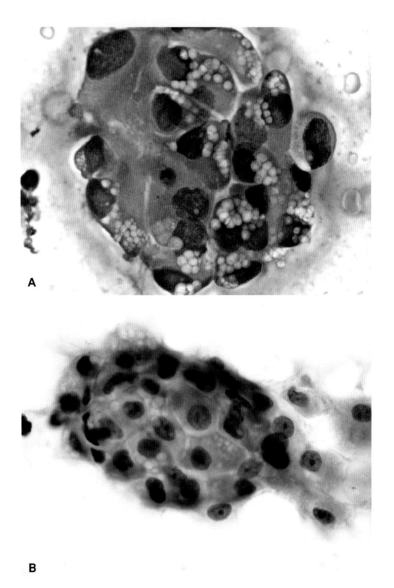

A

B

FIGURE 9.42 Epithelial cells with septate vacuoles may be seen in papillary carcinoma with cystic changes in both air dried, Diff Quik stain **(A)** and alcohol-fixed Papanicolaou-stained **(B)** preparations. These cells have pronounced dilation of their endoplasmic reticulum resulting in the appearance of septate cytoplasmic vacuoles.

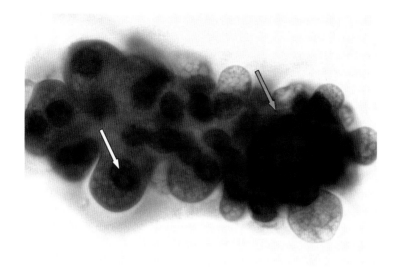

FIGURE 9.43 Histiocytoid cells are follicular epithelial cells with extensive cytoplasmic vacuolation that has progressed to a point that the epithelial cells resemble macrophages (histiocytes). These arise in papillary carcinomas that have undergone cystic change. Note the presence of the intranuclear inclusions (*white arrow*) and psammoma body (*orange arrow*) that help identify these cells as epithelial cells from a papillary carcinoma and not macrophages (ThinPrep, Papanicolaou stain).

Histiocytoid epithelial cells have also been described in FNA of papillary carcinoma and may be exaggerations of the septate vacuoles. These histiocytoid cells are epithelial cells with abundant and prominently vacuolated cytoplasm often seen in association with calcifications [53] (Fig. 9.43, e-Figs. 9.68 and 9.69). The importance of recognition of histiocytoid cells is to distinguish them from macrophages (e-Fig. 9.70) in a cystic lesion. The histiocytoid cells typically have less cytoplasm with a higher nuclear/cytoplasmic ratio than macrophages. The histiocytoid epithelial cells typically have larger nuclei, more prominent nucleoli, and have nuclear grooves and intranuclear inclusions, although the latter two features may be infrequent and difficult to identify. Unfortunately, their resemblance to macrophages may allow the histiocytoid cells to be overlooked in cystic papillary carcinomas.

Making the Diagnosis of Papillary Carcinoma

In an FNA of thyroid, no one feature is absolutely diagnostic of papillary carcinoma. A constellation or combination of nuclear features is required for the diagnosis. Of these features, the most important are oval and enlarged nuclei that contain altered chromatin and nucleoli, with nuclear grooves in a reasonable abundance and intranuclear inclusions. The presence of these features, even when found in a small population of cells

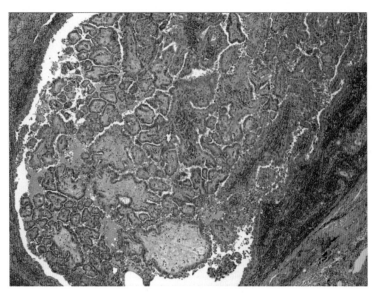

FIGURE 9.44 Chronic inflammation is commonly seen either within papillary carcinoma or in the adjacent thyroid parenchyma (hematoxylin & eosin stain).

whether it be a scanty or cellular aspirate, is associated with a high rate of papillary carcinoma at resection [55]. There are caveats and most important among these is that many of the nuclear features of papillary carcinoma may be seen in follicular epithelium of lymphocytic thyroiditis. Therefore, care must be exercised when a coexistent lymphoid infiltrate is identified and the features must be fully formed and clear-cut before a definitive diagnosis is issued.

Inflammatory infiltrates are relatively common with papillary carcinoma, either within the lesion or in the surrounding thyroid parenchyma [56,57] (Fig. 9.44, e-Fig. 9.71). Some have postulated that this inflammatory infiltrate may indicate host–tumor immune interactions that are responsible for the general indolence of this type of thyroid carcinoma [56]. Recent gene expression microarray studies of classical papillary carcinoma have identified that differentially expressed genes include members of cell differentiation, adhesion, immune response, and proliferation-associated pathways [58–62]. There is controversy surrounding the association of papillary carcinoma with chronic lymphocytic thyroiditis, but the immune response profile may account for the putative relationship.

Ancillary Studies

Ancillary studies can be helpful in the diagnosis of classical variant of papillary thyroid carcinoma (PTC), but they are not usually necessary.

IMMUNOHISTOCHEMISTRY

The role of immunohistochemistry is controversial, but some markers have proven helpful.

Cytokeratin 19 (CK19) is one of a family of keratin filaments that is expressed in glandular tissues. Papillary carcinomas express strong and diffuse immunoreactivity for CK7, CK18, and CK19 in more than 80% of cases [63,64] (Fig. 9.45, e-Fig. 9.72). High molecular weight cytokeratins identified by the antibody 34βE12 are also identified in PTC [65–67]. Normal thyroid follicular epithelium may be positive for CK19 and 34βE12, especially in compressed parenchyma surrounding nodules (Fig. 9.45, e-Fig 9.72), in follicular cells within lymphocytic thyroiditis [68], and in reactive follicular epithelium within degenerate thyroid nodules and at the site of previous biopsy. For this reason, positivity must be interpreted within the context of the location and surrounding parenchyma. While CK19 has been considered by many investigators to be a useful ancillary tool for the diagnosis of papillary carcinoma in FNAC, especially in cytologically suggestive but indeterminate cases [69–71], the well-known positivity of this marker in reactive atypia and chronic lymphocytic thyroiditis that can mimic PTC implies that the use of CK19 on cytologic specimens should be interpreted with great caution, and many diagnosticians, the authors included, do not endorse this application.

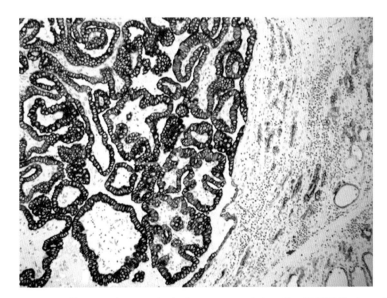

FIGURE 9.45 Papillary carcinomas typically express cytokeratin 19 (CK19) strongly and diffusely. Note that the compressed adjacent thyroid epithelium also shows weak immunoreactivity of CK19, which may also occur in the setting of lymphocytic thyroiditis and in reactive follicular epithelium arising within a degenerative nodule and following FNA (cytokeratin 19 & hematoxylin stain).

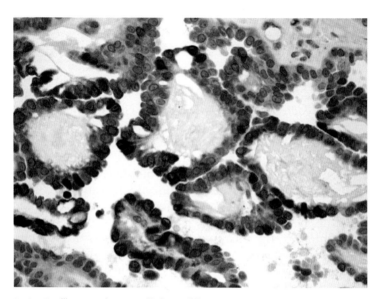

FIGURE 9.46 Papillary carcinoma will show diffuse cytoplasmic staining for galectin-3, but the expression of galectin-3 in the follicular epithelium of lymphocytic thyroiditis, follicular adenomas, and carcinomas limit its diagnostic specificity (galectin-3 & hematoxylin stain).

Galectin-3 is a member of a family of nonintegrin β-galactoside-binding lectins. Several reports have shown that galectin-3 is overexpressed in malignant thyroid tumors including papillary carcinomas [72–82]. Galectin-3 shows strong diffuse cytoplasmic and nuclear staining in most cases of PTC [72,75– 77,79,82,83] (Fig. 9.46, e-Fig. 9.73). Because positive staining is often identified in follicular epithelium affected by chronic lymphocytic thyroiditis [75,76,83], in follicular adenomas, and in follicular carcinomas [84], this is clearly not a diagnostic marker that can be relied upon in biopsies.

HBME-1 (Hector Battifora Mesothelial Epitope-1) is a monoclonal antibody that recognizes an unknown antigen in the microvilli of mesothelioma cells, normal tracheal epithelium, adenocarcinoma of the lung, pancreas, and breast [85,86]. HBME-1 is a useful marker of malignancy in thyroid nodules [64,66,69,78,79,86–89]. Most papillary carcinomas show diffuse positive staining for HBME-1, usually with a delicate luminal pattern of reactivity [64,66,69,78,79,86] (Fig. 9.47, e-Fig. 9.74), with cytoplasmic staining typical of the oncocytic variant. In most of the reports in which HBME-1 was also studied in normal, inflamed, and hyperplastic thyroid, these tissues were negative for this marker [64,79]. HBME-1 has occasionally been reported in lesions identified as adenomatous goiter and follicular adenoma [69,78,79,86]; however, the high specificity of this marker for malignancy in many series and the known observer variability in the diagnosis of nodular goiter and adenoma [47] raise the possibility that these cases with HBME-1 immunorea ctivity would have been considered malignant by some experts.

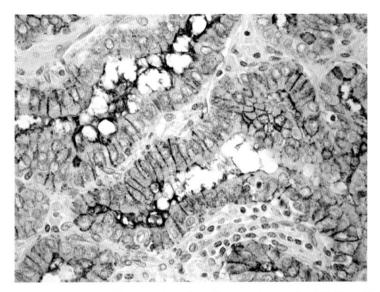

FIGURE 9.47 Immunoperoxidase staining of papillary carcinomas for HBME-1 will show a membranous staining pattern, with luminal accentuation (HBME-1 & hematoxylin stain).

Because of its apparent specificity for malignancy, HBME-1 detection has been considered to be a useful adjunct in the biopsy assessment of thyroid lesions [69,89,90]. The sensitivity, specificity, positive predictive value, and diagnostic accuracy of HBME-1 as a single marker in discriminating benign from malignant lesions are as high as 80%, 96%, 96.7%, and 86.4%, respectively [69].

MOLECULAR ALTERATIONS

In conventional papillary carcinoma, the most common form of thyroid cancer, specific mutations, or rearrangements involving MAPK pathway effectors appear pivotal for transformation. Indeed, exclusive, nonoverlapping activating events involving *RET*, *NTRK*, *BRAF*, or *RAS* are detectable in nearly 70% of all cases [91]. These molecular changes provide helpful ancillary tools for diagnosis on biopsy.

Mutations in *BRAF* are the most frequent genetic events in PTC. This proto-oncogene on 7q24 encodes a serine/threonine kinase that transduces regulatory signals through the RAS/RAF/MEK/ERK cascade. Gain-of-function *BRAF* mutation provides an alternative route for aberrant activation of ERK signaling implicated in tumorigenesis of several human cancers such as melanoma and colon carcinoma [91]. Several point mutations of exon 15 have been identified in thyroid cancers; BRAF^{V600E} is the most common alteration in sporadic PTC, found in 29% to 69% of PTCs, mainly in classical variant lesions [91]. This mutation is rare in other variants of papillary carcinoma and is not found in follicular thyroid carcinoma. While this is a highly specific marker of PTC, it is also present in up to 13% of poorly differentiated thyroid carcinoma and 35% of undifferentiated thyroid carcinomas [91], indicating that there is dedifferentiation from PTC to these more aggressive lesions. The identification of a *BRAF* mutation in a biopsy is diagnostic of malignancy but not only of PTC, and morphologic features that suggest a more aggressive carcinoma should be considered important in the differential diagnosis.

BRAF mutations have been reported in papillary microcarcinomas and are considered to be an early event in thyroid follicular cell transformation. However, in some studies, BRAF mutations correlate with distant metastasis and more advanced clinical stage [92] and occur at a significantly higher frequency in older patients; a gender difference is still controversial [91]. While the diagnostic value of the mutation is indisputable, its prognostic value remains uncertain. Recent studies suggest that additional molecular events are required to support more aggressive behavior [93]. The development of BRAF inhibitors has led to a need for predictive analysis for patients with advanced disease who may benefit from this therapy [94,95].

RET was the first activated receptor tyrosine kinase identified in thyroid cancer. The proto-oncogene on 10q11.2 encodes a transmembrane receptor tyrosine kinase with four cadherin-related motifs in the extracellular domain [91]. *RET* is normally expressed in the developing central and peripheral nervous systems and is essential for renal organogenesis and enteric neurogenesis. Glial-derived neurotrophic factor (GDNF) ligands and GDNF family receptor-α (GFRα) bind the extracellular domain of RET to form a trimeric complex that induces tyrosine kinase auto-phosphorylation and activates several signaling pathways including ERK, PI3K, p38, and JUNK. Gain-of-function mutations of *RET* are involved in sporadic and familial C-cell-derived medullary thyroid carcinoma including multiple endocrine neoplasia (MEN) 2A, MEN 2B, and familial medullary thyroid carcinoma [96–98]. In contrast, more than 15 chimeric oncogenes, designated *RET*/PTC, are implicated in the development of PTC [100]. Somatic chromosomal rearrangement leads to fusion of the 3′-terminal sequence of *RET* encoding the tyrosine kinase domain and 5′-terminal sequences of heterologous genes [99–101]. Although wild-type RET is not normally expressed in follicular cells, *RET*/PTC chimeric oncoproteins lacking a signal peptide and transmembrane domain are expressed in the cytoplasm of follicular cells under the control of the newly acquired promoters. The constitutive activation of the tyrosine domain in the carboxyl-terminal end of RET/PTC induces signaling pathways within thyrocytes and causes cellular transformation in transgenic mice [102–104]. RET/PTC has been implicated in the development of the characteristic nuclear features of papillary carcinoma through alteration of the nuclear envelope and chromatin structure [105].

There is wide variation in the reported frequency of *RET*/PTC rearrangements in PTCs, related to geographic location, radiation exposure, and detection methods [106]. The high incidence of *RET* rearrangements in childhood PTCs following the Chernobyl accident suggests a role for radiation damage in the genesis of these paracentric inversions [107,108]. Analysis of chromatin patterns in thyroid follicular cells identified physical proximity of the partners involved in the illegitimate recombination of these rearrangements [109], providing a plausible scenario for radiation-related susceptibility. In nonradiation-induced sporadic papillary carcinomas, RET/PTC-1 and RET/PTC-3 are the most common types of RET rearrangements, identified in approximately 40% and 15% of cases, respectively [106,110,111].

Although thyroid-targeted expression of *RET*/PTC1 or *RET*/PTC3 induces thyroid neoplasms in transgenic mice, it does not recapitulate the metastatic phenotype without additional alterations [112]. The high frequency of *RET* rearrangements in subclinical papillary thyroid microcarcinomas is also consistent with these changes representing early events in the neoplastic process [15]. Heterogeneity of *RET* rearrangements in a single tumor has been identified and was interpreted as indicative of a relatively late event; however, an alternative interpretation is that multiple and distinct rearrangements signify multifocal transforming events in benign clonal neoplasms [113].

The utility of aberrant *RET* expression by rearrangement as a diagnostic marker in borderline thyroid lesions and preoperative evaluation of thyroid aspirates is supported by its high specificity for PTC [114–116]. Several techniques have been applied. Immunohistochemistry for RET was proposed as a surrogate marker of translocation, since follicular epithelium is negative for this protein in the absence of a rearrangement. This tool is limited by the availability of appropriate reagents. Currently, a number of monoclonal antibodies directed against the RET carboxy-terminus are commercially available, but most fail to reproduce the diffuse cytoplasmic positivity observed with previous polyclonal antisera that are no longer commercially available [15,87,117,118]. Several reports have proposed RET immunohistochemistry in combination with other antibodies including cytokeratin 19, galectin-3, and HBME-1 for the assessment of thyroid specimens and aspirates [64,89,116,117), but these also have relied on sensitive and specific antisera.

DNA analysis of these rearrangements is technically difficult due to the large introns and variable breakpoints in individual lesions. Therefore, the gold standard for identification of a RET/PTC rearrangement has been by the application of RT-PCR for identification of mRNA [15,115]. This test is easily performed on formalin-fixed, paraffin-embedded tissue and on FNA specimens prepared in alcohol-based fixatives for thin-layer cytology [15,115]. However, the need for optimal preservation and the variable expression levels of mRNA make this a difficult technique to apply on routine specimens. Both RT-PCR and immunohistochemistry rely on expression of the rearrangements that is known to be highly variable; the development of a reliable FISH assay to more sensitively identify these rearrangements [119] may prove valuable to resolve some of the controversies around this molecular event. Moreover, the availability of novel ret inhibitors as therapeutic modalities for patients who fail conventional therapy predicts a potential need for accurate identification of these rearrangements [95,120].

RET/PTC rearrangements have also been reported in thyroids with Hashimoto's thyroiditis [121]. The possibility of identifying a ret/PTC rearrangement in thyroiditis has been the major criticism hampering the application of this molecular marker to biopsy diagnosis. However, these findings are controversial and may reflect either PCR contamination or the presence of microscopic nodules of PTC, since many studies that have excluded these possibilities do not confirm the data [15,122]. The presence of papillary microcarcinoma is not to be underestimated as a cause of this problem, since this is a common finding, in up to 36% of autopsy thyroids and in up to 24% of total thyroidectomies for disorders other than follicular-derived cancer [14]. However, the approach using FISH assays suggests that rearrangements in scattered nontumorous thyrocytes in thyroiditis [119] may represent early events that give rise to clonal proliferations of papillary carcinoma.

The receptor tyrosine kinase *NTRK1* was the second identified subject of chromosomal rearrangement in thyroid tumorigenesis. The *NTRK1* (*TRK*, *TRKA*) proto-oncogene on 1q22 encodes the transmembrane tyrosine kinase receptor for nerve growth factor. NTRK1 is typically restricted to neurons of the sensory spinal and cranial ganglia of neural crest origin and regulates neuronal growth and survival. *NTRK1* rearrangements, showing ectopic expression and constitutive activation of the tyrosine kinase analogous to *RET* rearrangements, have been noted in 5% to 13% of sporadic but in only 3% of post-Chernobyl childhood PTCs [91]. To date, *TPM3*, *TPR*, and *TFG* have been identified as fusion partners forming chimeric oncogenes designated as TRK, TRK-T1 and T2, and TRK-T3, respectively. The prevalence of each fusion type is nearly equal in sporadic PTCs, while *TPM3-NTRK* is more frequent than other *NTRK1* rearrangements in post-Chernobyl childhood PTCs. The relatively lower incidence of these rearrangements makes them less valuable as routine markers for diagnostic biopsies.

PAPILLARY CARCINOMA, PAPILLARY VARIANTS

Papillary carcinoma has a number of histologic variants. The need to recognize the exact variant on FNA or core biopsy is debatable as the immediate management of the nodule in question is not altered by the subtype of papillary carcinoma. Thus, the goal is to recognize these variants as papillary carcinomas, something that is typically achieved without difficulty as the same nuclear features are seen in the subtypes. Although there have been descriptions of the cytomorphology of many of the variants of papillary carcinoma, it may not be possible in all cases to recognize the exact histological variant of papillary carcinoma from the appearance of the fine needle aspirate [123]. A notable exception to this is oncocytic variant of papillary carcinoma that may be easily recognized in some cases.

The recognition of the variants of papillary carcinoma on the resected specimen is another matter as the histologic distinctions are characteristic [9,22,24,124–126] and are of prognostic value.

Papillary microcarcinoma [127] has a better prognosis than larger papillary carcinoma. Microcarcinomas are recognized solely by a size criteria and do not have a unique morphology. These tumors, defined as less than 1 cm (Fig. 9.48, e-Figs. 9.75–9.77), are common and appear to be different biologically than larger tumors [24,127–129]. The significance of this diagnosis on biopsy is controversial, since occult papillary microcarcinomas are identified in up to 24% of the population in thyroids that are removed for nonmalignant or unrelated disease [14]. However, with the increasing use of ultrasound, more of these lesions are being identified and biopsied.

Cystic papillary carcinoma is common, representing up to 10% of papillary carcinomas [20,21,22,130]. This diagnosis must be considered when evaluating a cystic lesion (Chapter 7). For this reason, ultrasound evaluation should be used when biopsying cystic lesions to identify any solid component that will yield diagnostic material. Although the histology of cystic papillary carcinomas will show retention of a focus with classical papillary architecture and nuclear features of papillary carcinoma, this may not be represented in an FNA. Typically, an FNA yields old

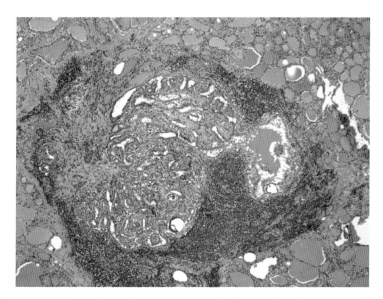

FIGURE 9.48 Papillary microcarcinomas are, by definition, smaller than 1 cm and identified in approximately 24% of the thyroids resected for nonmalignant reasons (hematoxylin & eosin stain).

blood, proteinaceous material, and hemosiderin-laden macrophages with a dearth of epithelium. When the epithelium is present, classical features of papillary carcinoma may be evident, but these lesions are the source of the metaplasticlike cells, cells with septate vacuoles, and histiocytoid cells described earlier in this chapter. Because the scarcity of epithelial cells and the subtly of nuclear abnormalities, cystic PTC has long been recognized as source of false-negative thyroid FNAs. It should be remembered that atypical cyst-lining cells can be seen in aspirate of benign cysts [131]. These reactive cells are arranged in sheets with enlarged nuclei, nucleoli, and they may have nuclear grooves. However, they often have more spindle cell morphology and lack nuclear crowding and intranuclear inclusions. It is important not to over-diagnose the atypical cyst lining cells without definitive nuclear features of PTC.

Oncocytic, oxyphilic, or Hürthle cell variant of papillary carcinoma has been reported to comprise from 1% to 11% of all papillary carcinomas [132–138]. These tumors have papillary architecture, but are composed predominantly or entirely of Hürthle cells [136,139] (Figs. 9.49 and 9.50, e-Figs. 9.78 and 9.79). The nuclei may exhibit the characteristics of usual papillary carcinoma [133,140] but the features may be camouflaged by the pleomorphism and hyperchromasia associated with oncocytic change [134,141]. The clinical behavior of this subtype is controversial. Some authors have reported that they behave like typical papillary carcinomas [137,139–142]. Others maintain that the oncocytic morphology confers a more aggressive behavior [143,144] with higher rates of 10-year tumor recurrence and cause-specific mortality [134]. This suggestion of

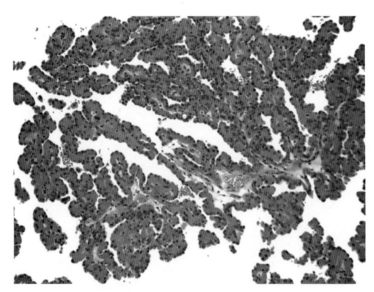

FIGURE 9.49 The oncocytic variant of papillary carcinoma displays a papillary architecture, but the papillae are lined by Hürthle cells (hematoxylin & eosin stain).

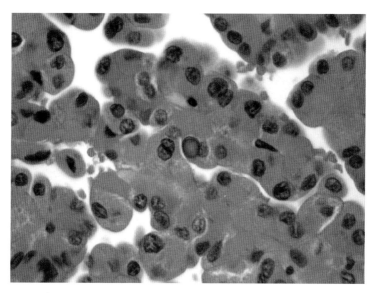

FIGURE 9.50 The nuclei of the oncocytic variant of papillary carcinoma typically show the classical features of papillary carcinoma. However, in some cases, the nuclear pleomorphism and hyperchromasia associated with oncocytic change may obscure the nuclear features of papillary carcinoma (hematoxylin & eosin stain).

aggressive behavior may be attributed to inclusion of tall cell variant of papillary carcinoma (see below) in the group of oncocytic papillary carcinomas. It is important to make a distinction between these two different papillary variants of PTC.

On aspiration, the oncocytic variant of papillary carcinoma will yield epithelium arranged in monolayered sheets, syncytial aggregates often with transgressing vessels, microfollicular structures, papillary fragments, or as scattered single cells [145,146] (Figs. 9.51 and 9.52, e-Figs. 9.80 and 9.81). One of the two possible diagnoses will be made when confronted with such an aspirate. If the characteristic nuclear features of papillary carcinoma are identified, a diagnosis of oncocytic variant of papillary carcinoma will be made. If, however, the nuclear features are missed or lacking, the lesion will be labeled as Hürthle cell neoplasm. Therefore, in all FNAs of oncocytic neoplasms, it is critical to carefully examine the nuclei for features of papillary carcinoma.

Mitochondrial DNA (mtDNA) deletion and/or point mutations have been identified in nonneoplastic and neoplastic thyroid cells displaying morphologic oncocytic changes, suggesting a contribution of mtDNA alterations to the oncocytic process [147–150]. However, it is not clear if this represents a separate and distinct process from neoplastic transformation. The coexistence of ret/PTC or BRAF mutations with oncocytic change and mtDNA alterations proves that the two processes may be independent. Several studies have demonstrated an impact of mtDNA mutation

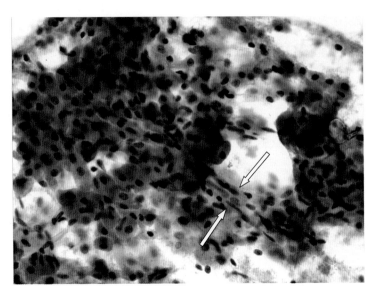

FIGURE 9.51   FNA of papillary oncocytic variant of papillary carcinoma often reveals a monotony of Hürthle (oncocytic) cells without evidence of papillary structures. As illustrated in this image, complex, thick fragments of Hürthle cells may be identified with transgressing vessels (between *white arrows*), indicative of a Hürthle cell neoplasm (direct smear, Papanicolaou stain).

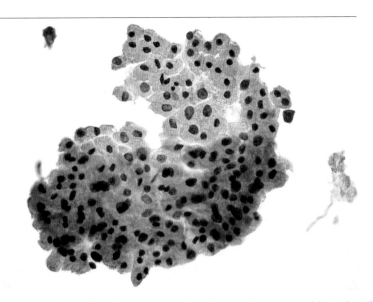

FIGURE 9.52   When the full nuclear features of papillary carcinoma are evident, the Hürthle (oncocytic) cell variant of papillary carcinoma is readily diagnosed on FNA. However, not all nuclear features may be apparent as in this case and it becomes impossible to achieve a more definitive diagnosis than Hürthle cell neoplasm (ThinPrep, Papanicolaou stain).

on cell growth and tumorigenicity [91]. The identification of somatic and germline missense mutations in the *GRIM-19* (19p13.2) gene in oncocytic follicular and PTCs suggests a possible dual function of this gene in mitochondrial metabolism and cell death [150]. Clearly, further investigations are necessary to clarify whether mtDNA mutation truly contributes to initiation and/or progression or principally to the oncocytic phenotype in thyroid neoplasia.

One morphologic subtype of oncocytic papillary carcinoma which, because of a characteristic cystic change and extensive lymphocytic infiltration into the cores of the papillae of the tumor, has a striking histological resemblance to papillary cystadenoma lymphomatosum of the salivary gland has been called "Warthin-like tumor of the thyroid" [151]. This lesion occurs in the setting of chronic lymphocytic thyroiditis, predominantly in women, and is associated with a similar prognosis to usual papillary carcinoma. In histologic sections, oncocytic cells with nuclear features of papillary carcinoma are arranged in papillary fragments with lymphocytes infiltrating the fibrovascular stalk of the papillae (Fig. 9.53, e-Figs. 9.82 and 9.83). Because this lesion is usually associated with thyroiditis, there may be areas of classical thyroiditis with focal clusters of tumor cells that must be recognized as distinct from the inflammatory process [152–154].

Aggressive variants of papillary carcinoma include the *tall cell variant* and probably related lesions, the *trabecular and columnar cell variant* [155–162]. The tall cell variant is defined as a tumor composed of cells

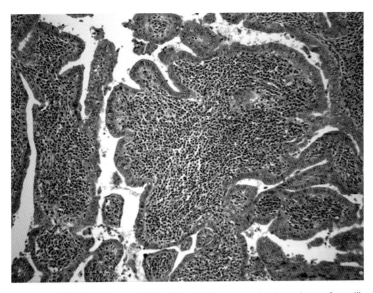

FIGURE 9.53 Warthin-like tumor of the thyroid is an oncocytic variant of papillary carcinoma characterized by infiltration of the papillary stalks by a lymphoplasmacytic population that is very reminiscent of Warthin's tumor of the salivary gland (hematoxylin & eosin stain).

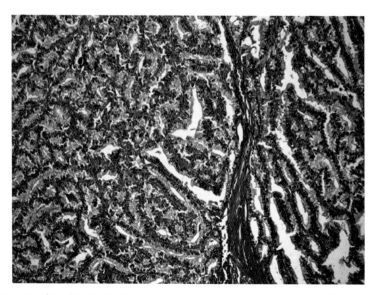

FIGURE 9.54 The tall cell variant of papillary carcinoma is composed of epithelial cells that have a height-to-width ratio that exceeds 3:1 with abundant eosinophilic cytoplasm. The tumors usually have a complex papillary architecture and necrosis may be present (hematoxylin & eosin stain).

that have a height-to-width ratio that exceeds 3:1 (Figs. 9.54 and 9.55, e-Figs. 9.84 and 9.85). They usually have complex papillary architecture and may show focal tumor cell necrosis. Tall cells generally have abundant eosinophilic cytoplasm.

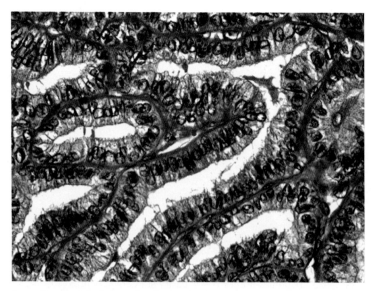

FIGURE 9.55 The nuclei of the tall cell variant of papillary carcinoma show all the classical features of papillary carcinoma (hematoxylin & eosin stain).

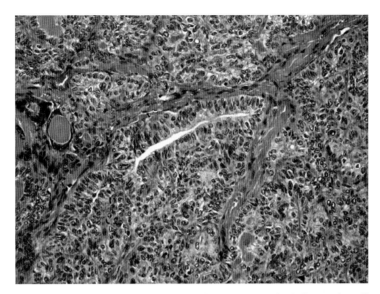

FIGURE 9.56   The columnar cell variant of papillary carcinoma is similar to the tall cell variant, but the nuclei tend to be more crowded with pseudostratification, resembling a colonic adenoma (hematoxylin & eosin stain).

As with the other variants of papillary carcinoma, the florid nuclear features make this variant recognizable as a papillary carcinoma on aspiration. However, achieving the definitive diagnosis of the tall cell variant may be hindered, as cytologic preparations may preclude recognition of the cellular elongation and polarity [163–165].

Columnar cells are similar to tall cells but are more crowded with pseudostratification, resembling respiratory epithelium or colonic adenomas (Figs. 9.56 and 9.57, e-Figs. 9.86 and 9.89), and they harbor subnuclear vacuoles, resembling secretory endometrium. The tumor cells exhibit nuclear features of PTC but often are more hyperchromatic [166]. The differential diagnosis includes metastatic carcinomas and when in doubt, immunolocalization of TTF-1 and thyroglobulin should be performed to verify the follicular cell differentiation of these lesions.

Tumors that exhibit tall or columnar cell morphology in more than 30% of the tumor mass generally tend to occur in older individuals with a median age at diagnosis of 20 years older than usual papillary carcinoma, are often large lesions greater than 5 cm, and often exhibit extrathyroidal extension at the time of diagnosis [161]. In addition to lymphatic invasion, vascular invasion is not uncommonly found in these lesions. Tumor mortality rates vary up to 25% for tall cell tumors and 90% for columnar cell carcinoma [155,157]. There is a high prevalence of *BRAF* mutations in tall cell PTCs, reported in 55% to 100% of cases [91]. However, this ancillary marker is rarely required, since the cytomorphology is highly characteristic.

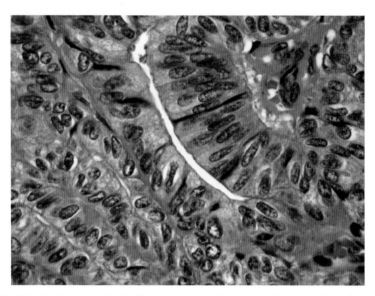

FIGURE 9.57   Nuclear pseudostratification characterizes the columnar cells variant of papillary carcinoma in which the classical nuclear features are also preserved. Subnuclear cytoplasmic vacuolation may also be seen, similar to that occurring in secretary endometrium (hematoxylin & eosin stain).

The *diffuse sclerosis variant* occurs in young individuals and often presents as goiter without a specific mass lesion [167–170]. This tumor microscopically involves thyroid lymphatics, exhibits squamous metaplasia, and forms numerous psammoma bodies, giving it a very gritty appearance when examined grossly (Figs. 9.58–9.60, e-Figs. 9.90–9.94). These tumors almost always have lymph node metastases at presentation and 25% have lung metastases as well. It is interesting that about 10% of the pediatric thyroid cancers that occurred following the Chernobyl nuclear accident in 1986 were of the diffuse sclerosis type [107].

An unusual variant of PTC known as the *cribriform-morular variant* has been identified in patients who harbor mutations of the APC gene that is responsible for familial adenomatous polyposis (FAP) syndrome [171–173]. These lesions have unusual architecture as their name implies; they exhibit intricate admixtures of cribriform, follicular, papillary, trabecular, and solid patterns of growth with morular or squamoid areas. Cribriform structures are prominent. The tumor cells are generally cuboidal or tall, with nuclear pseudostratification (Figs. 9.61 and 9.62, e-Figs. 9.95–9.97). Vascular and capsular invasion are common in these lesions, and while they may exhibit lymph node metastasis, there are no data to suggest that they have worse outcomes than other conventional forms of papillary carcinoma.

They harbor ret/PTC gene rearrangements and do not exhibit loss of heterozygosity of the normal allele of the APC gene to explain an independent mechanism of tumorigenesis. Alterations in the APC gene are not

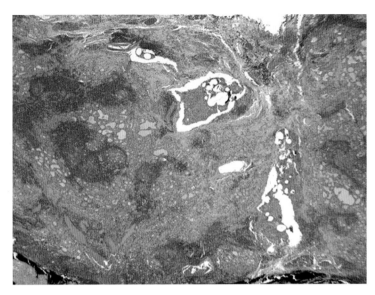

FIGURE 9.58   In the diffuse sclerosis variant of papillary carcinoma, a gross tumor mass is not typically apparent. Instead, the tumor diffusely infiltrates the lymphatics of the thyroid gland. This propensity for lymphatic invasion may account for the high frequency of nodal and pulmonary metastases (hematoxylin & eosin stain).

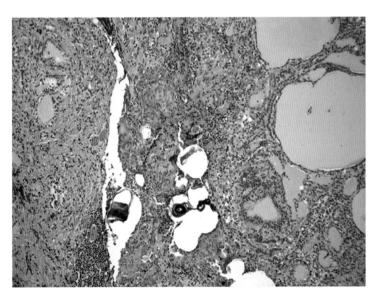

FIGURE 9.59   The stealthy lymphatic permeation by the diffuse sclerosis variant of papillary carcinoma might be difficult to appreciate if it were not for the profusion of psammoma bodies present in many cases (hematoxylin & eosin stain).

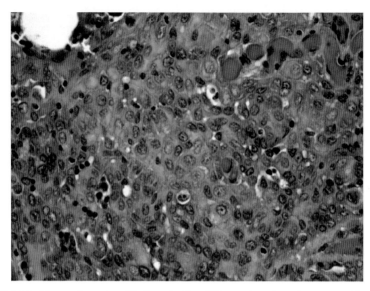

FIGURE 9.60 The malignant epithelium in the diffuse sclerosis variant of papillary carcinoma frequently grows in solid nests and sheets with foci of squamous metaplasia occasionally encountered (hematoxylin & eosin stain).

thought to underlie the more common sporadic thyroid carcinomas [174,175]; however, somatic mutations in exon 3 of the beta-catenin gene (CTNNB1) have been described in patients with this rare tumor variant who do not have germline mutations and FAP syndrome [176]. On biopsy,

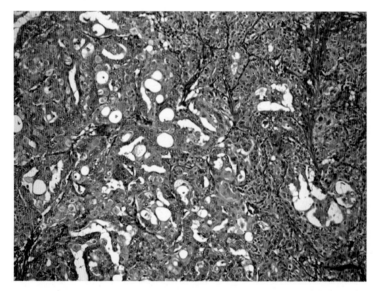

FIGURE 9.61 The cribriform-morular variant of papillary carcinoma reveals a variety of architectures including cribriform, follicular, papillary, trabecular, and solid patterns of growth. The cribriform architecture tends to predominate (hematoxylin & eosin stain).

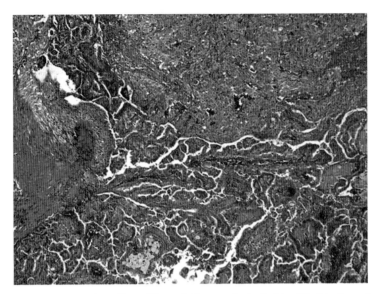

FIGURE 9.62 Regions of papillary differentiation are typically identified in the cribriform-morular variant of papillary carcinoma (hematoxylin & eosin stain).

the lesion is characterized by a cribriform pattern without colloid. The epithelial cells may lack the powdery chromatin pattern characteristic of papillary carcinoma, but they have been described to have scattered intranuclear cytoplasmic pseudoinclusions and grooved nuclei. In FNA samples, the epithelial morules or whorls have atypical enlarged nuclei with thickened nuclear membranes and entirely clear contents. Hyaline-like necrotic cells may also be observed in the cell clusters or in the background [177].

REFERENCES

1. Das DK. Marginal vacuoles (fire-flare appearance) in fine needle aspiration smears of thyroid lesions: does it represent diffusing out of thyroid hormones at the base of follicular cells? *Diagn Cytopathol* 2006;34:277–283.
2. Das DK, Jain S, Tripathi RP, et al. Marginal vacuoles in thyroid aspirates. *Acta Cytol* 1998;42:1121–1128.
3. Namba H, Ross JL, Goodman D, et al. Solitary polyclonal autonomous thyroid nodule: a rare cause of childhood hyperthyroidism. *J Clin Endocrinol Metab* 1991;72:1108–1112.
4. Lyons J, Landis CA, Harsh G. Two G protein oncogenes in human endocrine tumors. *Science* 1990;249:635–639.
5. Porcellini A, Ciullo I, Laviola L, et al. Novel mutations of thyrotropin receptor gene in thyroid hyperfunctioning adenomas. Rapid identification by fine needle aspiration biopsy. *J Clin Endocrinol Metab* 1994;79:657–661.
6. van Sande J, Parma J, Tonacchera M, et al. Genetic basis of endocrine disease. Somatic and germline mutations of the TSH receptor gene in thyroid disease. *J Clin Endocrinol Metab* 1995;80:2577–2585.

7. Parma J, Duprez L, Van Sandem H, et al. Diversity and prevalence of somatic mutations in the thyrotropin receptor and Gs alpha genes as a cause of toxic thyroid adenomas. *J Clin Endocrinol Metab* 1997;82:2695–2701.

8. Krohn D, Fuhrer D, Holzapfel H, et al. Clonal origin of toxic thyroid nodules with constitutively activating thyrotropin receptor mutations. *J Clin Endocrinol Metab* 1998;83:180–184.

9. Rosai J, Carcangiu ML, DeLellis RA. Tumors of the thyroid gland. In: *Atlas of tumor pathology*. 3rd series, fascicle 5. Washington, DC: Armed Forces Institute of Pathology, 1992.

10. Kini SR. *Thyroid*. New York: Igaku-Shoin Ltd., 1996.

11. Casey MB, Lohse CM, Lloyd RV. Distinction between papillary thyroid hyperplasia and papillary thyroid carcinoma by immunohistochemical staining for cytokeratin 19, galectin-3, and HBME-1. *Endocr Pathol* 2003;14:55–60.

12. Hay ID. Papillary thyroid carcinoma. *Endocrinol Metab Clin North Am* 1990;19:545–576.

13. Mazzaferri EL, Jhiang SM. Long-term impact of initial surgical and medical therapy on papillary and follicular thyroid cancer. *Am J Med* 1994;97:418–428.

14. Fink A, Tomlinson G, Freeman JL, et al. Occult micropapillary carcinoma associated with benign follicular thyroid disease and unrelated thyroid neoplasms. *Mod Pathol* 1996;9:816–820.

15. Sugg SL, Ezzat S, Rosen IB, et al. Distinct multiple *ret*/PTC gene rearrangements in multifocal papillary thyroid neoplasia. *J Clin Endocrinol Metab* 1998;83:4116–4122.

16. Shattuck TM, Valimaki S, Obara T, et al. Somatic and germ-line mutations of the HRPT2 gene in sporadic parathyroid carcinoma. *N Engl J Med* 2003;349:1722–1729.

17. Vickery AL. Thyroid papillary carcinoma. Pathological and philosophical controversies. *Am J Surg Pathol* 1983;7:797–807.

18. Vickery AL, Carcangiu ML, Johannessen JV, et al. Papillary carcinoma. *Semin Diagn Pathol* 1985;2:90–100.

19. Rosai J, Zampi G, Carcangiu ML, et al. Papillary carcinoma of the thyroid. *Am J Surg Pathol* 1983;7:809–817.

20. Carcangiu ML, Zampi G, Rosai J. Papillary thyroid carcinoma: a study of its many morphologic expressions and clinical correlates. *Pathol Annu* 1985;20(part 1):1–44.

21. Carcangiu ML, Zampi G, Pupi A, et al. Papillary carcinoma of the thyroid. A clinicopathologic study of cases treated at the University of Florence, Italy. *Cancer* 1985;805:822.

22. LiVolsi VA. *Surgical pathology of the thyroid*. Philadelphia: WB Saunders, 1990.

23. LiVolsi VA. Papillary neoplasms of the thyroid. Pathologic and prognostic features. *Am J Clin Pathol* 1992;97:426–434.

24. DeLellis RA, Lloyd RV, Heitz PU, et al. *Pathology and genetics of tumours of endocrine organs*. WHO Classification of Tumours. Lyons: IARC Press, 2004.

25. Kaneko C, Shamoto M, Niimi H, et al. Studies on intranuclear inclusions and nuclear grooves in papillary thyroid cancer by light, scanning electron and transmission electron microscopy. *Acta Cytol* 1996;40:417–422.

26. Papotti M, Manazza AD, Chiarle R, et al. Confocal microscope analysis and tridimensional reconstruction of papillary thyroid carcinoma nuclei. *Virchows Arch* 2004;444:350–355.

27. Deligeorgi-Politi H. Nuclear crease as a cytodiagnostic feature of papillary thyroid carcinoma in fine-needle aspiration biopsies. *Diagn Cytopathol* 1987;3:307–310.

28. Shurbaji MS, Gupta PK, Frost JK. Nuclear grooves: a useful criterion in the cytopathologic diagnosis of papillary thyroid carcinoma. *Diagn Cytopathol* 1988;4:91–94.

29. Rupp M, Ehya H. Nuclear grooves in the aspiration cytology of papillary carcinoma of the thyroid. *Acta Cytol* 1989;33:21–26.

30. Gould E, Watzak L, Chamizo W, et al. Nuclear grooves in cytologic preparations. A study of the utility of this feature in the diagnosis of papillary carcinoma. *Acta Cytol* 1989;33:16–20.

31. Francis IM, Das DK, Sheikh ZA, et al. Role of nuclear grooves in the diagnosis of papillary thyroid carcinoma. A quantitative assessment on fine needle aspiration smears. *Acta Cytol* 1995;39:409–415.

32. Yang YJ, Demirci SS. Evaluating the diagnostic significance of nuclear grooves in thyroid fine needle aspirates with a semiquantitative approach. *Acta Cytol* 2003;47:563–570.

33. Das DK, Sharma PN. Intranuclear cytoplasmic inclusions and nuclear grooves in fine needle aspiration smears of papillary thyroid carcinoma and its variants: advantage of the count under an oil-immersion objective over a high-power objective. *Anal Quant Cytol Histol* 2005;27:83–94.

34. Nassar A, Gupta P, LiVolsi VA, et al. Histiocytic aggregates in benign nodular goiters mimicking cytologic features of papillary thyroid carcinoma (PTC). *Diagn Cytopathol* 2003;29:243–245.

35. Chan JKC, Saw D. The grooved nucleus: a useful diagnostic criterion of papillary carcinoma of the thyroid. *Am J Surg Pathol* 1986;10:672–679.

36. Berho M, Suster S. Clear nuclear changes in Hashimoto's thyroiditis. A clinicopathologic study of 12 cases. *Ann Clin Lab Sci* 1995;25:513–521.

37. Zhang Y, Fraser JL, Wang HH. Morphologic predictors of papillary carcinoma on fine-needle aspiration of thyroid with ThinPrep preparations. *Diagn Cytopathol* 2001;24: 378–383.

38. Hapke MR, Dehner LP. The optically clear nucleus. A reliable sign of papillary carcinoma of the thyroid? *Am J Surg Pathol* 1979;3:31–38.

39. Naganuma H, Murayama H, Ohtani N, et al. Optically clear nuclei in papillary carcinoma of the thyroid: demonstration of one of the fixation artifacts and its practical usefulness. *Pathol Int* 2000;50:113–118.

40. Yang GC, Greenebaum E. Clear nuclei of papillary thyroid carcinoma conspicuous in fine-needle aspiration and intraoperative smears processed by ultrafast Papanicolaou stain. *Mod Pathol* 1997;10:552–555.

41. Yang GC. Clear nuclei are specific to papillary carcinoma in thyroid fine-needle aspirates processed by Ultrafast Papanicolaou stain. *Diagn Cytopathol* 2003;29:236–237.

42. Yang GC, Liebeskind D, Messina AV. Diagnostic accuracy of follicular variant of papillary thyroid carcinoma in fine-needle aspirates processed by ultrafast Papanicolaou stain: histologic follow-up of 125 cases. *Cancer* 2006;108:174–179.

43. Johannessen JV, Sobrinho-Simoes M. The origin and significance of thyroid psammoma bodies. *Lab Invest* 1980;43:287–296.

44. Das DK, Mallik MK, Haji BE, et al. Psammoma body and its precursors in papillary thyroid carcinoma: a study by fine-needle aspiration cytology. *Diagn Cytopathol* 2004; 31:380–386.

45. Sedivy R, Battistutti WB. Nanobacteria promote crystallization of psammoma bodies in ovarian cancer. *APMIS* 2003;111:951–954.

46. Hudelist G, Singer CF, Kubista E, et al. Presence of nanobacteria in psammoma bodies of ovarian cancer: evidence for pathogenetic role in intratumoral biomineralization. *Histopathology* 2004;45:633–637.

47. Lloyd RV, Erickson LA, Casey MB, et al. Observer variation in the diagnosis of follicular variant of papillary thyroid carcinoma. *Am J Surg Pathol* 2004;28:1336–1340.

48. Kini SR, Miller JM, Hamburger JI, et al. Cytopathology of papillary carcinoma of the thyroid by fine needle aspiration. *Acta Cytol* 1980;24:511–521.

49. Tsou PL, Hsiao YL, Chang TC. Multinucleated giant cells in fine needle aspirates. Can they help differentiate papillary thyroid cancer from benign nodular goiter? *Acta Cytol* 2002;46:823–827.

50. Guiter GE, DeLellis RA. Multinucleate giant cells in papillary thyroid carcinoma. A morphologic and immunohistochemical study. *Am J Clin Pathol* 1996;106:765–768.

51. Shabb NS, Tawil A, Gergeos F, et al. Multinucleated giant cells in fine-needle aspiration of thyroid nodules: their diagnostic significance. *Diagn Cytopathol* 1999;21:307–312.

52. Tabbara SO, Acoury N, Sidawy MK. Multinucleated giant cells in thyroid neoplasms. A cytologic, histologic and immunohistochemical study. *Acta Cytol* 1996;40:1184–1188.

53. Renshaw AA. "Histiocytoid" cells in fine-needle aspirations of papillary carcinoma of the thyroid: frequency and significance of an under-recognized cytologic pattern. *Cancer* 2002;96:240–243.

54. Hirokawa M, Carney JA, Goellner JR, et al. Observer variation of encapsulated follicular lesions of the thyroid gland. *Am J Surg Pathol* 2002;26:1508–1514.

55. Renshaw AA. Focal features of papillary carcinoma of the thyroid in fine-needle aspiration material are strongly associated with papillary carcinoma at resection. *Am J Clin Pathol* 2002;118:208–210.

56. Schröder S, Schwarz W, Rehpenning W, et al. Dendritic/Langerhans cells and prognosis in patients with papillary thyroid carcinomas. *Am J Clin Pathol* 1988;89:295–300.

57. Volpé R. Immunology of human thyroid disease. In: Volpé R, ed. *Autoimmune diseases of the endocrine system*. Boca Raton: CRC Press, 1990.

58. Huang Y, Prasad M, Lemon WJ, et al. Gene expression in papillary thyroid carcinoma reveals highly consistent profiles. *Proc Natl Acad Sci USA* 2001;98:15044–15049.

59. Wasenius VM, Hemmer S, Kettunen E, et al. Hepatocyte growth factor receptor, matrix metalloproteinase-11, tissue inhibitor of metalloproteinase-1, and fibronectin are up-regulated in papillary thyroid carcinoma: a cDNA and tissue microarray study. *Clin Cancer Res* 2003;9:68–75.

60. Yano Y, Uematsu N, Yashiro T, et al. Gene expression profiling identifies platelet-derived growth factor as a diagnostic molecular marker for papillary thyroid carcinoma. *Clin Cancer Res* 2004;10:2035–2043.

61. Chevillard S, Ugolin N, Vielh P, et al. Gene expression profiling of differentiated thyroid neoplasms: diagnostic and clinical implications. *Clin Cancer Res* 2004;10:6586–6597.

62. Jarzab B, Wiench M, Fujarewicz K, et al. Gene expression profile of papillary thyroid cancer: sources of variability and diagnostic implications. *Cancer Res* 2005;65:1587–1597.

63. Lam KY, Lui MC, Lo CY. Cytokeratin expression profiles in thyroid carcinomas. *Eur J Surg Oncol* 2001;27:631–635.

64. Cheung CC, Ezzat S, Freeman JL, et al. Immunohistochemical diagnosis of papillary thyroid carcinoma. *Mod Pathol* 2001;14:338–342.

65. Raphael SJ, Apel RL, Asa SL. Detection of high-molecular-weight cytokeratins in neoplastic and non-neoplastic thyroid tumors using microwave antigen retrieval. *Mod Pathol* 1995;8:870–872.

66. Choi YL, Kim MK, Suh JW, et al. Immunoexpression of HBME-1, high molecular weight cytokeratin, cytokeratin 19, thyroid transcription factor-1, and E-cadherin in thyroid carcinomas. *J Korean Med Sci* 2005;20:853–859.

67. Hirokawa M, Carney JA, Ohtsuki Y. Hyalinizing trabecular adenoma and papillary carcinoma of the thyroid gland express different cytokeratin patterns. *Am J Surg Pathol* 2000;24:877–881.

68. Baloch ZW, Abraham S, Roberts S, et al. Differential expression of cytokeratins in follicular variant of papillary carcinoma: an immunohistochemical study and its diagnostic utility. *Hum Pathol* 1999;30:1166–1171.

69. Saggiorato E, De PR, Volante M, et al. Characterization of thyroid "follicular neoplasms" in fine-needle aspiration cytological specimens using a panel of immunohistochemical markers: a proposal for clinical application. *Endocr Relat Cancer* 2005;12:305–317.

70. Khurana KK, Truong LD, LiVolsi VA, et al. Cytokeratin 19 immunolocalization in cell block preparation of thyroid aspirates. An adjunct to fine-needle aspiration diagnosis of papillary thyroid carcinoma. *Arch Pathol Lab Med* 2003;127:579–583.

71. Nasser SM, Pitman MB, Pilch BZ, et al. Fine-needle aspiration biopsy of papillary thyroid carcinoma: diagnostic utility of cytokeratin 19 immunostaining. *Cancer* 2000;90:307–311.

72. Fernandez PL, Merino MJ, Gomez M, et al. Galectin-3 and laminin expression in neoplastic and non-neoplastic thyroid tissue. *J Pathol* 1997;181:80–86.

73. Kawachi K, Matsushita Y, Yonezawa S, et al. Galectin-3 expression in various thyroid neoplasms and its possible role in metastasis formation. *Hum Pathol* 2000;31:428–433.

74. Cvejic D, Savin S, Golubovic S, et al. Galectin-3 and carcinoembryonic antigen expression in medullary thyroid carcinoma: possible relation to tumour progression. *Histopathology* 2000;37:530–535.
75. Herrmann ME, LiVolsi VA, Pasha TL, et al. Immunohistochemical expression of galectin-3 in benign and malignant thyroid lesions. *Arch Pathol Lab Med* 2002;126: 710–713.
76. Kovacs RB, Foldes J, Winkler G, et al. The investigation of galectin-3 in diseases of the thyroid gland. *Eur J Endocrinol* 2003;149:449–453.
77. Weber KB, Shroyer KR, Heinz DE, et al. The use of a combination of galectin-3 and thyroid peroxidase for the diagnosis and prognosis of thyroid cancer. *Am J Clin Pathol* 2004;122:524–531.
78. Papotti M, Rodriguez J, De PR, et al. Galectin-3 and HBME-1 expression in well-differentiated thyroid tumors with follicular architecture of uncertain malignant potential. *Mod Pathol* 2005;18:541–546.
79. Prasad ML, Pellegata NS, Huang Y, et al. Galectin-3, fibronectin-1, CITED-1, HBME1 and cytokeratin-19 immunohistochemistry is useful for the differential diagnosis of thyroid tumors. *Mod Pathol* 2005;18:48–57.
80. Oestreicher-Kedem Y, Halpern M, Roizman P, et al. Diagnostic value of galectin-3 as a marker for malignancy in follicular patterned thyroid lesions. *Head Neck* 2004;26: 960–966.
81. Ito Y, Yoshida H, Tomoda C, et al. Galectin-3 expression in follicular tumours: an immunohistochemical study of its use as a marker of follicular carcinoma. *Pathology* 2005;37:296–298.
82. Cvejic DS, Savin SB, Petrovic IM, et al. Galectin-3 expression in papillary thyroid carcinoma: relation to histomorphologic growth pattern, lymph node metastasis, extrathyroid invasion, and tumor size. *Head Neck* 2005;27:1049–1055.
83. Bartolazzi A, Gasbarri A, Papotti M, et al. Application of an immunodiagnostic method for improving preoperative diagnosis of nodular thyroid lesions. *Lancet* 2001;357: 1644–1650.
84. Maruta J, Hashimoto H, Yamashita H, et al. Immunostaining of galectin-3 and CD44v6 using fine-needle aspiration for distinguishing follicular carcinoma from adenoma. *Diagn Cytopathol* 2004;31:392–396.
85. Sheibani K, Esteban JM, Bailey A, et al. Immunopathologic and molecular studies as an aid to the diagnosis of malignant mesothelioma. *Hum Pathol* 1992;23:107–116.
86. Mase T, Funahashi H, Koshikawa T, et al. HBME-1 immunostaining in thyroid tumors especially in follicular neoplasm. *Endocr J* 2003;50:173–177.
87. Erickson LA, Lloyd RV. Practical markers used in the diagnosis of endocrine tumors. *Adv Anat Pathol* 2004;11:175–189.
88. Rezk S, Khan A. Role of immunohistochemistry in the diagnosis and progression of follicular epithelium-derived thyroid carcinoma. *Appl Immunohistochem Mol Morphol* 2005;13:256–264.
89. Rossi ED, Raffaelli M, Minimo C, et al. Immunocytochemical evaluation of thyroid neoplasms on thin-layer smears from fine-needle aspiration biopsies. *Cancer* 2005;105:87–95.
90. Sack MJ, Astengo-Osuna C, Lin BT, et al. HBME-1 immunostaining in thyroid fine-needle aspirations: a useful marker in the diagnosis of carcinoma. *Mod Pathol* 1997;10: 668–674.
91. Kondo T, Ezzat S, Asa SL. Pathogenetic mechanisms in thyroid follicular-cell neoplasia. *Nat Rev Cancer* 2006;6:292–306.
92. Nikiforova MN, Kimura ET, Gandhi M, et al. BRAF mutations in thyroid tumors are restricted to papillary carcinomas and anaplastic or poorly differentiated carcinomas arising from papillary carcinomas. *J Clin Endocrinol Metab* 2003;88:5399–5404.
93. Costa AM, Herrero A, Fresno MF, et al. BRAF mutation associated with other genetic events identifies a subset of aggressive papillary thyroid carcinoma. *Clin Endocrinol (Oxf)* 2008;68:618–634.
94. Groussin L, Fagin JA. Significance of BRAF mutations in papillary thyroid carcinoma: prognostic and therapeutic implications. *Nat Clin Pract Endocrinol Metab* 2006;2: 180–181.

95. Sherman SI. Early clinical studies of novel therapies for thyroid cancers. *Endocrinol Metab Clin North Am* 2008;37:511–524, xi.
96. Mulligan LM, Kwok JBJ, Healey CS, et al. Germ-line mutations of the *RET* proto-oncogene in multiple endocrine neoplasia type 2A. *Nature* 1993;363:458–460.
97. Mulligan LM, Eng C, Healey CS, et al. Specific mutations of the *RET* proto-oncogene are related to disease phenotype in MEN 2A and FMTC. *Nature Genet* 1994;6:70–74.
98. Mulligan LM, Ponder BAJ. Genetic basis of endocrine disease. Multiple endocrine neoplasia type 2. *J Clin Endocrinol Metab* 1995;80:1989–1995.
99. Tallini G, Asa SL. RET oncogene activation in papillary thyroid carcinoma. *Adv Anat Pathol* 2001;8:345–354.
100. Fenton CL, Lukes Y, Nicholson D, et al. The ret/PTC mutations are common in sporadic papillary thyroid carcinoma of children and adults. *J Clin Endocrinol Metab* 2000;85:1170–1175.
101. Bounacer A, Wicker R, Caillou B, et al. High prevalence of activating ret proto-oncogene rearrangements, in thyroid tumors from patients who had received external radiation. *Oncogene* 1997;15:1263–1273.
102. Jhiang SM, Sagartz JE, Tong Q, et al. Targeted expression of the ret/PTC1 oncogene induces papillary thyroid carcinomas. *Endocrinology* 1996;137:375–378.
103. Jhiang SM, Mazzaferri EL. The ret/PTC oncogene in papillary thyroid carcinoma [Review]. *J Lab Clin Med* 1994;123:331–337.
104. Powell DJ Jr, Russell J, Nibu K, et al. The RET/PTC3 oncogene: metastatic solid-type papillary carcinomas in murine thyroids. *Cancer Res* 1998;58:5523–5528.
105. Fischer AH, Bond JA, Taysavang P, et al. Papillary thyroid carcinoma oncogene (RET/PTC) alters the nuclear envelope and chromatin structure. *Am J Pathol* 1998;153:1443–1450.
106. Santoro M, Papotti M, Chiappetta G, et al. RET activation and clinicopathologic features in poorly differentiated thyroid tumors. *J Clin Endocrinol Metab* 2002;87:370–379.
107. Nikiforov Y, Gnepp DR. Pediatric thyroid cancer after the Chernobyl disaster: Pathomorphologic study of 84 cases (1991–1992) from the Republic of Belarus. *Cancer* 1994;74:748–766.
108. Nikiforov Y, Koshoffer A, Nikiforova M, et al. Chromosomal breakpoint positions suggest a direct role for radiation in inducing illegitimate recombination between the ELE1 and RET genes in radiation-induced thyroid carcinomas. *Oncogene* 1999;18:6330–6334.
109. Nikiforova MN, Stringer JR, Blough R, et al. Proximity of chromosomal loci that participate in radiation-induced rearrangements in human cells. *Science* 2000;290:138–141.
110. Elisei R, Romei C, Vorontsova T, et al. RET/PTC rearrangements in thyroid nodules: studies in irradiated and not irradiated, malignant and benign thyroid lesions in children and adults. *J Clin Endocrinol Metab* 2001;86:3211–3216.
111. Rhoden KJ, Johnson C, Brandao G, et al. Real-time quantitative RT-PCR identifies distinct c-RET, RET/PTC1 and RET/PTC3 expression patterns in papillary thyroid carcinoma. *Lab Invest* 2004;84:1557–1570.
112. La Perle KM, Jhiang SM, Capen CC. Loss of p53 promotes anaplasia and local invasion in ret/PTC1-induced thyroid carcinomas. *Am J Pathol* 2000;157:671–677.
113. Fusco A, Chiappetta G, Hui P, et al. Assessment of RET/PTC oncogene activation and clonality in thyroid nodules with incomplete morphological evidence of papillary carcinoma: a search for the early precursors of papillary cancer. *Am J Pathol* 2002;160:2157–2167.
114. Salvatore G, Giannini R, Faviana P, et al. Analysis of BRAF point mutation and RET/PTC rearrangement refines the fine-needle aspiration diagnosis of papillary thyroid carcinoma. *J Clin Endocrinol Metab* 2004;89:5175–5180.
115. Cheung CC, Carydis B, Ezzat S, et al. Analysis of ret/PTC gene rearrangements refines the fine needle aspiration diagnosis of thyroid cancer. *J Clin Endocrinol Metab* 2001;86:2187–2190.
116. Fusco A, Chiappetta G, Hui P, et al. Assessment of RET/PTC oncogene activation and clonality in thyroid nodules with incomplete morphological evidence of papillary

carcinoma: a search for the early precursors of papillary cancer. *Am J Pathol* 2002;160: 2157–2167.

117. Cerilli LA, Mills SE, Rumpel CA, et al. Interpretation of RET immunostaining in follicular lesions of the thyroid. *Am J Clin Pathol* 2002;118:186–193.

118. Shin E, Hong SW, Kim SH, et al. Expression of down stream molecules of RET (p-ERK, p-p38 MAPK, p-JNK and p-AKT) in papillary thyroid carcinomas. *Yonsei Med J* 2004;45:306–313.

119. Rhoden KJ, Unger K, Salvatore G, et al. RET/papillary thyroid cancer rearrangement in nonneoplastic thyrocytes: follicular cells of Hashimoto's thyroiditis share low-level recombination events with a subset of papillary carcinoma. *J Clin Endocrinol Metab* 2006;91:2414–2423.

120. Castellone MD, Santoro M. Dysregulated RET signaling in thyroid cancer. *Endocrinol Metab Clin North Am* 2008;37:363–74, viii.

121. Wirtschafter A, Schmidt R, Rosen D, et al. Expression of the RET/PTC fusion gene as a marker for papillary carcinoma in Hashimoto's thyroiditis. *Laryngoscope* 1997;107: 95–100.

122. Nikiforov YE, Rowland JM, Bove KE, et al. Distinct pattern of *ret* oncogene rearrangements in morphological variants of radiation-induced and sporadic thyroid papillary carcinomas in children. *Cancer Res* 1997;57:1690–1694.

123. Leung CS, Hartwick RWJ, Bédard YC. Correlation of cytologic and histologic features in variants of papillary carcinoma of the thyroid. *Acta Cytol* 1993;37:645–650.

124. Hawk WA, Hazard JB. The many appearances of papillary carcinoma of the thyroid. *Cleve Clin Q* 1976;43:207–216.

125. Chan JK. Papillary carcinoma of the thyroid: classical and variants. *Histol Histopathol* 1990;5:241–257.

126. Mizukami Y, Michigishi T, Nonomura A, et al. Mixed medullary-follicular carcinoma of the thyroid occurring in familial form. *Histopathology* 1993;22:284–287.

127. Yamashita H, Noguchi S, Murkama N, et al. Prognosis of minute carcinoma of the thyroid. Follow-up study of 48 patients. *Acta Pathol Jpn* 1986;36:1469–1475.

128. Harach HR, Franssila KO, Wasenius V-M. Occult papillary carcinoma of the thyroid. A "normal" finding in Finland. A systematic autopsy study. *Cancer* 1985;56:531–538.

129. Yamashita H, Nakayama I, Noguchi S, et al. Thyroid carcinoma in benign thyroid diseases. An analysis from minute carcinoma. *Acta Pathol Jpn* 1985;35:781–788.

130. Evans HL. Encapsulated papillary neoplasms of the thyroid. A study of 14 cases followed for a minimum of 10 years. *Am J Surg Pathol* 1987;11:592–597.

131. Faquin WC, Cibas ES, Renshaw AA. "Atypical" cells in fine-needle aspiration biopsy specimens of benign thyroid cysts. *Cancer* 2005;105:71–79.

132. Gardner LW. Hürthle-cell tumors of the thyroid. *Arch Pathol* 1955;59:372–381.

133. González-Campora R, Herrero-Zapatero A, Lerma E, et al. Hürthle cell and mitochondrion-rich cell tumors. A clinicopathologic study. *Cancer* 1986;57:1154–1163.

134. Herrera MF, Hay ID, Wu PS, et al. Hürthle cell (oxyphilic) papillary thyroid carcinoma: a variant with more aggressive biologic behavior. *World J Surg* 1992;16:669–675.

135. Meissner WA, Adler A. Papillary carcinoma of the thyroid. A study of the pathology of two hundred twenty-six cases. *Arch Pathol* 1958;66:518–525.

136. Sobrinho-Simoes M, Nesland JM, Holm R, et al. Hürthle cell and mitochondrion-rich papillary carcinomas of the thyroid gland: an ultrastructural and immunocytochemical study. *Ultrastruct Pathol* 1985;8:131–142.

137. Tscholl-Ducommun J, Hedinger C. Papillary thyroid carcinomas. Morphology and Prognosis. *Virchows Arch A Pathol Anat Histol* 1982;396:19–39.

138. Beckner ME, Heffess CS, Oertel JE. Oxyphilic papillary thyroid carcinoma. *Am J Clin Pathol* 1995;103:280–287.

139. Hill JH, Werkhaven JA, DeMay RM. Hürthle cell variant of papillary carcinoma of the thyroid gland. Otolaryngol. *Head Neck Surg* 1988;98:338–341.

140. Berho M, Suster S. The oncocytic variant of papillary carcinoma of the thyroid. A clinicopathologic study of 15 cases. *Hum Pathol* 1997;28:47–53.

141. Hedinger C, Williams ED, Sobin LH. *Histological typing of thyroid tumours*. World Health Organization International Histological Classification of Tumours. Berlin: Springer-Verlag, 1988.

142. Chen KTK. Fine-needle aspiration cytology of papillary Hürthle-cell tumors of thyroid: a report of three cases. *Diagn Cytopathol* 1991;7:53–56.

143. Barbuto D, Carcangiu ML, Rosai J. Papillary Hürthle cell neoplasms of the thyroid gland: a study of 20 cases [Abstract]. *Lab Invest* 1990;62:7A.

144. Wu PS-C, Hay ID, Herrmann MA, et al. Papillary thyroid carcinoma (PTC), oxyphilic cell type: a tumor misclassified by the World Health Organization (WHO)? [Abstract]. *Clin Res* 1991;39:279A.

145. Doria MI Jr., Attal H, Wang HH, et al. Fine needle aspiration cytology of the oxyphil variant of papillary carcinoma of the thyroid. A report of three cases. *Acta Cytol* 1996; 40:1007–1011.

146. Moreira AL, Waisman J, Cangiarella JF. Aspiration cytology of the oncocytic variant of papillary adenocarcinoma of the thyroid gland. *Acta Cytol* 2004;48:137–141.

147. Yeh JJ, Lunetta KL, van Orsouw NJ, et al. Somatic mitochondrial DNA (mtDNA) mutations in papillary thyroid carcinomas and differential mtDNA sequence variants in cases with thyroid tumours. *Oncogene* 2000;19:2060–2066.

148. Maximo V, Sobrinho-Simoes M. Hurthle cell tumours of the thyroid. A review with emphasis on mitochondrial abnormalities with clinical relevance. *Virchows Arch* 2000; 437:107–115.

149. Maximo V, Soares P, Lima J, et al. Mitochondrial DNA somatic mutations (point mutations and large deletions) and mitochondrial DNA variants in human thyroid pathology: a study with emphasis on Hurthle cell tumors. *Am J Pathol* 2002;160:1857–1865.

150. Maximo V, Botelho T, Capela J, et al. Somatic and germline mutation in GRIM-19, a dual function gene involved in mitochondrial metabolism and cell death, is linked to mitochondrion-rich (Hurthle cell) tumours of the thyroid. *Br J Cancer* 2005;92:1892–1898.

151. Apel RL, Asa SL, LiVolsi VA. Papillary Hürthle cell carcinoma with lymphocytic stroma. "Warthin-like tumor" of the thyroid. *Am J Surg Pathol* 1995;19:810–814.

152. Yousef O, Dichard A, Bocklage T. Aspiration cytology features of the Warthin tumor-like variant of papillary thyroid carcinoma. A report of two cases. *Acta Cytol* 1997;41: 1361–1368.

153. Vasei M, Kumar PV, Malekhoseini SA, et al. Papillary Hurthle cell carcinoma (Warthin-like tumor) of the thyroid. Report of a case with fine needle aspiration findings. *Acta Cytol* 1998;42:1437–1440.

154. Baloch ZW, LiVolsi VA. Warthin-like papillary carcinoma of the thyroid. *Arch Pathol Lab Med* 2000;124:1192–1195.

155. Evans HL. Columnar-cell carcinoma of the thyroid. A report of two cases of an aggressive variant of thyroid carcinoma. *Am J Clin Pathol* 1986;85:77–80.

156. Sobrinho-Simoes M, Nesland JM, Johannessen JV. Columnar cell carcinoma: another variant of poorly differentiated carcinoma of the thyroid. *Am J Clin Pathol* 1988;89: 264–267.

157. Johnson TL, Lloyd RV, Thompson NW, et al. Prognostic implications of the tall cell variant of papillary thyroid carcinoma. *Am J Surg Pathol* 1988;12:22–27.

158. Akslen L, Varhaug JE. Thyroid carcinoma with mixed tall cell and columnar cell features. *Am J Clin Pathol* 1990;94:442–445.

159. Flint A, Davenport RD, Lloyd RV. The tall cell variant of papillary carcinoma of the thyroid gland. *Arch Pathol Lab Med* 1991;115:169–171.

160. Hicks MJ, Batsakis JG. Tall cell carcinoma of the thyroid gland. *Ann Otol Rhinol Laryngol* 1993;102:402–403.

161. Van den Brekel MWM, Hekkenberg RJ, Asa SL, et al. Prognostic features in tall cell papillary carcinoma and insular thyroid carcinoma. *Laryngoscope* 1997;107:254–259.

162. Wenig BM, Thompson LD, Adair CF, et al. Thyroid papillary carcinoma of columnar cell type: a clinicopathologic study of 16 cases. *Cancer* 1998;82:740–753.

163. Bocklage T, DiTomasso JP, Ramzy I, et al. Tall cell variant of papillary thyroid carcinoma: cytologic features and differential diagnostic considerations. *Diagn Cytopathol* 1997;17:25–29.

164. Gamboa-Dominguez A, Candanedo-Gonzalez F, Uribe-Uribe NO, et al. Tall cell variant of papillary thyroid carcinoma. A cytohistologic correlation. *Acta Cytol* 1997;41: 672–676.

165. Solomon A, Gupta PK, LiVolsi VA, et al. Distinguishing tall cell variant of papillary thyroid carcinoma from usual variant of papillary thyroid carcinoma in cytologic specimens. *Diagn Cytopathol* 2002;27:143–148.

166. Jayaram G. Cytology of columnar-cell variant of papillary thyroid carcinoma. *Diagn Cytopathol* 2000;22:227–229.

167. Chan JKC, Tsui MS, Tse CH. Diffuse sclerosing variant of papillary carcinoma of the thyroid: a histological and immunohistochemical study of three cases. *Histopathology* 1987;11:191–201.

168. Carcangiu ML, Bianchi S. Diffuse sclerosing variant of papillary thyroid carcinoma: clinicopathologic study of 15 cases. *Am J Surg Pathol* 1989;13:1041–1049.

169. Soares J, Limbert E, Sobrinho-Simoes M. Diffuse sclerosing variant of papillary thyroid carcinoma. A clinicopathologic study of 10 cases. *Path Res Pract* 1989;185:200–206.

170. Fujimoto Y, Obara T, Ito Y, et al. Diffuse sclerosing variant of papillary carcinoma of the thyroid. *Cancer* 1990;66:2306–2312.

171. Cetta F, Toti P, Petracci M, et al. Thyroid carcinoma associated with familial adenomatous polyposis. *Histopathology* 1997;31:231–236.

172. Cameselle-Teijeiro J, Chan JK. Cribriform-morular variant of papillary carcinoma: a distinct variant representing the sporadic counterpart of familial adenomatous polyposis-associated with thyroid carcinoma. *Mod Pathol* 1999;12:400–411.

173. Soravia C, Sugg SL, Berk T, et al. Familial adenomatous polyposis-associated thyroid cancer. *Am J Pathol* 1999;154:127–135.

174. Zeki K, Spambalg D, Sharifi N, et al. Mutations of the adenomatous polyposis coli gene in sporadic thyroid neoplasms. *J Clin Endocrinol Metab* 1994;79:1317–1321.

175. Colletta G, Sciacchitano S, Palmirotta R, et al. Analysis of adenomatous polyposis coli gene in thyroid tumours. *Br J Cancer* 1994;70:1085–1088.

176. Xu B, Yoshimoto K, Miyauchi A, et al. Cribriform-morular variant of papillary thyroid carcinoma: a pathological and molecular genetic study with evidence of frequent somatic mutations in exon 3 of the beta-catenin gene. *J Pathol* 2003;199:58–67.

177. Kuma S, Hirokawa M, Xu B, et al. Cribriform-morular variant of papillary thyroid carcinoma. Report of a case showing morules with peculiar nuclear clearing. *Acta Cytol* 2004;48:431–436.

FOLLICULAR LESIONS

FOLLICULAR MULTINODULAR DISEASE

The most common disorder of the thyroid is the presence of numerous follicular nodules with heterogeneous architecture and cytology. These lesions may be small and clinically insignificant, or they may become large and complex, giving rise to the entity known as sporadic nodular goiter (Fig. 10.1, e-Figs. 10.1–10.5). The pathogenesis of this common disorder is unknown. The presence of multifocal, poorly delineated proliferative lesions has been interpreted as indicative of a hyperplastic phenomenon, and several pathogenetic mechanisms, including autoimmunity and altered hormonal regulation, have been proposed [1–4]. The features supporting a hyperplastic etiology include incomplete encapsulation, poor demarcation from internodular tissue, and heterogeneity of follicular architecture. However, the common identification of large encapsulated lesions with relatively monotonous architecture within these nodular glands makes distinction of hyperplasia from adenoma difficult. The confusion surrounding this disorder is reflected in the terminology applied to the diagnosis of the lesions. They are called "colloid nodules," but in many instances they are not colloid rich. They are called "hyperplastic" nodules, but molecular studies have indicated that they are monoclonal proliferations. Therefore, they represent benign neoplasms and may be more appropriately called adenomas [2,5], similar to solitary follicular nodules [6,7]. In fact, the hyperfunctioning nodules that give rise to Plummer's disease in multinodular thyroids are also now known to be clonal benign neoplasms with activating mutations of the TSH receptor or Gsα [8,9]. These lesions are discussed in the chapter on papillary lesions (Chapter 9) because they usually have papillary architecture. The terminology "adenomatous" or "adenomatoid" nodule, although vague and lacking conviction, may be the most appropriate at this point until further progress is made in the understanding of their pathogenesis. However, pathologists should be aware that the thyroid is a site where progression from hyperplasia to neoplasia occurs and where additional genetic events may give rise to malignant transformation. This is rarely recognized clinically, since the vast majority of nodular goiters remain entirely clinically benign, but the occasional emergence of malignancy in multinodular goiter supports this concept.

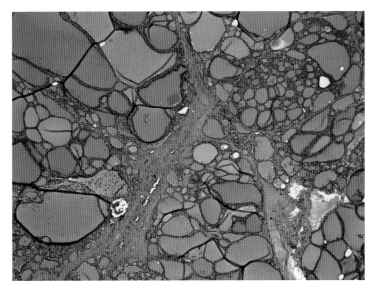

FIGURE 10.1 Sporadic nodular disease is the most common cause of thyroid nodules. The lesions tend to be incompletely encapsulated, poorly demarcated from the internodular tissue, and show heterogeneity of follicular architecture. "Hyperplasia" is a misnomer, since clonality studies have indicated that these are clonal lesions (hematoxylin & eosin stain).

Fine needle aspiration (FNA) and biopsy of these lesions identifies follicular epithelium in a combination of macro- and microfollicular architectures. The macrofollicular architecture in FNA is recognized by monolayered sheets and less commonly as intact macrofollicles. The amount of colloid is variable, but often abundant, and the colloid itself is often watery in consistency (Fig. 10.2, e-Figs. 10.6–10.7). Because of this, FNAs processed by ThinPrep usually show little colloid as it is sufficiently watery to be lost through the filter. When identified, the abundance of colloid suggests a benign process, but this can be misleading, since follicular variant papillary carcinomas can also have abundant colloid and the absence of colloid may be the result of processing techniques such as monolayer preparations. The critical feature is the presence of simple monolayered sheets of epithelium composed of evenly distributed and well-structured follicular epithelial cells with small nuclei, a fine chromatin pattern and relatively inconspicuous nucleoli [10,11] (Figs. 10.3–10.4, e-Figs. 10.8–10.11). In direct smears, the cytoplasm appears to be moderately abundant, but seems less voluminous in ThinPrep preparations as a result of rounding up of the cells during liquid fixation. Oncocytic change is relatively common and the cytoplasm may show numerous, small blue–black granules known as "paravacuolar granules" [11] (e-Fig. 10.12) that represent lysosomes containing hemosiderin and lipofuscin pigment.

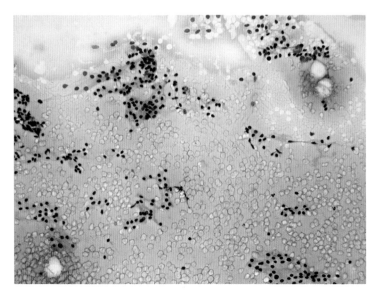

FIGURE 10.2 FNA of lesions in sporadic nodular disease often yields an abundance of thin watery colloid in which numerous red blood cells are entrapped with simple monolayered sheets of follicular epithelium (direct smear, Papanicolaou stain).

There are no cytologic features of the epithelial cells that allow distinction of "hyperplastic" follicular epithelium from normal "nonhyperplastic" epithelium. Thus, cytology has utilized two secondary findings that may occur in follicular nodular disease. The first of these is a relative abundance

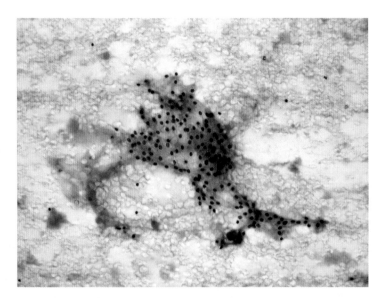

FIGURE 10.3 The epithelium in follicular nodular disease is typically seen as monolayered sheets and may also show oncocytic (Hürthle cell) change as in this example (direct smear, Papanicolaou stain).

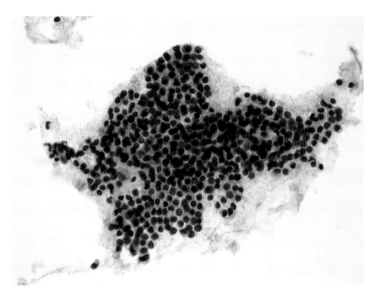

FIGURE 10.4 When thin and watery, the colloid in follicular nodular disease is frequently lost in ThinPrep processing, leaving behind the simple monolayered sheets of follicular epithelium (ThinPrep, Papanicolaou stain).

of colloid as discussed above. Again, it must be remembered that the colloid seen on the slides may underrepresent the colloid content of the lesion. The second is the finding of remote hemorrhage or "degenerative changes" as indicated by the presence of "old" red blood cells, resistant to erythrolytic agents and the presence of hemosiderin-laden macrophages. Nodular lesions may undergo hemorrhagic cystic change; therefore, the finding of remote hemorrhage may suggest the presence of a lesion rather than normal tissue, with the very significant caveat that the epithelium present must not be malignant (Fig. 10.5, e-Fig. 10.13). Sample cellularity has occasionally been suggested as a means to ascertain whether a lesion is hyperplastic. However, the cellularity of an FNA sample is far more dependent on the skill of the aspirator and the quality of the aspiration than on the nature of the lesion, so that sample cellularity cannot be used to reliably establish the pathological nature of the lesion. In fact, in many biopsies of thyroid follicular nodular disease, the FNA is simply labeled as "benign thyroid tissue."

Core biopsies also reveal variably sized follicles lined by a single layer of simple follicular epithelial cells with rounded nuclei that have vesicular chromatin and inconspicuous nucleoli (Figs. 10.6 and 10.7, e-Figs. 10.14 and 10.15). Macrophages, usually filled with hemosiderin, are also noted; however, their number depends upon the presence or absence of secondary degenerative changes or a cystic component [11–13].

The distinction of multinodular disease from follicular neoplasia is an area of controversy. The size of follicles is thought to be significant in the assessment of these nodules. Hyperplasia was thought to be characterized

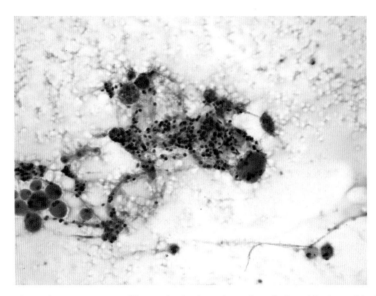

FIGURE 10.5   There are no specific cytologic alterations that distinguish the epithelium of follicular nodular disease from normal follicular epithelium. Thus the abundance of colloid and the presence of secondary changes such as old hemorrhage and hemosiderin-laden macrophages are used to suggest that this is a biopsy of lesional tissue (direct smear, Papanicolaou stain).

by macrofollicular lesions with abundant colloid, whereas neoplasia was thought to be a more cellular process with microfollicular architecture. Clonality studies have disproved this hypothesis and there is no correlation between clonality as a reflection of neoplasia and structural morphology of

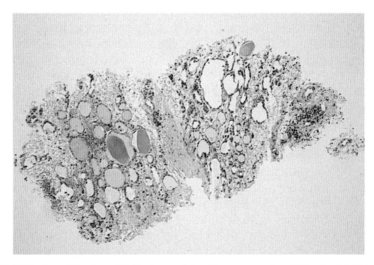

FIGURE 10.6   Core biopsies of follicular nodular disease reveal variably sized follicles lined by a single layer of simple follicular epithelial cells (hematoxylin & eosin stain)

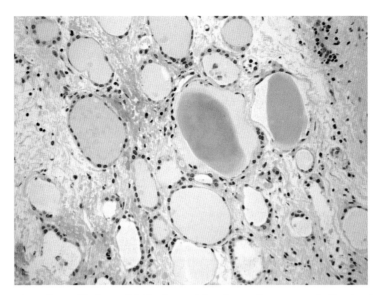

FIGURE 10.7 The epithelium of follicular nodular disease is composed of a simple single layer of flattened to cuboidal cells with small round nuclei, vesicular chromatin, and inconspicuous nucleoli (hematoxylin & eosin stain).

these follicular cell proliferations [5]. Indeed, on the basis of the clonality data, the distinction between follicular nodular disease and follicular adenoma is likely to be entirely academic. However, as discussed in the next section, the distinction between adenoma and carcinoma is not possible on the basis of cytologic features alone, resulting in a clinical dilemma about the correct approach to the diagnosis of what is clearly a proliferative lesion of thyroid follicular epithelium that has no clear features of malignancy. The various approaches are reviewed in Chapter 4 and summarized in Tables 4.1–4.3.

FOLLICULAR NEOPLASIA—ADENOMA AND CARCINOMA

Follicular adenomas and most well-differentiated follicular carcinomas are virtually indistinguishable with respect to their clinical presentation, radiographic appearance, cytologic findings, and microscopic features. In most cases, the parenchymal component of both tumor types is essentially the same histomorphologically. The distinction between these two conditions has been considered possible only by the recognition of capsular and/or vascular invasion or metastasis [14,15]. In the absence of such invasive behavior or of features of papillary carcinoma, these lesions are considered to be benign. It is well recognized that invasion cannot be reliably identified in FNA or core biopsy material and these lesions are diagnosed as follicular neoplasia. Therefore, the diagnosis of follicular adenoma or carcinoma cannot be rendered with confidence on a biopsy, and only thorough examination of a resection specimen can render a definitive diagnosis.

Follicular adenomas have been classified according the size of follicles, abundance of colloid, and degree of cellularity [14,16], but there is no clinical significance to the distinction of macrofollicular, microfollicular, fetal, or embryonal lesions as described in the older literature. Cytologic atypia in follicular neoplasms is always worrisome, but in this situation the major focus should be on the identification of follicular variant of papillary carcinoma through the recognition of the nuclear features of papillary carcinoma (see the next section). The presence of the cytologic features of papillary carcinoma should indicate that diagnosis; however, the identification of these nuclear features is inconsistently achieved and there has not been consensus on the minimum set of features that constitutes a definitive diagnosis, thus leading to a highly subjective area that exhibits the most inconsistency in diagnostic pathology [17]. The identification of mitotic figures, nuclear hyperchromasia, or other cellular atypia that does not fulfill the criteria for papillary carcinoma is considered to be inconsequential. This so-called "endocrine atypia" [14,18–21] has no implication for malignancy in well-differentiated thyroid follicular epithelium.

Follicular carcinomas are divided into groups that reflect the biology of tumor growth and metastasis. Widely invasive follicular carcinomas, which are usually identifiable as invasive grossly and certainly are not difficult to recognize as invasive microscopically, carry a poor prognosis with a 25% to 45% 10-year survival [22,23]. In our experience, these tend to be insular carcinomas (Chapter 11). Minimally invasive follicular carcinoma with invasion into and superficially through the capsule (Figs. 10.8–10.10,

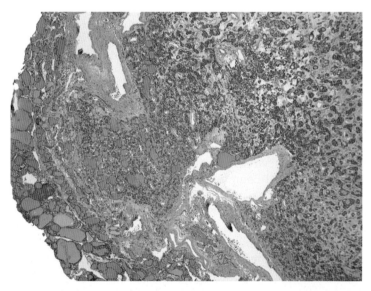

FIGURE 10.8 In this example of a minimally invasive follicular carcinoma, the tumor is caught in the act of penetration through the full thickness of the capsule and into the adjacent normal thyroid tissue (hematoxylin & eosin stain).

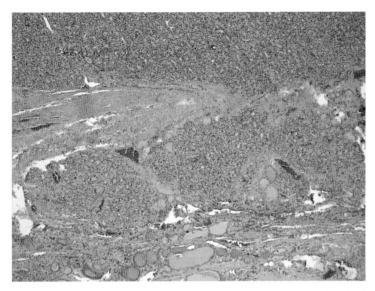

FIGURE 10.9   This minimally invasive follicular carcinoma invades the thyroid along the outer edge of the tumor capsule (hematoxylin & eosin stain).

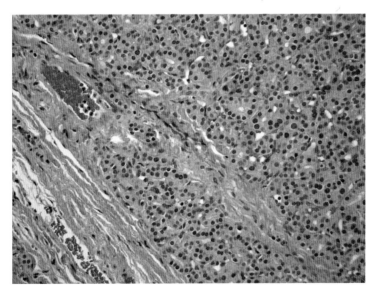

FIGURE 10.10   A follicular neoplasm may show an island of neoplastic cells surrounded by fibrous bands of the capsule that may constitute invasion into the tumor capsule. However, the irregular nature of the tumor capsule makes this assessment difficult and capsular invasion is often not accepted unless full thickness penetration is evident as in Figures 10.8 and 10.9 (hematoxylin & eosin stain).

e-Figs. 10.16–10.19) occurs in patients who are about 10 years younger than those with widely infiltrative carcinomas, and it has been suggested that encapsulated follicular carcinoma is a precursor of the widely invasive lesion [24]. Minimally invasive carcinomas have 10-year survival rates of 70% to 100% [25,26]. Clinically and radiologically they mimic follicular adenomas. The distinction between these two types of follicular carcinomas and follicular adenoma requires histologic evaluation with careful evaluation of the capsule [27] and, therefore, is not possible on FNA or core biopsy. Widely invasive lesions may be recognized radiologically or on ultrasound.

The concept of unencapsulated follicular carcinoma was raised by the identification of tumors that lack a capsule. In one report of four such cases, one patient developed metastases, and this gave rise to citations of a 25% metastatic rate by such lesions [28]. However, this has not been substantiated in larger series and this concept has largely been abandoned.

Vasculoinvasive follicular carcinomas are aggressive and require management accordingly. While vascular invasion is more reliable for the diagnosis of malignancy, again the criteria are vague. Vascular invasion cannot be evaluated within the tumor, and again the circumference of the lesion is the site that warrants careful examination for evidence of vascular invasion. Bulging of tumor under endothelium does not qualify as vascular invasion if the endothelium is intact. Nests of tumor cells within endothelial-lined lumens generally are accepted as representing invasion. However, it is recognized that artifactual implantation of tumor cells into blood vessels can occur during biopsy, surgery, or sectioning, particularly in endocrine tissues that have thin fenestrated endothelium. Therefore, the identification of tumor cells invading through a vessel wall and thrombus adherent to intravascular tumor is required to distinguish true invasion from artifact (Figs. 10.11–10.12, e-Figs. 10.20 and 10.21). This controversial area also requires complete histological evaluation and cannot be reliably determined on biopsy. The dominant determinant of cause-specific mortality in patients with follicular carcinoma is the presence of distant metastases [29–31].

The last few decades have seen a decrease in the incidence of follicular thyroid carcinoma. In areas of endemic goiter, this is may be due to dietary iodine supplementation [32]. However, there are other explanations for the change in incidence that are attributable to recognition of features that change the criteria for diagnosis. It is important to recognize these criteria to prevent misdiagnosis of this tumor. Since the incidence of follicular carcinoma is very low [32], the majority of patients with follicular lesions in biopsy will have benign disease.

The impact of biopsy on the subsequent evaluation of the lesion must be recognized [33]. Core biopsy and fine needle biopsy of a follicular lesion must, by definition, involve penetration of the capsule of the lesion. This results in one or several foci of capsular dehiscence that can be the site of subsequent artifactual penetration that can be mistaken for invasion.

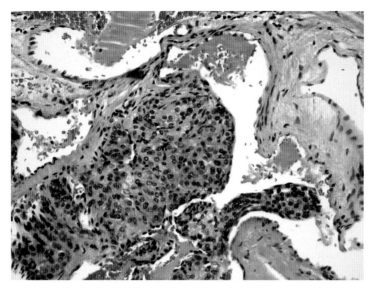

FIGURE 10.11 True vascular invasion is a reliable sign of malignancy and an ominous finding. Vascular invasion cannot be assessed within the tumor and, therefore, requires careful examination of the circumference of the lesion (hematoxylin & eosin stain).

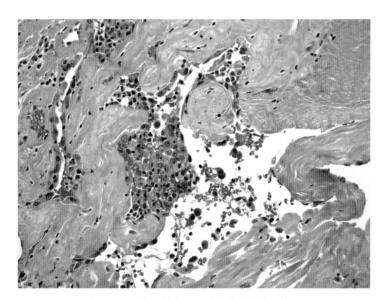

FIGURE 10.12 Nests of tumor cells within an endothelial-lined lumen may represent vascular invasion. However, this may also occur as an artifact caused by displacement of tumor cells occurring during biopsy, surgery, or handling. Therefore, the identification of tumor cells invading through a vessel wall and thrombus adherent to intravascular tumor is required to distinguish true invasion from artifact (hematoxylin & eosin stain).

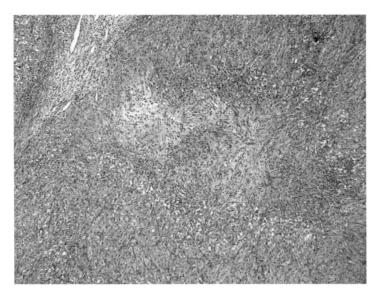

FIGURE 10.13   Both FNA and core biopsy may generate a needle tract injury. In this case, early fibrous tissue demarcates the needle tract (hematoxylin & eosin stain).

Injury to the lesion itself will result in the presence of needle tracts that will vary from immature granulation tissue to mature fibrotic regions, depending on the age of the injury (Figs. 10.13 and 10.14, e-Figs. 10.22 and 10.23). Rupture of small vessels can be the reason for thrombosis and

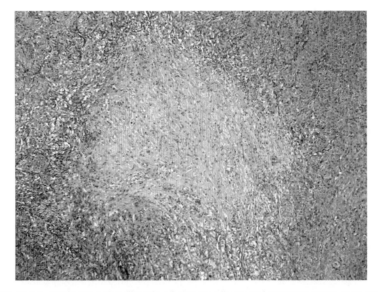

FIGURE 10.14   With time the fibrosis of the needle tract becomes more mature and a fibrous scar is left, still recognizable as a needle tract due to its circular demarcation from the surrounding tumor (hematoxylin & eosin stain).

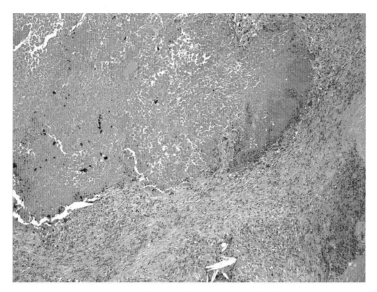

FIGURE 10.15 Rarely, previous needle sampling of a thyroid lesion may result in infarction of the lesion (hematoxylin & eosin stain).

when extensive, and particularly in oncocytic lesions with high vascular demand, can cause necrosis [33,34] (Figs. 10.15 and 10.16, e-Figs. 10.24–10.26). These changes must be interpreted appropriately on subsequent histological evaluation of material that has undergone biopsy.

Ancillary tools can be applied to aid in the distinction between benign and malignant follicular lesions. *Galectin-3* (Chapter 9) is overexpressed in malignant tumors, including follicular carcinomas [35–45]. Follicular carcinomas with minimal and extensive invasion express galectin-3 in 45% to 95% of cases [35,38–40,42,43]. Galectin-3 is less often detected in follicular adenomas (0% to 37.5% of cases) [35,38–40,42,43,46]. Hyperplastic nodules, nodular goiters, and normal follicular epithelium usually are negative for galectin-3 immunoreactivity [35,38,46]. However, one study reported galectin-3 positivity in more than 50% of hyperplastic nodules [42]. Interestingly, the galectin-3 expression level significantly increases with the degree of vascular or capsular invasion of follicular tumors [44]. In addition, galectin-3 has been studied in follicular-patterned lesions with uncertain malignant potential in which it was detected in 60% to 85% of cases [41,46]. Galectin-3 detection in FNA samples by immunohistochemistry has been used in preoperative evaluation of thyroid nodules [46–50]. This marker has been shown to have high (>90%) sensitivity, specificity, positive predictive value, and diagnostic accuracy [46] but has been reported to show reactivity in follicular adenomas as well [48]. It is evident from these data that galectin-3 may be a helpful tool, but it cannot be considered a diagnostic marker of malignancy.

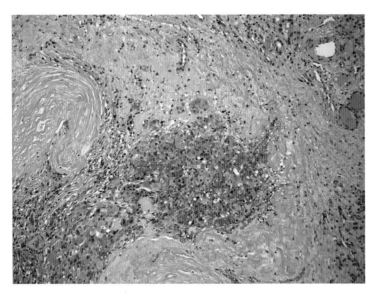

FIGURE 10.16   Lesion infarction post needle biopsy is more common in oncocytic tumors, presumably due to a more tenuous vascular supply. A careful search around the edge of the lesion from Figure 10.17 reveals some residual oncocytic tumor. However, as in this case, there may be too little tissue to allow definitive classification of the nodule (hematoxylin & eosin stain).

HBME-1 (Hector Battifora mesothelial epitope-1; Chapter 9) stains many follicular-derived malignant tumors, including follicular carcinomas, with a variable sensitivity and specificity in different series. HBME-1 detection in follicular carcinomas in different studies has varied between 50% and 100% [42,49,51–53]. Interestingly, membranous and apical-colloidal immunoreactivity for HBME-1 has been reported in follicular carcinomas with RAS mutations, either minimally or widely invasive [54]. In the same study, follicular carcinomas with PAX8–PPARγ rearrangements (see below) showed immunoreactivity for galectin-3, but not for HBME-1 [54]. A few studies have shown HBME-1 staining in follicular tumors of uncertain malignant potential that had questionable vascular or capsular invasion [41,42]. Reactivity for HBME-1 is not usually identified in normal thyroid, in nodules of sporadic nodular goiter, or in follicular adenomas [41,42,49,51,52]. Given the high specificity of this marker for malignancy in many series, and the known observer variability in the diagnosis of nodular goiter and adenoma, one wonders if the few reports of HBME-1 immunoreactivity in benign follicular nodules involved lesions that would have been considered malignant by some experts. Because of this high specificity, HBME-1 detection has been considered by some authors as a useful adjunct in the assessment of thyroid lesions by FNA [49,50,55].

The *peroxisome proliferator activated receptor gamma (PPARγ)* is the subject of a unique and interesting rearrangement in follicular thyroid carcinoma. PPARγ, encoded by PPARG (3p25), is a member of the steroid nuclear hormone receptor superfamily that forms heterodimers with retinoid X receptor. It is best known for its differentiating effects on adipocytes and insulin-mediated metabolic functions. PAX8–PPARG rearrangements were first identified in thyroid neoplasms with a cytogenetically detectable translocation t(2;3)(q13;p25) that generates a chimeric gene encoding the DNA binding domain of the thyroid-specific transcription factor paired-box gene (PAX8) and domains A–F of PPARγ [56]. The PPARG rearrangement acts through a dominant-negative effect on the transcriptional activity of wild-type PPARγ [56]. The fusion oncoprotein contributes to malignant transformation by targeting several cellular pathways, at least some of which are normally engaged by PPARγ. The PAX8–PPARγ1 rearrangement can be detected by RT-PCR for mRNA expression or by FISH [56], but this represents another example of how immunohistochemistry can be applied to identify altered protein products. While normal thyroid follicular cells express PPARγ, the levels are very low and strong nuclear reactivity has been proposed to reflect overexpression due to the high levels of Pax8 promoter activation in these cells. The rearrangement was initially reported to be restricted to follicular thyroid carcinoma with the initial suggestion that it correlates with a vasculoinvasive phenotype [57,58]. The presence of a PAX8–PPARG rearrangement in some follicular adenomas and in follicular variant of papillary thyroid carcinoma (PTC) is controversial [59–61]. Therefore, the application of this marker in differential diagnosis is unclear, but it has been suggested that it indicates a role for application of PPARγ agonists in the treatment of follicular types of thyroid cancer.

Flow cytometry is not helpful in the differential diagnosis of follicular neoplasms. Some encapsulated follicular adenomas exhibit evidence of aneuploidy. While these may represent in situ follicular carcinomas, and the data may be helpful in understanding the progression of thyroid neoplasia, this tool is not of practical value. Among histologically confirmed carcinomas, patients with thyroid tumors that have diploid DNA content tend to have a better prognosis than those with aneuploid values [62–64].

Variants

The subclassification of follicular neoplasms into simple, microfollicular, trabecular, and papillary types based on architecture and into oxyphil, clear cell, signet ring cell, or atypical cytologic variants has no prognostic significance. The molecular basis for the papillary variant is discussed in Chapter 9.

Oncocytic variants of follicular adenomas and carcinomas are diagnosed when more than 75% of a lesion is composed of oncocytic cells with abundant eosinophilic granular cytoplasm (Figs. 10.17 and 10.18, e-Figs. 10.27 and 10.28) due to accumulation of numerous and dilated or spherulated mitochondria. Clear cell adenomas or carcinomas are composed

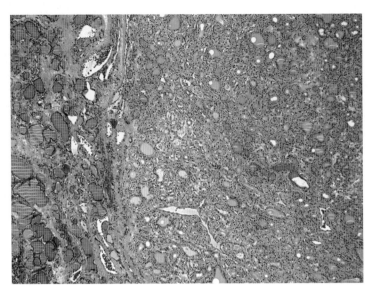

FIGURE 10.17   Although the classification of follicular adenomas on the basis of histomorphology is not of clinical significance, the appearances are sufficiently distinct to warrant attention. When more than 75% of the lesion shows oncocytic change, the lesion may be considered an oncocytic variant of follicular adenoma or carcinoma (hematoxylin & eosin stain).

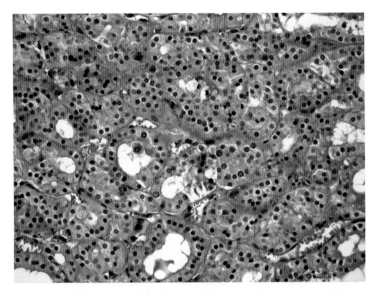

FIGURE 10.18   As in other oncocytic (Hürthle cell) lesions, the appearance of the cytoplasm of the cells in an oncocytic variant of follicular adenoma is the result of an accumulation of dilated mitochondria (hematoxylin & eosin stain).

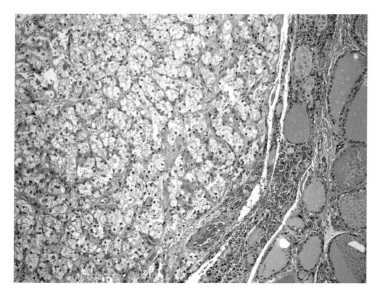

FIGURE 10.19 The accumulation of glycogen, lipid or dilated mtiochondria in some follic-ular neoplasms will impart a clear cell appearance to the tumor as in this example of a clear cell adenoma (hematoxylin & eosin stain).

of follicular cells with clear cytoplasm due to accumulation of glycogen, lipid, or, in some cases, dilated mitochondria (Figs. 10.19 and 10.20, e-Figs 10.29–10.31). There is often a mixed pattern of clear and oncocytic cells in tumors that have cytologic cytoplasmic changes, supporting a relationship

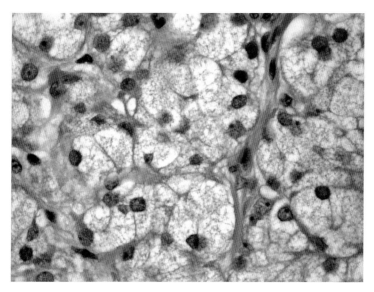

FIGURE 10.20 This high-power image shows the relatively abundant and markedly vacuo-lated cytoplasm of a clear cell adenoma (hematoxylin & eosin stain).

between these two cell types. These changes have no clinical significance on their own, and the criteria for the diagnosis of lesions that are composed predominantly of oncocytic or clear cells are the same as those applied to follicular lesions that do not exhibit these cytologic changes [65]. As indicated previously (Chapter 9), mutations in the mitochondrial DNA have been implicated in oncocytic change [66,67], whereas somatic or germline mutations in GRIM-19 may play dual roles in mitochondrial metabolism and cell death [68].

Numerous studies have indicated that the criteria that apply to all follicular neoplasms of the thyroid, namely capsular invasion and vascular invasion, also distinguish malignant from benign oncocytic neoplasms [65,69–75]. The larger the oncocytic neoplasm, however, the more likely it is to show invasive characteristics; an oncocytic neoplasm which is 4 cm or greater has an 80% chance of showing histologic evidence of malignancy [65]. Nuclear atypia, which is the hallmark of the oncocytic follicular cell, multinucleation, and mitotic activity are not useful to predict prognosis and, therefore, should not be used as diagnostic criteria for malignancy.

Small series of oncocytic follicular carcinomas have demonstrated positive *HBME-1* staining [42,51,53]; however, this marker is less reliable in oncocytic lesions than in those without oncocytic change [49].

Flow cytometric analyses document aneuploid cell populations in 10% to 25% of oncocytic follicular neoplasms that are clinically and histologically classified as adenomas [62,63,76]. Virtually, all of these tumors behave in a benign fashion after excision. Oncocytic neoplasms show frequent chromosomal DNA imbalance, with numerical chromosomal alterations being the dominant feature [77]. Activating ras mutations are infrequent in oncocytic tumors [77].

FOLLICULAR VARIANT OF PAPILLARY CARCINOMA

The follicular variant of papillary carcinoma has been recognized histologically with increasing frequency [16,78–80]. However, this diagnosis remains one of the most controversial areas of pathology [17,81].

On FNA, many follicular variant papillary carcinomas may be recognized as papillary carcinoma, but not necessarily of the follicular subtype [82–85]. In fact, in the follicular variant of papillary carcinoma, the nuclear features of papillary carcinoma are often more subtle [86] and, in particular, intranuclear inclusions may be less common [87,88]. This may account for a high frequency of diagnoses of "suspicious for papillary carcinoma" [86] or "follicular neoplasm" [83,86,88–90] and a propensity for misdiagnosis as a benign lesion [91–93]. As the cytologic recognition of the specific subtype of papillary carcinoma does not bear any significance on the immediate management of the lesion, the value of subtyping cytologically is questionable and the obvious goal is to recognize the lesion as a papillary carcinoma. There have been suggestions that the follicular variant of papillary carcinoma might be recognizable on FNA [82,94,95]. To

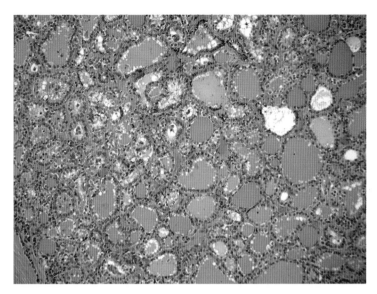

FIGURE 10.21   The follicular variant of papillary carcinoma is one of the most controversial diagnoses in pathology. Potential misidentification as a follicular carcinoma may have little clinical consequence, but when the subtle nuclear features of papillary carcinoma are missed in an encapsulated lesion, the potential for misidentification as a follicular adenoma is substantial with significant clinical consequences (hematoxylin & eosin stain).

date, no features to specifically identify the follicular variant have received acceptance and the literature suggests that, in practice, identification of this subtype of papillary carcinoma is difficult [85,89,96–98].

On examination of the excised lesion, the follicular variant of papillary carcinoma may be misdiagnosed as follicular carcinoma, in which case the clinical significance of the error is negligible. However, it may be underdiagnosed as follicular adenoma or atypical adenoma, potentially resulting in under treatment of the patient and medicolegal action directed against a pathologist if a previous FNA or core biopsy was diagnosed as suspicious or diagnostic of papillary carcinoma. Any lesion with follicular architecture and characteristic nuclear features of papillary carcinoma should be classified as papillary carcinoma (Figs. 10.21–10.23, e-Figs. 10.32–10.36). Infiltrating areas and metastases may exhibit a more striking papillary appearance and may even have psammoma bodies.

The true biological and clinical behavior of follicular variant is not entirely clear. Initial reports included aggressive lesions that developed metastases, leading to the impression that this variant is more aggressive than the classical form. However, prior to the 1980s, most of these lesions were diagnosed as follicular adenomas and atypical adenomas, and most patients did well with no long-term sequelae following limited surgery. This suggests that this variant may be more indolent than classical PTC.

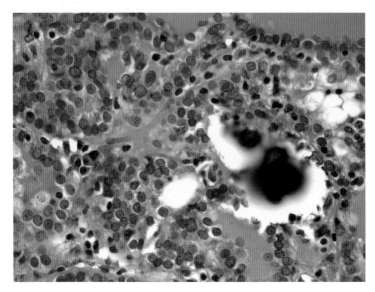

FIGURE 10.22 The absence of papillary architecture makes the low-power appearance of the follicular variant of papillary carcinoma more difficult to recognize, but the occasional presence of psammoma bodies, as in this image, may be of substantial aid. Paradoxically, papillary architecture and psammoma body production may be more pronounced in metastatic deposits of follicular variant of papillary carcinoma (hematoxylin & eosin stain).

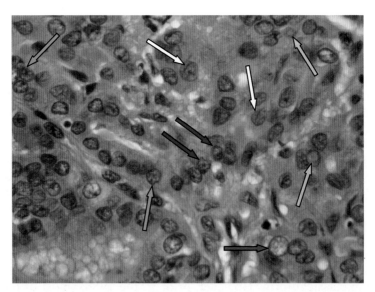

FIGURE 10.23 As with the other variants of papillary carcinoma, the follicular variant is recognized by the characteristic nuclear features of papillary carcinoma including nuclear grooves (white arrows) and notches (green arrows), intranuclear inclusions (orange arrows), chromatin clearing (red arrow) and micronucleoli with bare nucleoli (blue arrows) (hematoxylin & eosin stain).

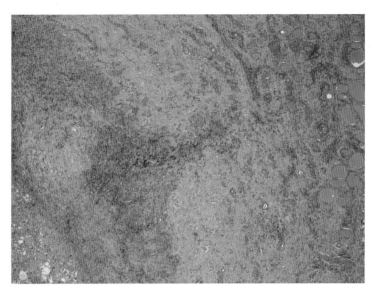

FIGURE 10.24 Various histologic alterations may occur following needle sampling of the thyroid and have been described as "worrisome histological alterations following FNA of thyroid (WHAFFT)" and are seen adjacent to needle tracts as identified in this image by the granulation tissue, inflammation, and hemosiderin-laden macrophages seen in a region of capsular disruption (hematoxylin & eosin stain).

The presence of cytologic atypia in a tissue section may raise the possibility of papillary carcinoma without being sufficiently convincing for an unequivocal diagnosis. In some cases, the changes may be induced by previous FNA or core needle biopsy. The presence of hemorrhage, granulation tissue and hemosiderin laden-macrophages, inflammation and foreign body giant cells, and even foreign material should point to this possibility. There may be calcification that can be mistaken for psammoma bodies. Various metaplastic changes occur. These changes have been described with the acronym WHAFFT, which stands for "worrisome histological alterations following FNA of thyroid" [33] (Figs. 10.24–10.25, e-Figs. 10.37–10.42). The diagnosis of papillary carcinoma should not be made in any situation where reactive changes can be implicated unless the lesion is entirely unequivocal.

In cases where the features are suggestive of papillary carcinoma but not entirely diagnostic, specific markers of this tumor as well as other markers if malignancy may be useful. A proportion of follicular variant of papillary carcinomas stain for *HBME-1* [55,99,100] and *galectin-3* [101–104]. In contrast to the 70% of classical PTC that stain for HBME-1, only 45% of follicular variant of PTCs stain for this marker, but this represents a highly specific marker of malignancy [51] and it is, therefore, useful for lesions with incomplete nuclear features of PTC [41,42].

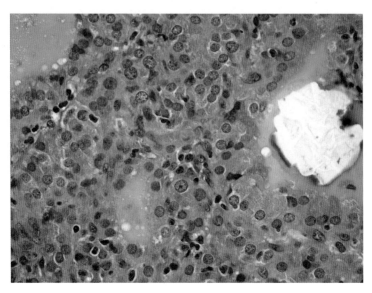

FIGURE 10.25 This epithelium adjacent to a needle tract shows nuclear atypia that approaches but does not meet criteria for papillary carcinoma and is one manifestation of WHAFFT. In the situation wherein nuclear atypia is identified in proximity to a needle tract, only unequivocal nuclear changes should be accepted as diagnostic. Notice the foreign material in a multinucleated giant cell that represents talc from a biopsy procedure (hematoxylin & eosin stain).

Stains for *high molecular weight cytokeratins* and *CK19* may be useful. Because CK19 detection in follicular adenomas and follicular carcinomas is often negative or only focal, this keratin has become one of the most commonly used to investigate follicular thyroid lesions where the differential diagnosis includes follicular variant of PTC [51,105–107]. The staining pattern is similar but less intense than in classical variant of PTC using CK19 as well as CK17 and CK20 antibodies [106]. Several authors emphasize the importance of the distribution and intensity of CK19 staining as the most critical aspect of accurate interpretation [51,107–109]. Normal thyroid follicular epithelium is often positive for CK19 and 34βE12, especially in the compressed thyroid parenchyma surrounding nodules and in follicular cells within lymphocytic thyroiditis [106]. This pattern of staining is consistent with the intense pattern of staining seen in reactive follicular epithelium within thyroid nodules around the site of degeneration, especially at the site of previous needle biopsy. However, the finely dispersed positivity seen in the cells of PTC is distinctive. While this feature is usually diffuse throughout the lesion, focal staining for CK19 does not rule out a diagnosis of PTC, particularly in nodules with nuclear features of PTC that are seen focally [107].

Follicular variant of PTCs rarely harbor the common BRAFV600E mutation of classical PTC but they have been reported to display

BRAFK601E mutations, suggesting possible phenotype–genotype correlations [110–112].

The *ret/PTC oncogenes* are found in follicular variant of PTCs including radiation-induced tumors [113–117] and sporadic papillary carcinomas [118–121]. The use of RT-PCR or FISH is most reliable, but as indicated above for classical PTC, immunohistochemical staining with antisera directed against the carboxy terminus of ret allows rapid and clinically useful detection of this marker of papillary carcinoma which can be helpful in follicular lesions that are controversial. RT-PCR has been applied to FNA specimens when collected in suspension [122].

PTCs harboring *ras mutations* generally have follicular architecture [123,124]. Although, sufficient nuclear features for the diagnosis of PTC are present, nuclear crowding/overlapping and nuclear irregularities are less pronounced [123]. They have a female preponderance and are characterized by large size. However, currently ras mutations are not readily identified for diagnostic purposes.

Macrofollicular Variant

The macrofollicular variant of PTC is rare and is defined histologically as a PTC in which over 50% of the follicles are macrofollicles (i.e., $\geq$250 μm) [125]. On FNA, monolayered two-dimensional sheets of atypical epithelium or large follicles are found with abundant colloid. As with other follicular variant of papillary carcinomas, the diagnostic nuclear features may be subtle [84,126,127] and the cytologic recognition can be extremely difficult. The differential diagnosis includes nodular goiter and macrofollicular adenoma due to the abundance of thin colloid, low cellularity, and subtle and focal nuclear atypia.

Oncocytic Variant

The diagnosis of Hürthle cell or oncocytic follicular variant of papillary carcinoma remains controversial. Many of these lesions have been diagnosed in the past as Hürthle cell adenoma; however, reports of aggressive behavior suggested that this diagnosis could not be trusted [73,128]. The application of ret/PTC analysis by RT-PCR allowed the recognition of a follicular variant of Hürthle cell papillary carcinoma as a group of lesions with no invasive behavior at the time of diagnosis but that harbored a ret/PTC gene rearrangement [129,130]. By definition, these lesions exhibit nuclear features of papillary carcinoma; they also frequently have irregularity of architecture with hypereosinophilic colloid [131,132]. In addition, they may have nuclear hyperchromasia and the prominent large nucleoli of oncocytic change (Figs. 10.26–10.28, e-Figs. 10.43–10.47). Nevertheless, they can be recognized when there is a high index of suspicion and with the addition of immunohistochemistry for HBME-1, galectin-3, CK19, and ret or by RT-PCR studies of ret/PTC rearrangements. These tumors have the potential to metastasize [133], explaining the occurrence of malignancy in patients with a histopathological diagnosis of adenoma.

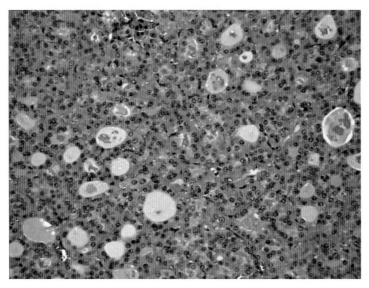

FIGURE 10.26   On low-power examination, the oncocytic follicular variant of papillary carcinoma may resemble an oncocytic follicular adenoma composed of microfollicles of oncocytic cells (hematoxylin & eosin stain).

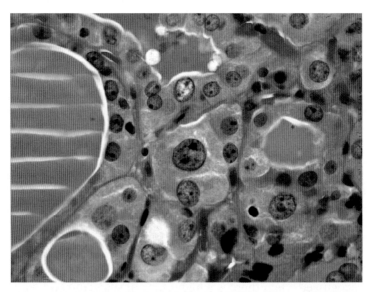

FIGURE 10.27   The oncocytic follicular variant of papillary carcinoma displays the nuclear atypia of Hürthle cells with more coarse and hyperchromatic chromatin with prominent nucleoli, but also exhibits nuclear enlargement, irregularity of nuclear contours that may result in grooves, and clearing of nucleoplasm with peripheral margination of chromatin and multiple micronucleoli (hematoxylin & eosin stain).

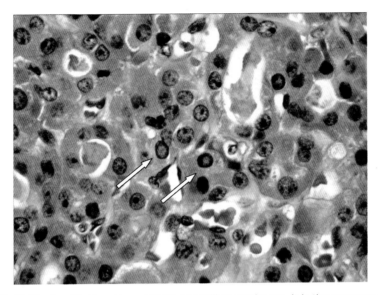

FIGURE 10.28   As with the other variants of papillary carcinoma, it is the presence of the nuclear features of papillary carcinoma (*arrows* demonstrate intranuclear inclusions) that allows the diagnosis of the oncocytic follicular variant of papillary carcinoma (hematoxylin & eosin stain).

REFERENCES

1. Studer H, Peter H-J, Gerber H. Natural heterogeneity of thyroid cells: the basis for understanding thyroid function and nodular goiter growth. *Endocr Rev* 1989;10:125–135.
2. Aeschimann S, Kopp PA, Kimura ET, et al. Morphological and functional polymorphism within clonal thyroid nodules. *J Clin Endocrinol Metab* 1993;77:846–851.
3. Studer H, Ramelli F. Simple goiter and its variants: euthyroid and hyperthyroid multinodular goiters. *Endocr Rev* 1982;3:40–61.
4. Peter HJ, Gerber H, Studer H, et al. Pathogenesis of heterogeneity in human multinodular goiter. A study on growth and function of thyroid tissue transplanted onto nude mice. *J Clin Invest* 1985;76:1992–2002.
5. Apel RL, Ezzat S, Bapat B, et al. Clonality of thyroid nodules in sporadic goiter. *Diag Mol Pathol* 1995;4:113–121.
6. Hicks DG, LiVolsi VA, Neidich JA, et al. Clonal analysis of solitary follicular nodules in the thyroid. *Am J Pathol* 1990;137:553–562.
7. Namba H, Matsuo K, Fagin JA. Clonal composition of benign and malignant human thyroid tumors. *J Clin Invest* 1990;86:120–125.
8. Parma J, Duprez L, Van Sandem H, et al. Diversity and prevalence of somatic mutations in the thyrotropin receptor and Gs alpha genes as a cause of toxic thyroid adenomas. *J Clin Endocrinol Metab* 1997;82:2695–2701.
9. Krohn D, Fuhrer D, Holzapfel H, et al. Clonal origin of toxic thyroid nodules with constitutively activating thyrotropin receptor mutations. *J Clin Endocrinol Metab* 1998;83:180–184.
10. Kini SR. *Thyroid.* New York: Igaku-Shoin, 1996.
11. Layfield LJ, Wax T, Jones C. Cytologic distinction of goiterous nodules from morphologically normal thyroid: analyses of cytomorphologic features. *Cancer* 2003;99:217–222.
12. Baloch ZW, Sack MJ, Yu GH, et al. Fine-needle aspiration of thyroid: an institutional experience. *Thyroid* 1998;8:565–569.

13. Nassar A, Gupta P, LiVolsi VA, et al. Histiocytic aggregates in benign nodular goiters mimicking cytologic features of papillary thyroid carcinoma (PTC). *Diagn Cytopathol* 2003;29:243–245.

14. LiVolsi VA. *Surgical pathology of the thyroid*. Philadelphia: WB Saunders, 1990.

15. Baloch ZW, LiVolsi VA. Follicular-patterned lesions of the thyroid: the bane of the pathologist. *Am J Clin Pathol* 2002;117:143–150.

16. Rosai J, Carcangiu ML, DeLellis RA. Tumors of the thyroid gland. In: *Atlas of tumor pathology*. 3rd Series, fascicle 5. Washington, DC: Armed Forces Institute of Pathology, 1992.

17. Lloyd RV, Erickson LA, Casey MB, et al. Observer variation in the diagnosis of follicular variant of papillary thyroid carcinoma. *Am J Surg Pathol* 2004;28:1336–1340.

18. Baloch ZW, LiVolsi VA. Pathology of thyroid gland. In: LiVolsi VA, Asa SL, eds. *Endocrine pathology*. Philadelphia: Churchill Livingstone, 2002.

19. LiVolsi VA, Baloch ZW. Follicular neoplasms of the thyroid: view, biases, and experiences. *Adv Anat Pathol* 2004;11:279–287.

20. Goldstein RE, Netterville JL, Burkey B, et al. Implications of follicular neoplasms, atypia, and lesions suspicious for malignancy diagnosed by fine-needle aspiration of thyroid nodules. *Ann Surg* 2002;235:656–662.

21. Kelman AS, Rathan A, Leibowitz J, et al. Thyroid cytology and the risk of malignancy in thyroid nodules: importance of nuclear atypia in indeterminate specimens. *Thyroid* 2001;11:271–277.

22. Treseler PA, Clark OH. Prognostic factors in thyroid carcinoma. *Surg Oncol Clin N Am* 1997;6:555–598.

23. Clark OH. Predictors of thyroid tumor aggressiveness. *West J Med* 1996;165:131–138.

24. Jorda M, Gonzalez-Campora R, Mora J, et al. Prognostic factors in follicular carcinoma of the thyroid. *Arch Pathol Lab Med* 1993;117:631–635.

25. Van Heerden JA, Hay ID, Goellner JR, et al. Follicular thyroid carcinoma with capsular invasion alone: a nonthreatening malignancy. *Surgery* 1992;112:1130–1138.

26. Harness JK, Thompson NW, McLeod MK, et al. Follicular carcinoma of the thyroid gland: trends and treatment. *Surgery* 1984;96:972–980.

27. Yamashina M. Follicular neoplasms of the thyroid. Total circumferential evaluation of the fibrous capsule. *Am J Surg Pathol* 1992;16:392–400.

28. Kahn NF, Perzin KH. Follicular carcinoma of the thyroid: an evaluation of the histologic criteria used for diagnosis. *Pathol Annu* 1983;1:221–253.

29. Samaan NA, Schultz PN, Haynie TP, et al. Pulmonary metastasis of differentiated thyroid carcinoma: treatment results in 101 patients. *J Clin Endocrinol Metab* 1985;65:376–380.

30. DeGroot LJ, Kaplan EL, Shukla MS, et al. Morbidity and mortality in follicular thyroid cancer. *J Clin Endocrinol Metab* 1995;80:2946–2953.

31. Mizukami Y, Michigishi T, Nonomura A, et al. Distant metastases in differentiated thyroid carcinomas: a clinical and pathologic study. *Hum Pathol* 1990;21:283–290.

32. LiVolsi VA, Asa SL. The demise of follicular carcinoma of the thyroid gland. *Thyroid* 1994;4:233–235.

33. LiVolsi VA, Merino MJ. Worrisome histologic alterations following fine needle aspiration of the thyroid. *Pathol Annu* 1994;29:99–120.

34. Baloch ZW, LiVolsi VA. Post fine-needle aspiration histologic alterations of thyroid revisited. *Am J Clin Pathol* 1999;112:311–316.

35. Fernandez PL, Merino MJ, Gomez M, et al. Galectin-3 and laminin expression in neoplastic and non-neoplastic thyroid tissue. *J Pathol* 1997;181:80–86.

36. Kawachi K, Matsushita Y, Yonezawa S, et al. Galectin-3 expression in various thyroid neoplasms and its possible role in metastasis formation. *Hum Pathol* 2000;31:428–433.

37. Cvejic D, Savin S, Golubovic S, et al. Galectin-3 and carcinoembryonic antigen expression in medullary thyroid carcinoma: possible relation to tumour progression. *Histopathology* 2000;37:530–535.

38. Herrmann ME, LiVolsi VA, Pasha TL, et al. Immunohistochemical expression of galectin-3 in benign and malignant thyroid lesions. *Arch Pathol Lab Med* 2002;126: 710–713.

39. Kovacs RB, Foldes J, Winkler G, et al. The investigation of galectin-3 in diseases of the thyroid gland. *Eur J Endocrinol* 2003;149:449–453.

40. Weber KB, Shroyer KR, Heinz DE, et al. The use of a combination of galectin-3 and thyroid peroxidase for the diagnosis and prognosis of thyroid cancer. *Am J Clin Pathol* 2004;122:524–531.

41. Papotti M, Rodriguez J, De PR, et al. Galectin-3 and HBME-1 expression in well-differentiated thyroid tumors with follicular architecture of uncertain malignant potential. *Mod Pathol* 2005;18:541–546.

42. Prasad ML, Pellegata NS, Huang Y, et al. Galectin-3, fibronectin-1, CITED-1, HBME1 and cytokeratin-19 immunohistochemistry is useful for the differential diagnosis of thyroid tumors. *Mod Pathol* 2005;18:48–57.

43. Oestreicher-Kedem Y, Halpern M, Roizman P, et al. Diagnostic value of galectin-3 as a marker for malignancy in follicular patterned thyroid lesions. *Head Neck* 2004;26: 960–966.

44. Ito Y, Yoshida H, Tomoda C, et al. Galectin-3 expression in follicular tumours: an immunohistochemical study of its use as a marker of follicular carcinoma. *Pathology* 2005;37:296–298.

45. Cvejic DS, Savin SB, Petrovic IM, et al. Galectin-3 expression in papillary thyroid carcinoma: relation to histomorphologic growth pattern, lymph node metastasis, extrathyroid invasion, and tumor size. *Head Neck* 2005;27:1049–1055.

46. Bartolazzi A, Gasbarri A, Papotti M, et al. Application of an immunodiagnostic method for improving preoperative diagnosis of nodular thyroid lesions. *Lancet* 2001;357: 1644–1650.

47. Gasbarri A, Martegani MP, Del PF, et al. Galectin-3 and CD44v6 isoforms in the preoperative evaluation of thyroid nodules. *J Clin Oncol* 1999;17:3494–3502.

48. Maruta J, Hashimoto H, Yamashita H, et al. Immunostaining of galectin-3 and CD44v6 using fine-needle aspiration for distinguishing follicular carcinoma from adenoma. *Diagn Cytopathol* 2004;31:392–396.

49. Saggiorato E, De PR, Volante M, et al. Characterization of thyroid "follicular neoplasms" in fine-needle aspiration cytological specimens using a panel of immunohistochemical markers: a proposal for clinical application. *Endocr Relat Cancer* 2005;12: 305–317.

50. Rossi ED, Raffaelli M, Minimo C, et al. Immunocytochemical evaluation of thyroid neoplasms on thin-layer smears from fine-needle aspiration biopsies. *Cancer* 2005; 105:87–95.

51. Cheung CC, Ezzat S, Freeman JL, et al. Immunohistochemical diagnosis of papillary thyroid carcinoma. *Mod Pathol* 2001;14:338–342.

52. Mase T, Funahashi H, Koshikawa T, et al. HBME-1 immunostaining in thyroid tumors especially in follicular neoplasm. *Endocr J* 2003;50:173–177.

53. Choi YL, Kim MK, Suh JW, et al. Immunoexpression of HBME-1, high molecular weight cytokeratin, cytokeratin 19, thyroid transcription factor-1, and E-cadherin in thyroid carcinomas. *J Korean Med Sci* 2005;20:853–859.

54. Nikiforova MN, Lynch RA, Biddinger PW, et al. RAS point mutations and PAX8-PPAR gamma rearrangement in thyroid tumors: evidence for distinct molecular pathways in thyroid follicular carcinoma. *J Clin Endocrinol Metab* 2003;88:2318–2326.

55. Sack MJ, Astengo-Osuna C, Lin BT, et al. HBME-1 immunostaining in thyroid fine-needle aspirations: a useful marker in the diagnosis of carcinoma. *Mod Pathol* 1997; 10:668–674.

56. Kroll TG, Sarraf P, Pecciarini L, et al. PAX8-PPARgamma1 fusion oncogene in human thyroid carcinoma. *Science* 2000;289:1357–1360.

57. Nikiforova MN, Biddinger PW, Caudill CM, et al. PAX8-PPARgamma rearrangement in thyroid tumors: RT-PCR and immunohistochemical analyses. *Am J Surg Pathol* 2002;26:1016–1023.

58. Marques AR, Espadinha C, Catarino AL, et al. Expression of PAX8-PPAR gamma 1 rearrangements in both follicular thyroid carcinomas and adenomas. *J Clin Endocrinol Metab* 2002;87:3947–3952.

59. Cheung L, Messina M, Gill A, et al. Detection of the PAX8-PPAR gamma fusion oncogene in both follicular thyroid carcinomas and adenomas. *J Clin Endocrinol Metab* 2003;88:354–357.

60. Dwight T, Thoppe SR, Foukakis T, et al. Involvement of the PAX8/peroxisome proliferator-activated receptor gamma rearrangement in follicular thyroid tumors. *J Clin Endocrinol Metab* 2003;88:4440–4445.

61. Castro P, Rebocho AP, Soares RJ, et al. PAX8-PPARγ rearrangement is frequently detected in the follicular variant of papillary thyroid carcinoma. *J Clin Endocrinol Metab* 2006;91:213–220.

62. Galera-Davidson H, Bobbo M, Bartels PH, et al. Correlation between automated DNA ploidy measurements of Hürthle cell tumors and their histopathologic and clinical features. *Anal Quant Cytol Histol* 1986;8:158–167.

63. McLeod MK, Thompson NW, Hudson JL, et al. Flow cytometric measurements of nuclear DNA and ploidy analysis in Hürthle cell neoplasms of the thyroid. *Arch Surg* 1988;123:849–854.

64. Klemi PJ, Joensuu H, Eerola E. DNA aneuploidy in anaplastic carcinoma of the thyroid gland. *Am J Clin Pathol* 1988;89:154–159.

65. Bronner MP, LiVolsi VA. Oxyphilic (Askenasy/Hürthle cell) tumors of the thyroid. Microscopic features predict biologic behavior. *Surg Pathol* 1988;1:137–150.

66. Yeh JJ, Lunetta KL, van Orsouw NJ, et al. Somatic mitochondrial DNA (mtDNA) mutations in papillary thyroid carcinomas and differential mtDNA sequence variants in cases with thyroid tumours. *Oncogene* 2000;19:2060–2066.

67. Maximo V, Soares P, Lima J, et al. Mitochondrial DNA somatic mutations (point mutations and large deletions) and mitochondrial DNA variants in human thyroid pathology: a study with emphasis on Hurthle cell tumors. *Am J Pathol* 2002;160:1857–1865.

68. Maximo V, Botelho T, Capela J, et al. Somatic and germline mutation in GRIM-19, a dual function gene involved in mitochondrial metabolism and cell death, is linked to mitochondrion-rich (Hurthle cell) tumours of the thyroid. *Br J Cancer* 2005;92:1892–1898.

69. Johnson TL, Lloyd RV, Burney RE, et al. Hürthle cell thyroid tumors: an immunohistochemical study. *Cancer* 1987;59:107–112.

70. Arganini M, Behar R, Wi TC, et al. Hürthle cell tumors: a twenty-five year experience. *Surgery* 1986;100:1108–1114.

71. Gosain AK, Clark OH. Hürthle cell neoplasms: malignant potential. *Arch Surg* 1984; 119:515–519.

72. Har-El G, Hadar T, Segal K, et al. Hurthle cell carcinoma of the thyroid gland. A tumor of moderate malignancy. *Cancer* 1986;57:1613–1617.

73. Thompson NW, Dunn EL, Batsakis JG, et al. Hürthle cell lesions of the thyroid gland. *Surg Gynecol Obstet* 1974;139:555–560.

74. Flint A, Lloyd RV. Hürthle cell neoplasms of the thyroid gland. *Pathol Annu* 1990;25: 37–52.

75. Carcangiu ML, Bianchiu S, Savino D, et al. Follicular Hürthle cell tumors of the thyroid gland. *Cancer* 1991;68:1944–1953.

76. Ryan JJ, Hay ID, Grant CS, et al. Flow cytometric DNA measurements in benign and malignant Hürthle cell tumors of the thyroid. *World J Surg* 1988;12:482–487.

77. Tallini G, Hsueh A, Liu S, et al. Frequent chromosomal DNA unbalance in thyroid oncocytic (Hürthle cell) neoplasms detected by comparative genomic hybridization. *Lab Invest* 1999;79:547–555.

78. Chen KTK, Rosai J. Follicular variant of thyroid papillary carcinoma: a clinicopathologic study of six cases. *Am J Surg Pathol* 1977;1:123–130.

79. Tielens ET, Sherman SI, Hruban RH, et al. Follicular variant of papillary thyroid carcinoma: a clinicopathologic study. *Cancer* 1994;73:424–431.

80. DeLellis RA, Lloyd RV, Heitz PU, et al. *Pathology and genetics of tumours of endocrine organs.* WHO Classification of Tumours. Lyons: IARC Press, 2004.

81. Hirokawa M, Carney JA, Goellner JR, et al. Observer variation of encapsulated follicular lesions of the thyroid gland. *Am J Surg Pathol* 2002;26:1508–1514.
82. Aron M, Mallik A, Verma K. Fine needle aspiration cytology of follicular variant of papillary carcinoma of the thyroid: morphologic pointers to its diagnosis. *Acta Cytol* 2006;50:663–668.
83. Goodell WM, Saboorian MH, Ashfaq R. Fine-needle aspiration diagnosis of the follicular variant of papillary carcinoma. *Cancer* 1998;84:349–354.
84. Mesonero CE, Jugle JE, Wilbur DC, et al. Fine-needle aspiration of the macrofollicular and microfollicular subtypes of the follicular variant of papillary carcinoma of the thyroid. *Cancer* 1998;84:235–244.
85. Shih SR, Shun CT, Su DH, et al. Follicular variant of papillary thyroid carcinoma: diagnostic limitations of fine needle aspiration cytology. *Acta Cytol* 2005;49:383–386.
86. Jain M, Khan A, Patwardhan N, et al. Follicular variant of papillary thyroid carcinoma: a comparative study of histopathologic features and cytology results in 141 patients. *Endocr Pract* 2001;7:79–84.
87. Fulciniti F, Benincasa G, Vetrani A, et al. Follicular variant of papillary carcinoma: cytologic findings on FNAB samples-experience with 16 cases. *Diagn Cytopathol* 2001;25:86–93.
88. Gallagher J, Oertel YC, Oertel JE. Follicular variant of papillary carcinoma of the thyroid: fine-needle aspirates with histologic correlation. *Diagn Cytopathol* 1997;16:207–213.
89. Nair M, Kapila K, Karak AK, et al. Papillary carcinoma of the thyroid and its variants: a cytohistological correlation. *Diagn Cytopathol* 2001;24:167–173.
90. Logani S, Gupta PK, LiVolsi VA, et al. Thyroid nodules with FNA cytology suspicious for follicular variant of papillary thyroid carcinoma: follow-up and management. *Diagn Cytopathol* 2000;23:380–385.
91. Baloch ZW, Gupta PK, Yu GH, et al. Follicular variant of papillary carcinoma. Cytologic and histologic correlation. *Am J Clin Pathol* 1999;111:216–222.
92. Amrikachi M, Ramzy I, Rubenfeld S, et al. Accuracy of fine-needle aspiration of thyroid. *Arch Pathol Lab Med* 2001;125:484–488.
93. Sangalli G, Serio G, Zampatti C, et al. Fine needle aspiration cytology of the thyroid: a comparison of 5469 cytological and final histological diagnoses. *Cytopathology* 2006;17:245–250.
94. Wu HH, Jones JN, Grzybicki DM, et al. Sensitive cytologic criteria for the identification of follicular variant of papillary thyroid carcinoma in fine-needle aspiration biopsy. *Diagn Cytopathol* 2003;29:262–266.
95. Powari M, Dey P, Saikia UN. Fine needle aspiration cytology of follicular variant of papillary carcinoma of thyroid. *Cytopathology* 2003;14:212–215.
96. Leung CS, Hartwick RWJ, Bédard YC. Correlation of cytologic and histologic features in variants of papillary carcinoma of the thyroid. *Acta Cytol* 1993;37:645–650.
97. Martinez-Parra D, Campos FJ, Hierro-Guilmain CC, et al. Follicular variant of papillary carcinoma of the thyroid: to what extent is fine-needle aspiration reliable? *Diagn Cytopathol* 1996;15:12–16.
98. Lin HS, Komisar A, Opher E, et al. Follicular variant of papillary carcinoma: the diagnostic limitations of preoperative fine-needle aspiration and intraoperative frozen section evaluation. *Laryngoscope* 2000;110:1431–1436.
99. Miettinen M, Karkkainen P. Differential reactivity of HBME-1 and CD15 antibodies in benign and malignant thyroid tumours. Preferential reactivity with malignant tumours. *Virchows Arch* 1996;429:213–219.
100. Van Hoeven KH, Kovatich AJ, Miettinen M. Immunocytochemical evaluation of HBME-1, CA 19-9, and CD-15 (Leu-M1) in fine-needle aspirates of thyroid nodules. *Diagn Cytopathol* 1997;18:93–97.
101. Fernandez PL, Merino MJ, Gomez M, et al. Galectin-3 and laminin expression in neoplastic and non-neoplastic thyroid tissue. *J Pathol* 1997;181:80–86.
102. Orlandi F, Saggiorato E, Pivano G, et al. Galectin-3 is a presurgical marker of human thyroid carcinoma. *Cancer Res* 1998;58:3015–3020.

103. Inohara H, Honjo Y, Yoishii T, et al. Expression of galectin-3 in fine-needle aspirates as a diagnostic marker differentiating benign from malignant thyroid neoplasms. *Cancer* 1999;85:2475–2484.

104. Cvejic D, Savin S, Paunovic I, et al. Immuhohistochemical localization of galectin-3 in malignant and benign human thyroid tissue. *Anticancer Res* 1998;18:2637–2642.

105. Cerilli LA, Mills SE, Rumpel CA, et al. Interpretation of RET immunostaining in follicular lesions of the thyroid. *Am J Clin Pathol* 2002;118:186–193.

106. Baloch ZW, Abraham S, Roberts S, et al. Differential expression of cytokeratins in follicular variant of papillary carcinoma: an immunohistochemical study and its diagnostic utility. *Hum Pathol* 1999;30:1166–1171.

107. Sahoo S, Hoda SA, Rosai J, et al. Cytokeratin 19 immunoreactivity in the diagnosis of papillary thyroid carcinoma: a note of caution. *Am J Clin Pathol* 2001;116:696–702.

108. Asa SL, Cheung CC. The mind's eye. *Am J Clin Pathol* 2001;116:635–636.

109. Asa SL. My approach to oncocytic tumours of the thyroid. *J Clin Pathol* 2004;57:225–232.

110. Trovisco V, Vieira DC I, Soares P, et al. BRAF mutations are associated with some histological types of papillary thyroid carcinoma. *J Pathol* 2004;202:247–251.

111. Trovisco V, Soares P, Soares R, et al. A new BRAF gene mutation detected in a case of a solid variant of papillary thyroid carcinoma. *Hum Pathol* 2005;36:694–697.

112. Trovisco V, Soares P, Preto A, et al. Type and prevalence of BRAF mutations are closely associated with papillary thyroid carcinoma histotype and patients' age but not with tumour aggressiveness. *Virchows Arch* 2005;446:589–595.

113. Klugbauer S, Lengfelder E, Demidchik EP, et al. High prevalence of RET rearrangement in thyroid tumors of children from Belarus after the Chernobyl reactor accident. *Oncoogene* 1995;11:2459–2467.

114. Nishisho I, Rowland JM, Bove KE, et al. Distinct pattern of ret oncogene rearrangements in morphological variants of radiation-induced and sporadic thyroid papillary carcinoma in children. *Cancer Res* 1997;57:1690–1694.

115. Klugbauer S, Lengfelder E, Demidchik EP, et al. A new form of RET rearrangement in thyroid carcinomas of children after the Chernobyl reactor accident. *Oncogene* 1996; 13:1099–1102.

116. Fugazzola L, Pierotti MA, Vigano E, et al. Molecular and biochemical analysis of RET/PTC4, a novel oncogenic rearrangement between RET and ELE1 genes, in a post-Chernobyl papillary thyroid cancer. *Oncogene* 1996;13:1093–1097.

117. Klugbauer S, Demidchik EP, Lengfelder E, et al. Detection of a novel type of RET rearrangement (PTC5) in thyroid carcinomas after Chernobyl and analysis of the involved RET-fused gene RFG5. *Cancer Res* 1998;58:198–203.

118. Williams GH, Rooney S, Thomas GA, et al. RET activation in adult and childhood papillary thyroid carcinoma using a reverse transcriptase-polymerase chain reaction approach on archival-nested material. *Br J Cancer* 1996;74:585–589.

119. Jhiang SM, Caruso DR, Gilmore E, et al. Detection of the PTC/retTPC oncogene in human thyroid cancers. *Oncogene* 1992;7:1331–1337.

120. Sugg SL, Zheng L, Rosen IB, et al. ret/PTC-1,-2 and -3 oncogene rearrangements in human thyroid carcinomas: Implications for metastatic potential? *J Clin Endocrinol Metab* 1996;81:3360–3365.

121. Mayr B, Brabant G, Goretzki P, et al. ret/Ptc-1, -2, and -3 oncogene rearrangements in human thyroid carcinomas: implications for metastatic potential? [letter; comment]. *J Clin Endocrinol Metab* 1997;82:1306–1307.

122. Cheung CC, Carydis B, Ezzat S, et al. Analysis of ret/PTC gene rearrangements refines the fine needle aspiration diagnosis of thyroid cancer. *J Clin Endocrinol Metab* 2001;86:2187–2190.

123. Adeniran AJ, Zhu Z, Gandhi M, et al. Correlation between genetic alterations and microscopic features, clinical manifestations, and prognostic characteristics of thyroid papillary carcinomas. *Am J Surg Pathol* 2006;30:216–222.

124. Zhu Z, Gandhi M, Nikiforova MN, et al. Molecular profile and clinical-pathologic features of the follicular variant of papillary thyroid carcinoma. An unusually high prevalence of ras mutations. *Am J Clin Pathol* 2003;120:71–77.

125. Albores-Saavedra J, Gould E, Vardaman C, et al. The macrofollicular variant of papillary thyroid carcinoma: a study of 17 cases. *Hum Pathol* 1991;22:1195–1205.

126. Hirokawa M, Shimizu M, Terayama K, et al. Macrofollicular variant of papillary thyroid carcinoma. Report of a case with fine needle aspiration biopsy findings. *Acta Cytol* 1998;42:1441–1443.

127. Chung D, Ghossein RA, Lin O. Macrofollicular variant of papillary carcinoma: a potential thyroid FNA pitfall. *Diagn Cytopathol* 2007;35:560–564.

128. Grant CS, Barr D, Goellner JR, et al. Benign Hürthle cell tumors of the thyroid: a diagnosis to be trusted? *World J Surg* 1988;12:488–495.

129. Cheung CC, Ezzat S, Ramyar L, et al. Molecular basis of Hurthle cell papillary thyroid carcinoma. *J Clin Endocrinol Metab* 2000;85:878–882.

130. Chiappetta G, Toti P, Cetta F, et al. The RET/PTC oncogene is frequently activated in oncocytic thyroid tumors (Hurthle cell adenomas and carcinomas), but not in oncocytic hyperplastic lesions. *J Clin Endocrinol Metab* 2002;87:364–369.

131. Moreira AL, Waisman J, Cangiarella JF. Aspiration cytology of the oncocytic variant of papillary adenocarcinoma of the thyroid gland. *Acta Cytol* 2004;48:137–141.

132. Doria MI Jr., Attal H, Wang HH, et al. Fine needle aspiration cytology of the oxyphil variant of papillary carcinoma of the thyroid. A report of three cases. *Acta Cytol* 1996; 40:1007–1011.

133. Belchetz G, Cheung CC, Freeman J, et al. Hurthle cell tumors: using molecular techniques to define a novel classification system. *Arch Otolaryngol Head Neck Surg* 2002;128:237–240.

11

SOLID AND TRABECULAR LESIONS

PAPILLARY CARCINOMA: SOLID VARIANT

The solid variant of papillary carcinoma is characterized by solid nests of epithelial cells that have well-defined borders but fail to form follicles and lack colloid storage [1]. The tumor cells remain well differentiated and exhibit the nuclear features of papillary carcinoma (Fig. 11.1, e-Figs. 11.1 and 11.2). Solid variant papillary carcinoma must be distinguished from insular carcinoma, which is composed of smaller, less well-differentiated cells and exhibits tumor cell necrosis (Fig. 11.2, e-Figs. 11.3 and 11.4). Although somewhat controversial, it appears that this variant of papillary carcinoma is associated with more aggressive behavior than classical papillary thyroid carcinoma (PTC) [2,3].

The fine needle aspiration (FNA) appearance of the solid variant is not necessarily recognized as a distinct entity, but tends to show a clean background with only scant or no colloid, and marked cellularity. The follicular epithelial cells are arranged in cohesive clusters with nuclear overlapping and crowding [4,5]. The nuclear changes of papillary carcinoma are identified with prominent grooves and micronucleoli and occasional intranuclear inclusions.

The histologic diagnosis can be confirmed by the identification of specific markers. These tumors stain for HBME-1 and galectin-3 [6] and are known to harbor ret/PTC rearrangements, as shown particularly in children exposed to radiation after the Chernobyl disaster [2,7]. Although the classical activating BRAF mutations are not found in this variant, the in-frame VK600-1E deletion (BRAFVK600-1E) has been detected in aggressive solid variant PTCs [8,9].

PAPILLARY CARCINOMA: HYALINIZING TRABECULAR VARIANT

An unusual tumor known as the *hyalinizing trabecular tumor* was originally described by pioneers such as Zipkin in 1905 [10], Masson in 1922 [11], and Ward et al. in 1982 [12]. The terminology "hyalinizing trabecular adenoma" (HTA) was defined by Carney et al. in 1987 [13]. This lesion has also been designated "paragangliomalike adenoma of thyroid" (PLAT) by Bronner et al. [14] because of its unusual histologic pattern that resembles

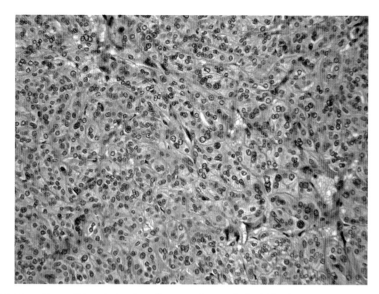

FIGURE 11.1 The solid variant of papillary carcinoma lacks follicular and papillary architecture and colloid production, but remains well differentiated with the classical nuclear features of papillary carcinoma evident (hematoxylin & eosin stain).

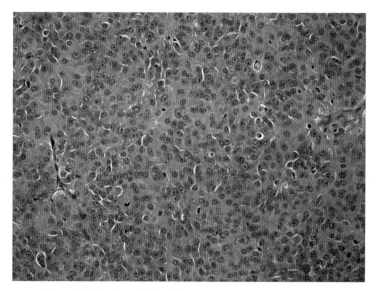

FIGURE 11.2 Superficially, the solid variant of papillary carcinoma may mimic insular carcinoma. However, as seen in this image, insular carcinoma is characterized by less well-differentiated follicular epithelial cells, lacking the nuclear features of papillary carcinoma and often betraying their aggressive nature with foci of necrosis and readily identified mitoses (hematoxylin & eosin stain).

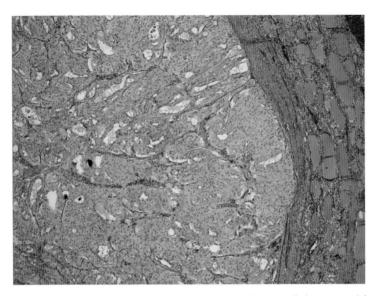

FIGURE 11.3 Hyalinizing trabecular tumors of the thyroid are well demarcated from the surrounding thyroid parenchyma, which may be appreciated grossly as well as microscopically (hematoxylin & eosin stain).

a neuroendocrine tumor. Since the original descriptions, a malignant counterpart, hyalinizing trabecular carcinoma (HTC), has been described [15–17] and both HTA and HTC are now incorporated under the umbrella of hyalinizing trabecular tumors (HTT) [1].

HTTs share many features with papillary carcinoma. Both lesions are of thyroid follicular epithelial origin and therefore both express thyroglobulin. HTTs have been associated with Hashimoto's thyroiditis and are reported in patients who have a history of neck irradiation [18]. HTT can coexist with papillary carcinoma [19] and they exhibit papillary carcinomalike histologic features such as psammoma-body formation, and characteristic nuclear changes including elongation and irregularity with grooves and pseudoinclusions and nuclear hypochromasia [13]. On the basis of these observations, as well as molecular genetic alterations that are shared by both entities [20,21], many experts and the authors consider these to be variants of PTC [1,22,23].

These lesions are generally well-delineated tumors characterized architecturally by solid trabecular and nesting architecture (Figs. 11.3 and 11.4, e-Figs. 11.5–11.7). The tumor cells are elongated with abundant pale eosinophilic cytoplasm and scattered "yellow bodies" [13,14,18,24]. There is perivascular hyaline fibrosis and the cytoplasmic hyaline is usually identified as cytoplasmic filaments of cytokeratin. Occasional cases are immunoreactive for S100 protein. Most importantly, the tumor cells harbor large clear nuclei with irregular and elongated contours, grooves, and inclusions as well as micronucleoli, which are the features of papillary carcinoma (Figs. 11.5–11.7, e-Figs. 11.8–11.11).

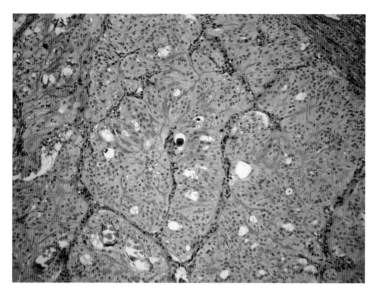

FIGURE 11.4 Hyalinizing trabecular tumors are composed of solid trabeculae, cords, and nests of cells with interposed hyalinized stroma (hematoxylin & eosin stain).

The morphologic key to the recognition of hyalinizing trabecular tumor on FNA is the identification of the aggregates of the hyalinized stroma with radially oriented, elongated/spindle epithelial cells with abundant cytoplasm (Figs. 11.8 and 11.9, e-Figs. 11.12–11.17). The cytoplasm is

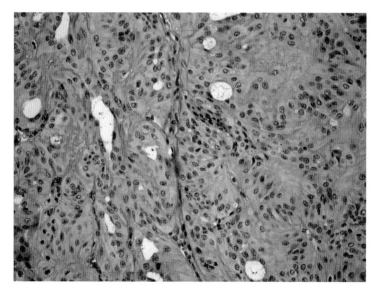

FIGURE 11.5 The epithelial cells of hyalinizing trabecular tumors are elongated with abundant eosinophilic cytoplasm and often show an organoid arrangement around the hyalinized stromal tissue (hematoxylin & eosin stain).

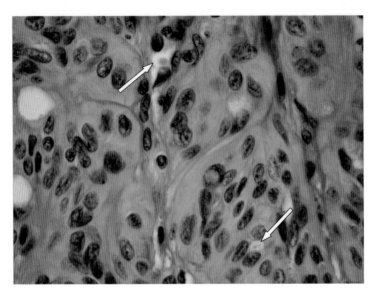

FIGURE 11.6   Hyalinizing trabecular tumors display all of the classical nuclear features of papillary carcinoma and usually to an exuberant degree. In addition, cytoplasmic inclusions containing a central body surrounded by a halo are seen in many cases (*arrows*) (hematoxylin & eosin stain).

often somewhat filamentous and cell borders indistinct. Romanowsky staining highlights the metachromatic hyaline material, perinucleolar clearing, and cytoplasmic bodies. Intranuclear cytoplasmic inclusions, nuclear grooves, and nuclear overlapping are the rule and well visualized on

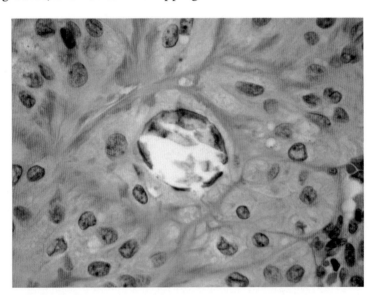

FIGURE 11.7   Psammoma bodies, often numerous, typify hyalinizing trabecular tumors (hematoxylin & eosin stain).

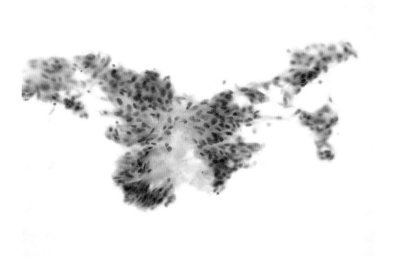

FIGURE 11.8 Fine needle aspirations of hyalinizing trabecular tumors are characterized by aggregates of hyaline stroma with radial arrangements of spindle epithelial cells (direct smear, Papanicolaou stain).

Papanicolaou staining [25–28] (Fig. 11.10, e-Figs. 11.17 and 11.18). As these lesions display all of the nuclear features of papillary carcinoma, the presence of the hyaline stroma may be overlooked and the sample diagnosed as "papillary carcinoma" [29].

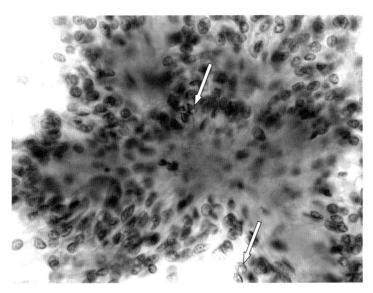

FIGURE 11.9 The epithelial cells of hyalinizing trabecular tumor are elongated, spindle cells, with indistinct cell borders. Even at this power, intranuclear inclusions are readily apparent (*white arrows*) (direct smear, Papanicolaou stain).

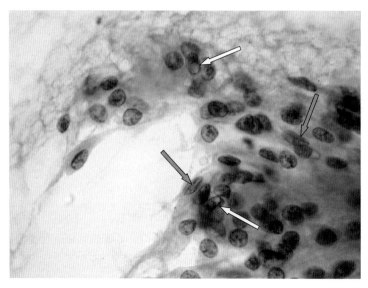

FIGURE 11.10 All of the classical nuclear features of papillary carcinoma are evident in hyalinizing trabecular tumor and these are typically found in abundance including nuclear grooves (*orange arrows*) and intranuclear inclusions (*white arrows*) (direct smear, Papanico-laou stain).

On histology, the differential diagnosis of these tumors includes paraganglioma or medullary carcinoma [13]. Immunohistochemical stains for neuroendocrine markers easily distinguish HTT from paraganglioma or medullary carcinoma. HTTs are negative for synaptophysin, chromo-granin, and CD56, whereas the neuroendocrine tumors stain for these markers. HTTs stain for thyroglobulin, whereas paraganglioma and medullary carcinoma are negative. CK7 and CK18 have been detected in a high percentage of HTT [30]. Variable expression of CK19 (50% to 100%) in HTA (e-Figs. 11.19 and 11.20) has been interpreted by some in-vestigators as proof that these tumors are benign, while others use this as evidence that they should be classified as a variant of papillary carcinoma [31,32]. The identification of anomalous membranous MIB-1 staining in these lesions has been suggested to be of diagnostic assistance [33,34] (Figs. 11.11 and 11.12, e-Figs. 11.21 and 11.22). It has been recognized that this staining result is unique to the MIB-1 clone of Ki-67 and is found only if the staining is performed at room temperature. This staining is not present if the procedure is performed at 37°C or other clones for Ki-67 are used [35]. The actual epitope recognized and the biological significance of this unusual staining pattern remains to be clarified.

The marked morphologic similarities between papillary carcinoma and hyalinizing trabecular tumor strongly suggest that HTT is simply a variant of papillary carcinoma. Furthermore, application of ret/PTC analysis has identified rearrangements in these lesions at a rate identical

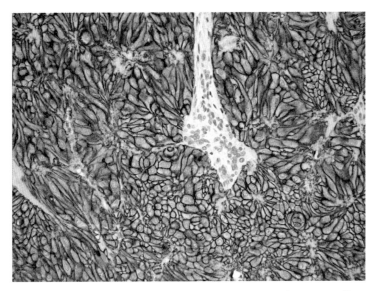

FIGURE 11.11   Hyalinizing trabecular tumor has been noted to show a peculiar membranous staining pattern for MIB-1 (MIB-1 immunoperoxidase stain & hematoxylin).

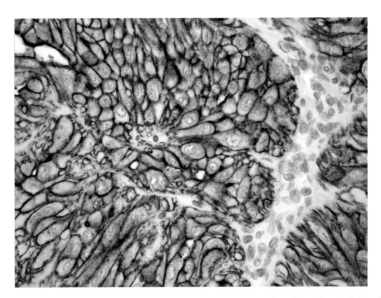

FIGURE 11.12   This anomalous staining for MIB-1 occurs only when the staining is performed at room temperature and with the use of this particular clone and has not been found with other clones of Ki-67 antibodies. This staining pattern has been suggested as a possible aid to the diagnosis of HTT; however, the actual epitope recognized and the biological significance of this finding have not been established. Note the absence of nuclear staining (MIB-1 immunoperoxidase stain & hematoxylin).

to that found in other papillary carcinomas [20,21], providing further evidence that this entity is a variant of papillary carcinoma. However, some continue to maintain that these are distinct lesions [33,36] and the matter remains open to debate.

POORLY DIFFERENTIATED CARCINOMA OF FOLLICULAR EPITHELIAL DERIVATION

Poorly differentiated carcinoma is a tumor of follicular cell origin that occupies a position both morphologically and biologically between well-differentiated papillary or follicular carcinoma and anaplastic thyroid carcinoma [1,37–39]. These lesions behave in an aggressive fashion and are often lethal. They do not respond well to treatment with radioactive iodine, since their uptake of this targeted therapy is reduced. This is the lesion that most often is identified as "widely invasive follicular carcinoma." Vascular invasion and metastases are frequent at the time of diagnosis. On complete histological evaluation, there is usually a focus of well-differentiated carcinoma (either papillary or follicular) with progression to dedifferentiation; however, some tumors are entirely composed of a poorly differentiated lesion. These tumors may have a central encapsulated nidus, and smaller lesions may not be widely invasive, but usually the lesion exhibits frank capsular invasion and forms satellite nodules in the surrounding thyroid.

The majority of these lesions have an architectural growth pattern that is characterized by large, well-defined solid nests (Fig. 11.13, e-Figs. 11.23 and 11.24) that mimics neuroendocrine tumors such as medullary

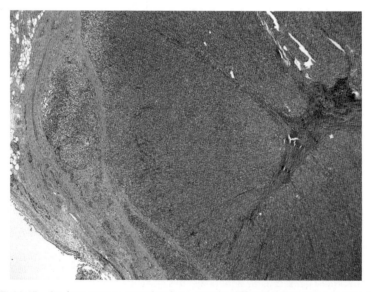

FIGURE 11.13 On low-power examination, poorly differentiated carcinomas show a growth pattern composed of solid nests of cells, resembling neuroendocrine tumors and giving origin to the designation of "insular" carcinomas (hematoxylin & eosin stain).

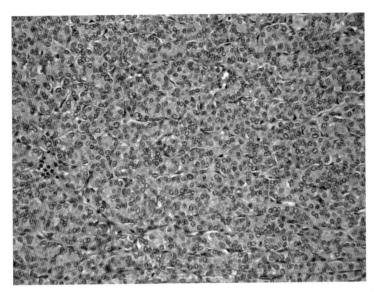

FIGURE 11.14 Colloid is typically absent in poorly differentiated carcinomas and the constituent cells are comparatively smaller and uniform in their appearance (hematoxylin & eosin stain).

carcinoma; this architecture has given rise to the terminology "insular" carcinoma. Other tumors have trabecular growth patterns. They are largely devoid of follicular architecture or colloid. The tumor cells are usually small and uniform in size (Fig. 11.14, e-Figs. 11.25 and 11.26) and there is mitotic activity with 3 or more mitoses per 10 high power fields [40,41] (Fig. 11.15, e-Figs. 11.27 and 11.28). Tumor necrosis is usually identified as single cell necrosis rather than the geographic necrosis that is characteristic of anaplastic carcinoma. In contrast to anaplastic carcinomas, there is little pleomorphism and no bizarre, giant, or multinucleated cells are found.

FNA of these lesions yields extremely cellular smears that are devoid of colloid [42–45]. The tumor is composed of small- to medium-sized epithelial cells seen individually and in small groups and solid clusters (Figs. 11.16–11.19, e-Figs. 11.29–11.34). Occasionally, a necrotic background is present. The cytoplasm is pale and may contain fine vacuoles. Nuclei are round and monomorphic with fine, hyperchromatic chromatin, and variable, but often small, nucleoli. Although demonstrating a "neoplastic" appearance, there is only mild nuclear atypia. In some cases, nuclear inclusions and grooves may be seen and indicate dedifferentiation of a papillary carcinoma.

The differential diagnosis includes well differentiated carcinomas with a solid growth pattern, medullary carcinoma of the thyroid and low-grade lymphoma. Sclerosis can mimic amyloid; however, Congo red stains are negative and immunohistochemical stains for calcitonin, chromogranin, and carcinoembryonic antigen (CEA) are negative. Markers of

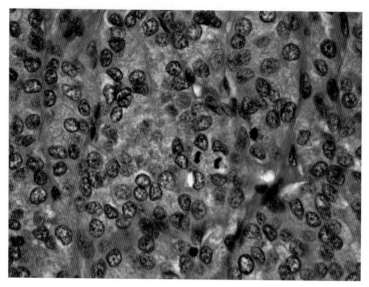

FIGURE 11.15 Mitotic activity is easily identified in poorly differentiated carcinomas, and tumor necrosis in the form of individual cell death is commonplace (hematoxylin & eosin stain).

hematologic differentiation are negative. In contrast, the tumors are uniformly positive for keratins and staining for thyroglobulin, although often weak and sometimes focal, confirms the follicular cell differentiation of this neoplasm [46].

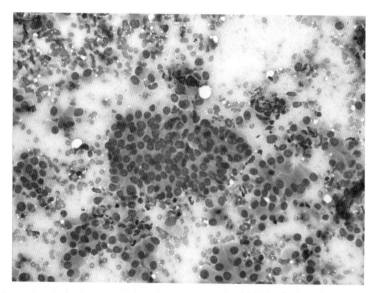

FIGURE 11.16 FNAs of poorly differentiated (insular) carcinomas are typically cellular with the epithelial cells seen individually, in small groups and as solid cell masses (direct smear, air-dried Diff Quik stain).

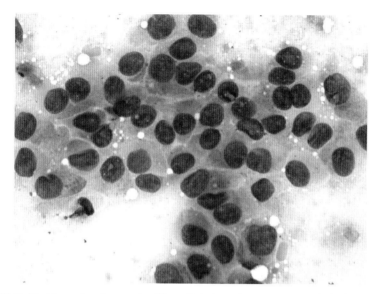

FIGURE 11.17 The cells of a poorly differentiated carcinoma appear relatively monomorphic with cytoplasm containing fine vacuoles, round nuclei, fine, hyperchromatic chromatin, and variable, but often small nucleoli. Although demonstrating a "neoplastic" appearance, there is only mild nuclear atypia (direct smear, air-dried Diff Quik stain).

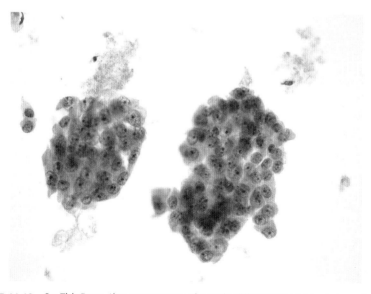

FIGURE 11.18 On ThinPrep, the appearance of poorly differentiated (insular) carcinoma is similar to direct smears with a cellular sample and numerous epithelial cells seen as individual cells and in complex groups. Note the necrotic background (ThinPrep, Papanicolaou stain).

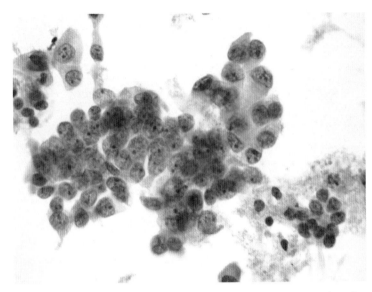

FIGURE 11.19   The cellular monomorphism is apparent on ThinPrep samples of poorly differentiated carcinoma and help distinguish these tumors from anaplastic carcinoma of the thyroid (ThinPrep, Papanicolaou stain).

Molecular studies have identified a high incidence of ras mutations in these lesions [47], and up to 25% harbor mutations of the *CTNNB1* gene, resulting in nuclear translocation of β-catenin and activation of a number of downstream targets of the WNT signaling pathway [48]. These mutations are not found in well-differentiated thyroid carcinomas and are more common in anaplastic carcinomas, suggesting that they play a role in progression of these lesions [49]. APC mutations, another cause of nuclear translocation of β-catenin, are not reported in thyroid carcinomas [49]. The loss of membranous staining for β-catenin can be seen by immunohistochemistry, and nuclear translocation is a marker of dedifferentiation. This mechanism also may account for the dehiscence that is characteristic of poorly differentiated carcinoma.

Poorly differentiated carcinomas often express HBME-1 [50–53], but the diagnosis of malignancy that is supported by this stain is not usually controversial in this entity. The expression of CK7, CK18, and CK19 is reduced in poorly differentiated carcinomas [54]. These tumors exhibit a low prevalence of expression of *RET* rearrangements [49,55]. This finding has been used as evidence that *RET*/PTC rearrangements predict indolent behavior; however, it is known that the promoters of the upstream genes involved in the translocations determine variable levels of expression and dedifferentiation results in down-regulation of expression with loss of RET/PTC gene expression by RT-PCR as well as protein expression by immunohistochemistry. A better understanding of this will require FISH analysis.

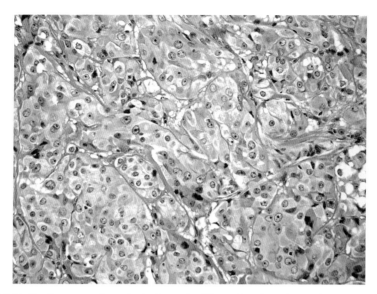

FIGURE 11.20 An oncocytic variant of poorly differentiated carcinoma is recognized, but in our experience, most aggressive oncocytic or Hürthle cell lesions show insular growth and focal tumor cell necrosis (hematoxylin & eosin stain).

Variants

Aggressive solid tumors that have widely invasive growth and are composed of oncocytic cells represent an *oncocytic variant* of poorly differentiated carcinoma (Fig. 11.20, e-Fig. 11.35). In our experience, most aggressive oncocytic or Hürthle cell lesions show insular growth and focal tumor cell necrosis; this may explain the poor outcome of tumors diagnosed as Hürthle cell carcinomas. As with other oncocytic lesions, these tumors likely have mutations of mitochondrial DNA in addition to the known mutations of poorly differentiated thyroid carcinomas [56].

Clear cell carcinoma is rare in the thyroid but often has solid growth, and when primary, often represents a *clear cell variant* of poorly differentiated carcinoma with accumulation of glycogen, lipid, or even mucin [19] (Fig. 11.21, e-Figs. 11.36 and 11.37). The term "clear cell tumor" should be restricted to lesions in which more than 75% of the tumor cells show this change. Clear cell change may occur focally within oncocytic lesions. The finding of a clear cell tumor raises an important differential diagnosis, since a common differential diagnosis is metastasis, particularly from renal or adrenal tumors [19], or biopsy of adjacent parathyroid tissue. Parathyroid nodules can be adjacent to or within the thyroid and can mimic a primary thyroid lesion [57]. A novel approach using Fourier transform infrared spectroscopic (FTIR) interrogation of touch imprint cytology that provides detailed spectra can be used to distinguish various tissue pathologies. FTIR spectral profiles of thyroid tissues differ visually when compared with parathyroid tissue

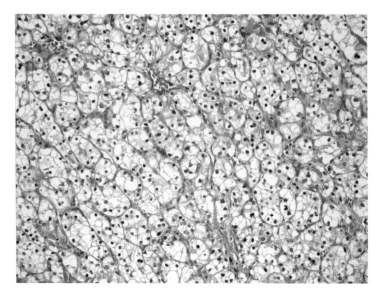

FIGURE 11.21   Focal clear cell change is common in oncocytic neoplasms, but when an excess of 75% of the tumor shows clear cell differentiation, they are classified as clear cell carcinoma of thyroid as seen in this illustration. It is imperative to exclude metastatic clear cell carcinoma (adrenal, renal) and the remote possibility of a clear cell parathyroid lesion (hematoxylin & eosin stain).

[58]. In more routine studies, proof of follicular cell derivation is obtained from thyroglobulin and TTF-1 staining, while other tissues have distinct immunoprofiles.

MEDULLARY CARCINOMA

Medullary carcinoma of the thyroid comprises approximately 5% of all thyroid carcinomas [19] but is responsible for 13.4% of the total deaths [59]. This lesion is usually readily recognized because of its unusual cytologic and histologic features but sometimes special investigation is required to distinguish it from follicular lesions or other tumors, including lymphomas and/or anaplastic carcinomas. The importance of distinguishing this tumor from follicular lesions is twofold. The first is for diagnostic classification and management considerations of the individual patient. These tumors do not preferentially take up iodine and therapy with radioactive iodine is not indicated; in contrast, expression of somatostatin receptors by some of these tumors [60] makes the OctreoScan a feasible diagnostic tool to localize the primary lesion and to identify metastatic deposits [61] and somatostatin analogues may have applications in the management of disseminated disease [62]. The other aspect of management involves the implications for both the patient and members of his/her family, since many of these tumors are hereditary [63].

The inherited forms of medullary carcinoma are of three types: familial medullary thyroid carcinoma alone (FMTC), multiple endocrine neoplasia

(MEN) type IIA in which MTC is associated with pheochromocytomas, and MEN IIB in which the thyroid and adrenal proliferative disorders are associated with mucosal ganglioneuromas and a marfanoid habitus. The inheritance of all three syndromes was mapped to the pericentromeric region of chromosome 10 by linkage analysis [64–66]. Subsequently, mutations in exons 10 and 11 of the *ret* proto-oncogene in patients with FMTC or MEN IIA and at codon 918 in MEN IIB [67,68] have provided a more accurate marker of germline mutation and predisposition to this disease [59,69,70]. Current recommendations suggest that family members of FMTC and MEN IIA kindreds have genetic screening early in life and affected members should undergo prophylactic thyroidectomy in childhood [59]. The ages recommended vary depending on the mutation and family history; the goal is to prevent the earliest possible onset of medullary thyroid carcinoma in these familial forms of the disease, since metastatic tumor has been found in patients as young as 6 years of age. Children affected with MEN IIB undergo surgery even earlier than those with MEN IIA and FMTC [71].

Familial forms of medullary thyroid carcinoma usually result in multicentric disease as well as multicentric C-cell hyperplasia [72,73]. C cells are usually limited to the central portion of the junction between the upper and middle thirds of the lateral lobes where they are generally distributed singly rather than in clusters. Increased numbers of C cells (more than seven cells per cluster), complete follicles surrounded by C cells, and distribution of cells beyond this geographic location are indicative of C-cell hyperplasia (Fig. 11.22, e-Figs. 11.38–11.40). The presence of C-cell hyperplasia usually indicates an inherited disorder rather than a sporadic lesion; however, C-cell hyperplasia can also be associated with chronic hypercalcemia, thyroid follicular nodular disease, and thyroiditis [74–76]. Patients with PTEN hamartoma tumor syndrome (PHTS), characterized by a predominance of non-thyroidal tumors, have a predisposition to develop multiple adenomatous follicular nodules but have also been reported to have a diffuse form of C-cell hyperplasia [77], but this has not been associated with medullary carcinoma.

Sporadic medullary carcinomas may also have mutations of ret in the same codons as the familial disorders, most frequently in codon 918 encoding the cytoplasmic tyrosine kinase domain [59,68,70,78]; the mutation involved may have prognostic value [79] and provide a target for novel therapeutic approaches. The presence of somatic *ret* mutations in sporadic tumors indicates the importance of analyzing DNA from white blood cells to establish that a mutation is germline, therefore potentially hereditary. Other oncogenes and tumor suppressor genes have not been implicated in the pathogenesis of MCT: *ras* mutations are rare, c-*myc* and c-*erb* B are not amplified [80,81], and p53 mutations are not found in these tumors [82].

Aspirates from medullary carcinoma have a variable appearance [83–85]. The most classical cytomorphology is that of a dyshesive or weakly cohesive, biphasic tumor composed of varying degrees of spindle and epithelioid cells (Fig. 11.23, e-Fig. 11.41). However, medullary carcinoma adopts a number of disguises and may appear as a pure population

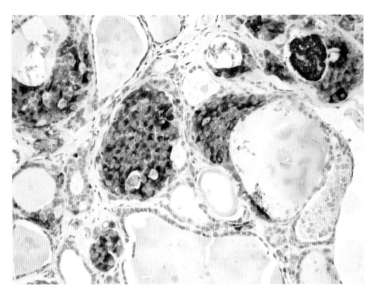

FIGURE 11.22 C-cell hyperplasia is defined by clusters consisting of more than seven C cells, complete follicles surrounded by C cells, and the identification of C cells outside of the central portion of the junction between the upper and middle thirds of the lateral lobes. The presence of C-cell hyperplasia usually indicates an inherited disorder rather than a sporadic lesion; however, C-cell hyperplasia can also be associated with chronic hypercalcemia, thyroid follicular nodular disease, and thyroiditis (calcitonin & hematoxylin stain).

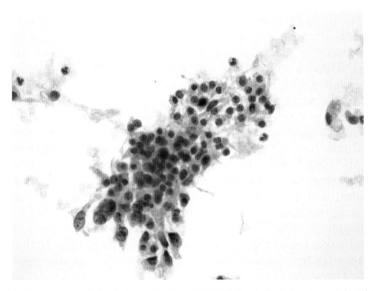

FIGURE 11.23 The prototypical FNA appearance of medullary carcinoma is a biphasic tumor with both epithelioid and spindle cell elements (ThinPrep, Papanicolaou stain).

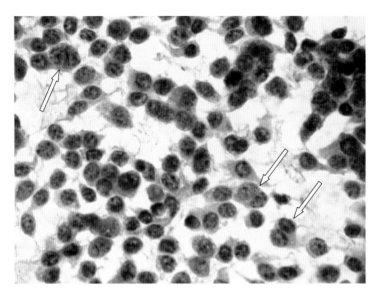

FIGURE 11.24 The epithelioid component of a medullary carcinoma is dyshesive and composed of plasmacytoid cells that are frequently binucleate (*white arrows*). The chromatin is granular, imparting a "neuroendocrine appearance" to the nuclei that contain small nucleoli (direct smear, Papanicolaou stain).

of epithelioid cells, in which a plasmacytoid appearance typically dominates (Fig. 11.24, e-Figs. 11.42–11.44) to the other extreme of a pure spindle cell tumor (Fig. 11.25, e-Figs. 11.45 and 11.46). Bizarre tumor cells may be encountered (Fig. 11.26, e-Fig. 11.47) as well as tumor giant cells

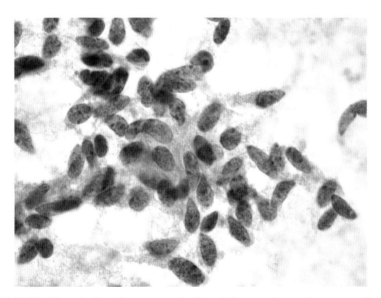

FIGURE 11.25 The spindle cell component of medullary carcinoma is composed of relatively bland spindle cells with scant cytoplasm. Similar to the epithelioid cells, the chromatin is granular and has a "neuroendocrine" appearance (direct smear, Papanicolaou stain).

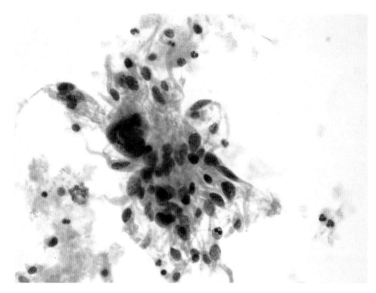

FIGURE 11.26 Large and frankly bizarre cells are occasionally identified in the epithelial cell groups of medullary carcinoma, but unlike anaplastic carcinoma do not dominate the lesion (direct smear, Papanicolaou stain).

and a variety of epithelial differentiations including oncocytic cells, squamoid cells, clear cells, mucinous cells, and even a small cell carcinomalike appearance. Fortunately, most of these variations are uncommon and usually there is a population of plasmacytoid cells admixed with a number of nondescript spindle cells. The plasmacytoid cells have moderately abundant cytoplasm (e-Figs. 11.43 and 11.44) and may contain azurophilic granules that are seen as red, perinuclear cytoplasmic granules on air dried, May–Grünwald–Giemsa-stained preparations (Fig. 11.27, e-Figs. 11.48–11.50). The nuclei are eccentrically placed and show increased chromatin granularity, imparting a typical "neuroendocrine" look to the nucleus. Binucleation is fairly common and nucleoli are typically present. Intranuclear pseudoinclusions may be found (Fig. 11.28, e-Figs. 11.51–11.53) and psammoma bodies are seen in some cases (Fig. 11.29, e-Fig. 11.54), creating a diagnostic mimic of papillary carcinoma. Beyond the presence of neoplastic vascularization (Fig. 11.30, e-Figs. 11.55–11.59) and occasional epithelial rosettes (Fig. 11.31, e-Fig. 11.60), other architectural differentiation is typically lacking.

Amyloid is present in many aspirates, but is either overlooked or misidentified as colloid. Amyloid is an amorphous material that on Papanicolaou staining appears translucent or weakly cyanophilic (Figs. 11.32–11.34, e-Figs. 11.61–11.63). It often has a waxy or fibrillar appearance and typically shows rounded, smooth edges. Unlike colloid, amyloid does not appear to crack and may seem to have cells embedded within its substance. Amyloid shows its characteristic apple-green birefringence

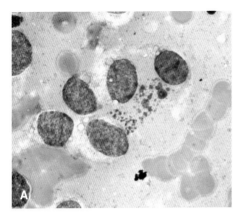
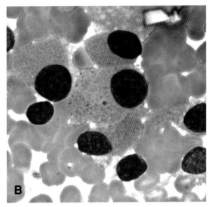

FIGURE 11.27 On rare occasions, red cytoplasmic granules may be seen within the epithelioid cells of medullary carcinoma on air-dried, May–Grünwald–Giemsa-stained material. The morphology of the granules may be vary from coarse aggregates (A) to fine particulate granules (B). (direct smear, May–Grünwald–Giemsa stain).

with polarized light after Papanicolaou staining and is highlighted by Congo red staining. It should be remembered that amyloid may be present in situations other than medullary carcinoma such as systemic amyloidosis or amyloid goiter and occasionally something that is thought to be amyloid is actually hyalinized stroma, as in a hyalinizing trabecular tumor.

When considered, the diagnosis of medullary carcinoma can be verified by immunolocalization of calcitonin (which may be weak and focal in its

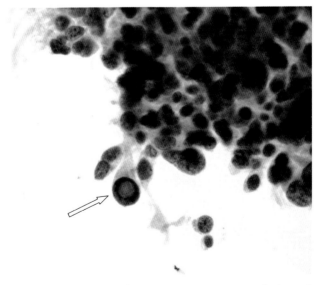

FIGURE 11.28 Intranuclear inclusions (*white arrow*) are not common, but may be identified in cases of medullary carcinoma (direct smear, Papanicolaou stain).

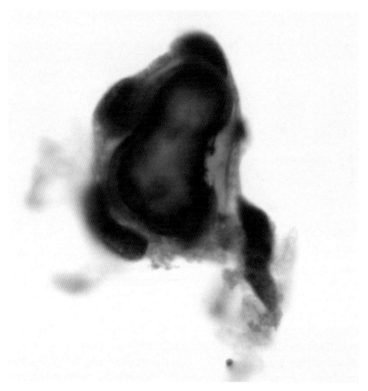

FIGURE 11.29 Calcification of amyloid may occur and rarely true psammoma bodies can be found in cases of medullary carcinoma as seen in this illustration (direct smear, Papanicolaou stain).

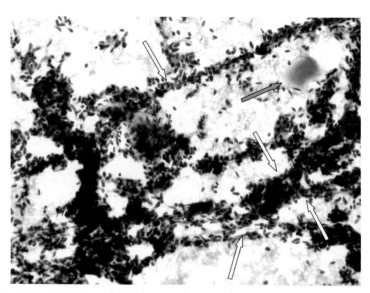

FIGURE 11.30 Neoplastic vascularization is often prominent in aspirates of medullary carcinoma. In this example, numerous capillary-sized vessels (*white arrows*) are evident with adherent neoplastic spindle cells. Note the presence of amyloid (*orange arrow*) (direct smear, Papanicolaou stain).

202

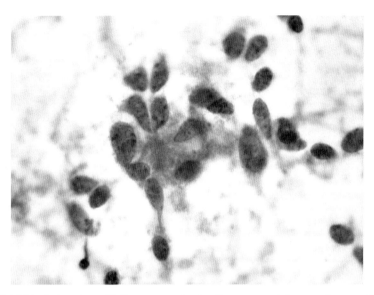

FIGURE 11.31 In keeping with its neuroendocrine lineage, medullary carcinoma will occasionally demonstrate rosettes on FNA (direct smear, Papanicolaou stain).

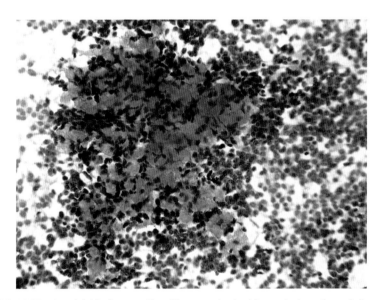

FIGURE 11.32 Amyloid is frequently either overlooked in aspirates of medullary carcinoma or misidentified as colloid. In this case, the amyloid superficially resembles colloid, but on closer examination, it has a fine fibrillary nature and appears to have cells embedded within its matrix, two features that are not seen with colloid (direct smear, Papanicolaou stain).

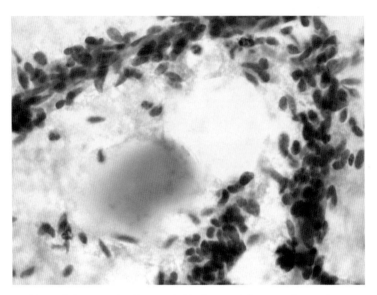

FIGURE 11.33 In this example, the amyloid of a medullary carcinoma is more waxy in appearance than colloid and shows smooth rounded edges (direct smear, Papanicolaou stain).

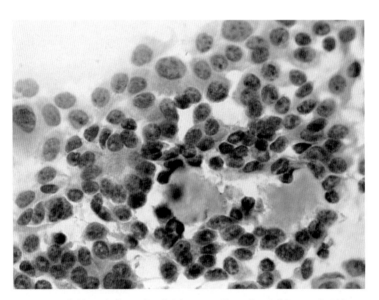

FIGURE 11.34 Amyloid's mimicry of colloid may at times be striking, as in this case where the amyloid and neoplastic cells of a medullary carcinoma produce pseudofollicles. In these situations, only through the use of polarized light, Congo red staining, and immunoperox-idase studies will it be possible to determine if the substance in question is colloid or amy-loid (direct smear, Papanicolaou stain).

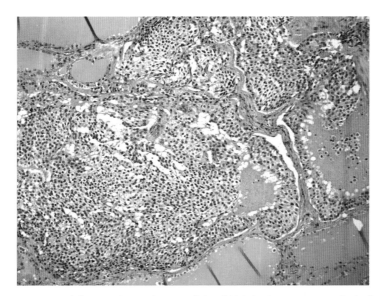

FIGURE 11.35 Medullary carcinoma has a variety of histologic appearances including large sheetlike growths of tumor (hematoxylin & eosin stain).

staining characteristics), chromogranin, and/or CEA. In some tumors, not all of these markers are positive, hence the need for more than one marker. However, caution must be exercised, especially with oncocytic tumors, in which nonspecific binding of the antibodies may falsely appear to indicate the presence of a marker and lead to a misdiagnosis of medullary carcinoma. For this reason, it is recommended that thyroglobulin immunostains also be performed, for which medullary carcinoma is expected to be negative.

When the thyroid is the target of aspiration, the possibility of medullary carcinoma often enters the list of differential diagnoses. However, this is not the case when a lymph node is the target of aspiration. Medullary carcinoma is too often forgotten when dealing with the "carcinoma of unknown primary." This is unfortunate, as it is relatively common for medullary carcinoma to present as a nodal metastasis prior to discovery of the primary thyroid tumor, and failure to consider this possibility may delay diagnosis.

Medullary carcinoma also has a wide range of histologic appearances [1] that have been the basis of subtype classification that is of pathologic interest, but does not have clinical relevance. Typically, the tumors are composed of sheets, or more usually, nests of round, polyhedral, or spindle-shaped cells which may exhibit palisading at the periphery (Figs. 11.35–11.42, e-Figs. 11.64–11.73). The stroma is vascular, accounting for the neoplastic vascular seen in aspirates. There may be prominent amyloid in the stroma (Figs. 11.43–11.47, e-Figs. 11.74–11.81) that, when present, provides a helpful diagnostic marker. However, although amyloid is present in more than half of these tumors, it may be intracytoplasmic and difficult to identify without a high index of suspicion. In addition, as previously

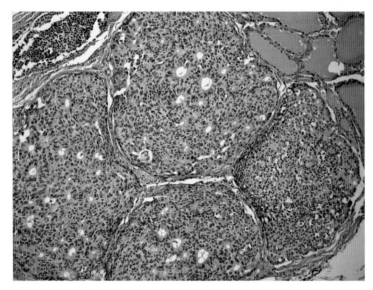

FIGURE 11.36   A nesting pattern is commonly identified in medullary carcinoma. Note the rosette and pseudofollicular structures in this example (hematoxylin & eosin stain).

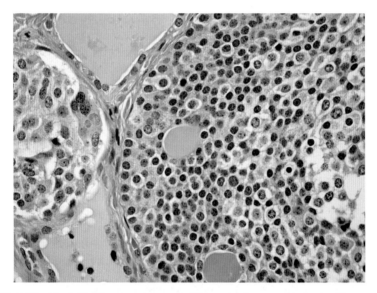

FIGURE 11.37   Much like the appearance in FNA, medullary carcinoma is often seen as a biphasic tumor where the epithelioid cells are round and often plasmacytoid or polyhedral (hematoxylin & eosin stain).

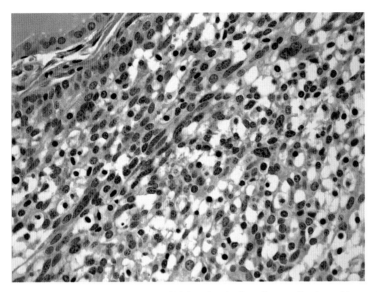

FIGURE 11.38 Foci showing both epithelioid and spindle cells may be found in medullary carcinoma (hematoxylin & eosin stain).

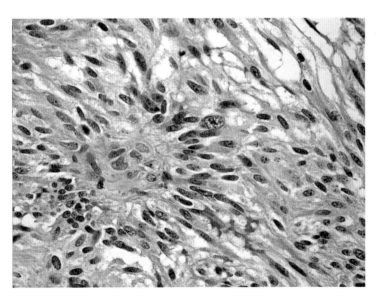

FIGURE 11.39 **Pure spindle cell regions may be identified in medullary carcinoma.** Note the perivascular arrangements of the spindle cells that give origin to the neoplastic vascularization seen in the FNA of Figure 11.30 (hematoxylin & eosin stain).

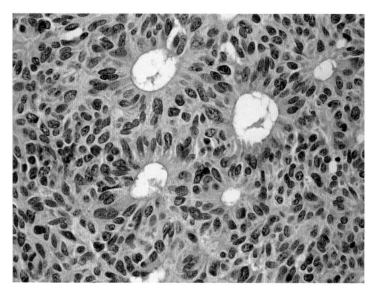

FIGURE 11.40 The pseudofollicular arrangement in medullary carcinoma may generate a false impression of a follicular neoplasm and with the nuclear grooves, as seen in this example, may raise the differential diagnosis of a follicular variant of papillary carcinoma (hematoxylin & eosin stain).

mentioned, amyloid may be present in situations in which a medullary carcinoma is not present and in other nonmedullary thyroid carcinomas [86]. The identification of amyloid is aided by its characteristic apple-green birefringence seen under polarized light. This birefringence is a

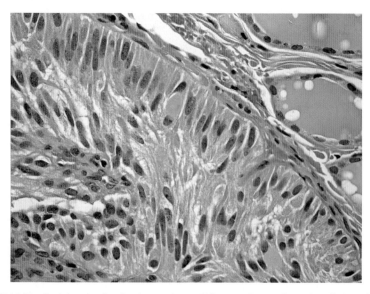

FIGURE 11.41 Peripheral palisading is seen in medullary carcinoma (hematoxylin & eosin stain).

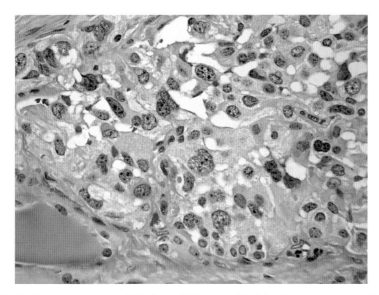

FIGURE 11.42 Just as seen in FNA, foci of bizarre epithelial cells may be encountered in the histology of medullary carcinoma (hematoxylin & eosin stain).

property inherent to the amyloid and can be seen on unstained sections, hematoxylin and eosin stained slides as well as slides stained with Congo red. Foreign body giant cells may be associated with amyloid deposits and calcification may be identified (Fig. 11.48, e-Fig. 11.82). True psammoma bodies are uncommon, but have been reported.

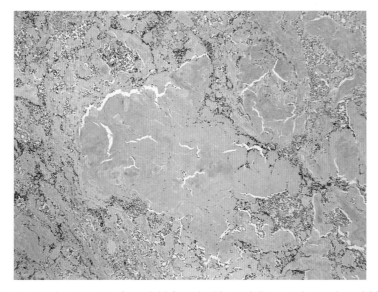

FIGURE 11.43 The amount of amyloid found with medullary carcinoma is variable, but often there is prominent stromal amyloid that with regular light microscopy appears as amorphous, eosinophilic material (hematoxylin & eosin stain).

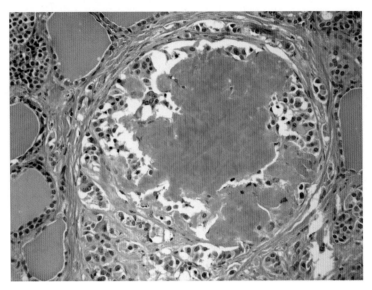

FIGURE 11.44   A nodular mass of amyloid in a section of a medullary carcinoma (hematoxylin & eosin stain).

Fixation artifact rarely produces a pseudopapillary appearance and true papillary architecture has been found in some cases. When present, the papillary architecture may make it difficult to distinguish from papillary carcinoma [87]. The presence of nuclear grooves and intranuclear

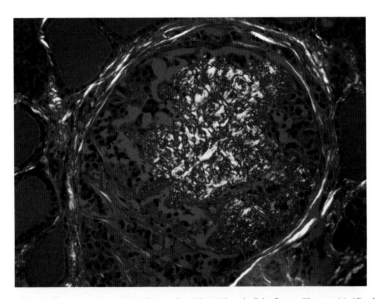

FIGURE 11.45   The same hematoxylin and eosin stained slide from Figure 11.45, showing the same mass of nodular amyloid, but visualized with polarized light. Note the apple-green birefringence of the amyloid and the white birefringence of the collagen. This slide has not been stained with Congo red (hematoxylin & eosin stain, polarized light).

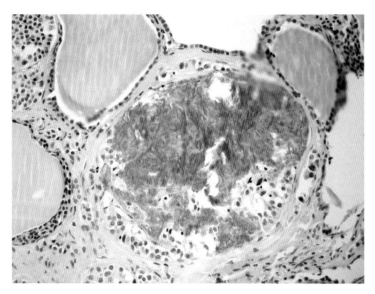

FIGURE 11.46 A separate section, stained with Congo red, shows the same mass of amyloid as in Figures 11.45 and 11.46. Note the red color of the amyloid and the pale orange color of the collagen (Congo red stain).

inclusions (Fig. 11.49, e-Figs. 11.83 and 11.84) may further medullary carcinoma's mimicry of papillary carcinoma. A pseudofollicular appearance frequently results from entrapped nonneoplastic thyroid follicles or rounded masses of amyloid and true glandular variants have been described.

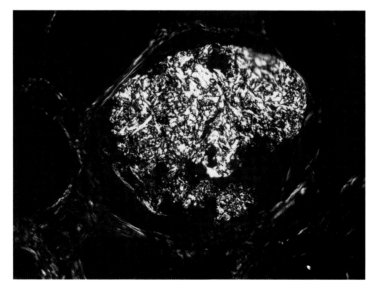

FIGURE 11.47 The same Congo red stained slide as in Figure 11.47, showing the same mass of nodular amyloid, but visualized with polarized light (Congo red stain, polarized light).

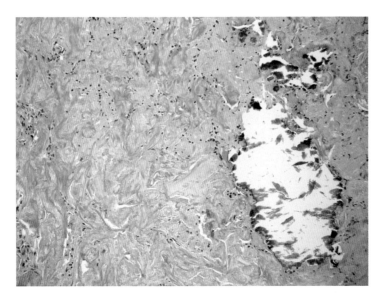

FIGURE 11.48 Calcification of the amyloid stroma of medullary carcinoma is relatively common and must not be mistaken for psammomatous calcifications. True psammoma bodies are occasionally found in medullary carcinoma (hematoxylin & eosin stain).

Dedifferentiation results in a small cell tumor morphology, which can mimic lymphoma (Chapter 13). Oncocytic features may predominate and make the distinction of medullary from oncocytic follicular carcinoma difficult.

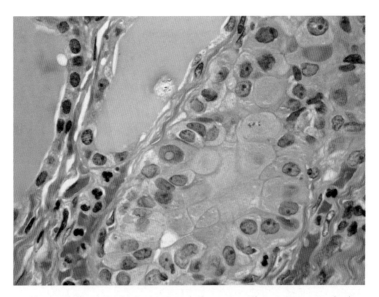

FIGURE 11.49 Medullary carcinoma may mimic many other tumors, and when nuclear grooves and intranuclear inclusions are present, as in this example, the possibility of a papillary carcinoma may be entertained (hematoxylin & eosin stain).

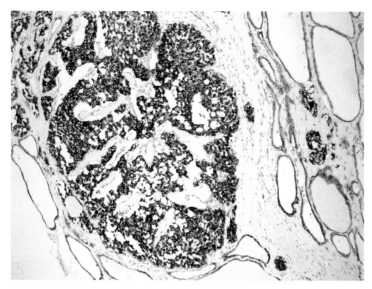

FIGURE 11.50 Immunoperoxidase staining of medullary carcinoma will show expression of low molecular weight keratins as well as cytokeratin 7, whereas mixed keratins (AE1:AE3) tends to mark the normal thyroid epithelium, but stains medullary carcinoma poorly (Cam 5.2 and hematoxylin stain).

Immunohistochemical staining represents the gold standard for the diagnosis of medullary thyroid carcinoma. These tumors express cytokeratins (mainly CK7 and CK18 [88]), TTF-1, and chromogranin A (Figs. 11.50–11.52, e-Figs. 11.85–11.91), but the most specific diagnostic marker

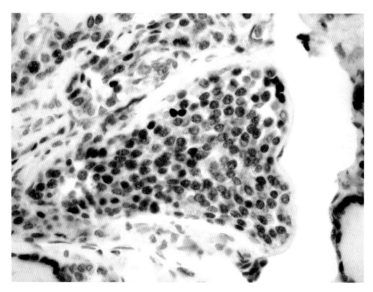

FIGURE 11.51 Immunoperoxidase staining of medullary carcinoma will show nuclear expression of thyroid transcription factor-1 (TTF-1) (TTF-1 and hematoxylin stain).

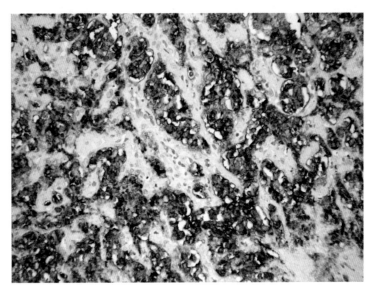

FIGURE 11.52 Medullary carcinoma shows expression of chromogranin as well as other markers of neuroendocrine differentiation including synaptophysin and CD56 (chromogranin & hematoxylin stain).

is calcitonin (Fig. 11.53, e-Fig. 11.92). The number of calcitonin-positive cells varies from case to case and may be low, but the diagnosis should be questioned in the absence of calcitonin staining. The amyloid in these tumors often stains for calcitonin (Fig. 11.54, e-Fig. 11.93), likely because the amyloid protein represents deposition of a precursor of the calcitonin molecule. These tumors also stain for CEA (Fig. 11.55, e-Fig. 11.94), and an inverse relationship exists between the intensity of staining for calcitonin and that for CEA. This may be prognostically significant as tumors containing few calcitonin-positive cells and abundant CEA immunoreactivity are said to have a worse prognosis than the well-differentiated tumors with strong calcitonin immunoreactivity [89,90]. CEA is not identified in follicular thyroid tumors; occasional reports of positivity are attributable to use of antibodies that react with nonspecific cross-reacting antigens [91]. The application of monoclonal antibodies to CEA overcomes this problem. Specific CEA positivity excludes a follicular cell tumor and indicates the presence of medullary thyroid carcinoma or other lesions such as metastatic carcinomas or thymic carcinomas.

Medullary thyroid carcinomas also produce a number of other peptides including somatostatin, derivatives of the proopiomelanocortin molecule (ACTH, MSH, β-endorphin, and enkephalin), serotonin, glucagon, gastrin, cholecystokinin, vasoactive intestinal polypeptide, bombesin, and α-HCG [19,92–94]. Calcitonin gene-related peptide (CGRP) is also identified in normal C cells as well as medullary thyroid carcinomas. Individual tumors may express a variety of these various hormones and some give

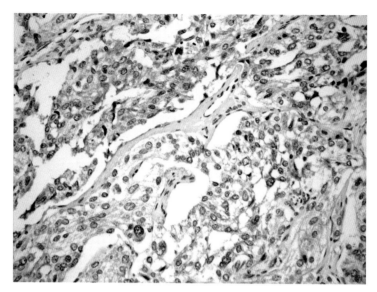

FIGURE 11.53 Calcitonin expression is the most specific marker for medullary carcinoma. However, calcitonin staining may be weak and focal. In the complete absence of calcitonin expression, the diagnosis of medullary carcinoma should be questioned (calcitonin & hematoxylin stain).

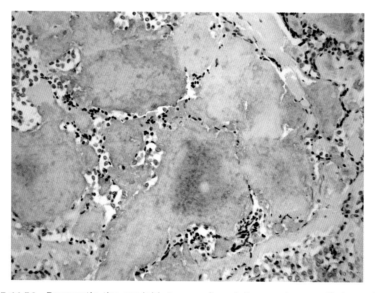

FIGURE 11.54 Frequently, the amyloid stroma of medullary carcinoma will show staining for calcitonin, as the amyloid is composed of a calcitonin precursor protein (calcitonin & hematoxylin stain).

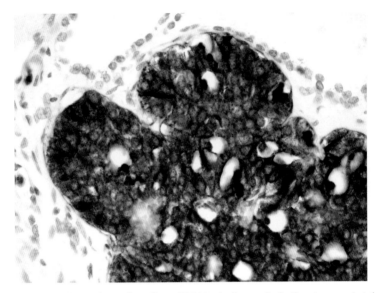

FIGURE 11.55   Carcinoembryonic antigen (CEA) typically results in the strongest staining of medullary carcinoma. CEA is not expressed by thyroid neoplasms of follicular epithelial derivation, thus the express of CEA excludes these entities from the differential diagnosis. However, the expression of CEA is not pathognomic of medullary carcinoma as metastatic tumors may express this marker (hematoxylin & eosin stain).

rise to atypical presentations, such as Cushing syndrome in patients with ectopic ACTH production.

Ultrastructural examination confirms the presence of cells that do not form desmosomes but do show complex interdigitations of cell membranes. The cytoplasm contains characteristic membrane-bound secretory granules that usually are numerous and variable in size.

MIXED FOLLICULAR–C-CELL LESIONS

Although controversial, mixed follicular–parafollicular cell carcinomas are reported [95]; Rare monomorphous tumors are composed of cells showing dual differentiation [96,97]. Composite tumors composed of two intermixed well-differentiated components are more common. In these lesions, one population is composed of thyroglobulin-immunoreactive follicular cells, usually with cytologic features of papillary carcinoma, and another population of admixed cells has calcitonin and CEA immunopositivity [98,99]. Some of these may represent coincidental collision tumors within thyroid, especially since papillary carcinomas are relatively common [100]. Rarely, composite tumors can metastasize together. Moreover, the two tumors may occur separately in the same gland and metastasize together to a regional node [101,102].

Biopsy of such lesions can be confusing and challenging [103]. The identification of atypical C cells associated with thyroid follicular cells in a thyroid aspirate should lead to the diagnosis of medullary carcinoma; in the absence of nuclear atypia of PTC, there can be no justification for concern about the follicular elements. Many of the reported cases have had a papillary carcinoma component and can be diagnosed on the basis of the nuclear atypia. Clearly, when identified in a lymph node together, a biopsy diagnosis can be more convincing.

THYMIC CARCINOMA

Rare tumors with thymuslike differentiation occur in the thyroid; there are two variants, the spindle cell tumor with thymuslike differentiation (SETTLE) (discussed in Chapter 12) and carcinoma showing thymuslike differentiation of the thyroid (CASTLE). In both cases, although the tumors arise within the thyroid gland, the cell of origin is not of follicular epithelial or C-cell derivation. Instead, it has been suggested that they derive from ectopic thymic tissue that is often seen in the thyroid or from the branchial pouch developmental remnants in the thyroid that are known as solid cell nests or ultimobranchial body rests (Chapter 2) [104–107].

The tumor known as CASTLE is a rare, low-grade malignant neoplasm arising within the thyroid gland that has a solid architectural growth pattern resembling medullary or squamous cell carcinoma. There are usually lymphoid cells infiltrating a dominant solid epithelial component arranged in tubules, papillae, cords, and solid nests with scattered glandular spaces. The epithelial cells are cuboidal to columnar and may be mucinous or ciliated with foci of squamous metaplasia occasionally seen. They are positive for cytokeratins, but lack expression of TTF-1, thyroglobulin, calcitonin, chromogranin, and S-100; in contrast, they exhibit diffuse p63 and HMWK staining and are positive for CD5 [107,108]. Positivity for CEA can lead to confusion with medullary thyroid carcinoma [105,107]; therefore, it is important to perform additional immunohistochemical stains.

MUCOEPIDERMOID CARCINOMA

Mucoepidermoid carcinoma is a common neoplasm of the salivary glands. It is composed of squamous cells, mucus-secreting cells, and "intermediate" cells. The squamous (epidermoid) cells have abundant eosinophilic or even oncocytic cytoplasm and rare keratin pearl formation or dyskeratosis. Mucous cells ("mucocytes") occur singly or in clusters; they have pale, foamy cytoplasm, a distinct cell border, and small, peripherally placed, compressed nuclei. These cells often form the lining of cysts or ductlike structures. The intermediate cells frequently predominate. Their appearance ranges from small basal cells with scanty basophilic cytoplasm to larger and more oval cells with more abundant pale eosinophilic cytoplasm that appears to merge into epidermoid or mucous cells.

Mucoepidermoid carcinomas occur rarely as primary intrathyroidal lesions, where they have been thought to derive from ultimobranchial

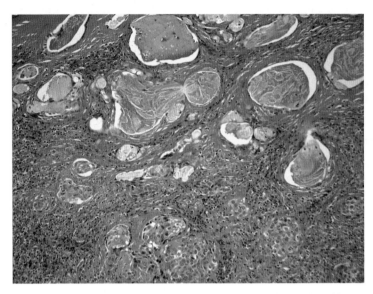

FIGURE 11.56   Mucoepidermoid carcinomas occur rarely as a primary thyroid tumor. In this example, the nests of intermediate and squamous cells are evident in the lower portion of the image with lakes of mucin evident that are partially lined by the mucous cells (hematoxylin & eosin stain).

body rests [109], but the reported presence of TTF-1 and thyroglobulin staining [110–112] raises the possibility that they derive from follicular epithelium, and indeed some have been associated with papillary carcinoma [110]. They are most common in women and are often associated with thyroiditis. They are usually indolent tumors, even when metastatic to local lymph nodes [110]. Reports of diagnosis on a preoperative biopsy are rare, but in at least one case, aspiration identified a highly bimorphic cellular lesion with a background rich in a neutrophilic, inflammatory infiltrate, and necrotic debris. Polygonal squamoid cells had well-defined borders and dense cytoplasm, clumped nuclear chromatin, and prominent nucleoli. They were admixed with ring-shaped mucus-secreting cells that contained a large vacuole, with condensed acid and neutral mucins, and a peripherally displaced nucleus [113] (Figs. 11.56–11.59, e-Figs. 11.95–11.99).

An unusual variant of mucoepidermoid carcinoma that occurs in the thyroid is *sclerosing mucoepidermoid carcinoma with eosinophilia (SMECE)*. This lesion is characterized by extensive sclerosis, squamous and glandular differentiation, a concomitant inflammatory infiltrate rich in eosinophils, and a background of lymphocytic thyroiditis. The tumor cells are positive for cytokeratin and negative for calcitonin, and they express TTF-1 [111], but unlike classical mucoepidermoid carcinomas SMECE are negative for thyroglobulin [110,111]. On FNAB, the lesions are composed of malignant cells with definite glandular and squamoid differentiation in small cohesive aggregates; eosinophils associated with the tumor cells distinguish these from other mucoepidermoid carcinomas [114].

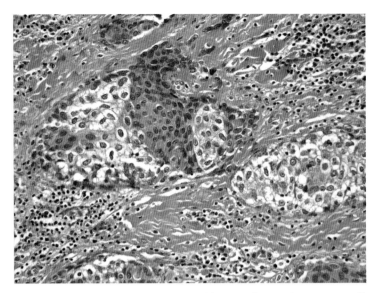

FIGURE 11.57   High power image of the nests of intermediate and squamous cells of a primary mucoepidermoid carcinoma of the thyroid (hematoxylin & eosin stain).

METASTATIC CARCINOMA

The identification of a solid or trabecular epithelial neoplasm on a thyroid biopsy raises the possibility of a metastasis from another site. In patients with a history of a prior nonthyroid malignancy and a thyroid nodule, the diagnosis is considered; a more difficult scenario arises when there is no

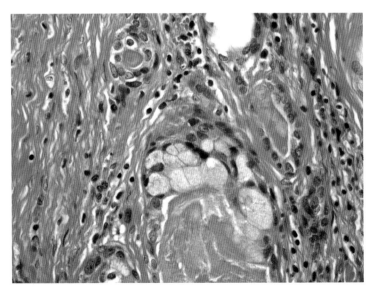

FIGURE 11.58   High power image of the nests of mucous cells of a primary mucoepidermoid carcinoma of the thyroid (hematoxylin & eosin stain).

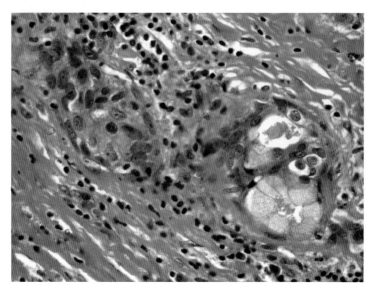

FIGURE 11.59 Mucous cells and a nest of squamous (epidermoid) cells of a primary mucoepidermoid carcinoma of the thyroid (hematoxylin & eosin stain).

known history of malignancy elsewhere. The most common lesion to present with thyroid metastasis is renal cell carcinoma, a tumor that can mimic thyroid follicular neoplasia [1,19,115] and produce colloidlike material or form blood filled folliclelike structures. Other carcinomas that frequently spread to thyroid include breast and colon (e-Figs. 11.100–11.103).

In such cases, the diagnosis may be obvious when the lesion has features characteristic of tumors at other sites. However, immunohistochemical staining may be required. Tumors that are negative for TTF-1, thyroglobulin, and calcitonin are potentially suggestive of metastatic carcinoma and further analysis may be required as a helpful adjunct in the evaluation of thyroid nodules in patients with a past history of malignancy or those in whom metastasis is suspected [116].

Metastasis to a thyroid nodule is a well-described phenomenon that can complicate the diagnosis of metastatic malignancy, particularly on biopsy [117,118], when two cell populations are identified. Again, immunohistochemistry can be critical in reaching a correct diagnosis.

THYROID PARAGANGLIOMA AND OTHER NEUROENDOCRINE TUMORS

Primary intrathyroid paragangliomas have been reported. The tumors occur in women and present as a solitary nodule that has ranged from 1.5 - 10 cm in size. Extrathyroidal extension into the neighboring structures has been reported. These lesions exhibit the characteristic nesting or "Zellballen" architecture seen in paragangliomas elsewhere in the body. They stain for NSE, chromogranin and synaptophysin, and they have S-100 positive sustentacular cells. They are negative for keratins, thyroglobulin, calcitonin and CEA.[119,120]. Very rarely, well differentiated neuroendocrine tumors occur in the thyroid that have epithelial differentiation with cytokeratin, synaptophysin and chromogranin positivity and have features resembling medullary carcinoma, but they do not stain for calcitonin. In the absence of this marker, the possibility of a metastatic neuroendocrine carcinoma must be excluded [121]. Immunohistochemistry can be useful if the lesion stains for markers of gastroenteropancreatic differentiation, such as CDX2, cytokeratins 7 and 20, or specific hormones that are associated with origin in the gastrointestinal tract. In this setting, TTF-1 is not helpful, since lung endocrine tumors and occasional prostate endocrine tumors also express this transcription factor. If no other primary site is identified, the tumor can be considered an unusual primary neuroendocrine tumor of thyroid. The biological behavior of these extremely rare tumors is not known.

REFERENCES

1. DeLellis RA, Lloyd RV, Heitz PU, et al. *Pathology and genetics of tumours of endocrine organs*. WHO Classification of Tumours. Lyons: IARC Press, 2004.
2. Nikiforov YE, Erickson LA, Nikiforova MN, et al. Solid variant of papillary thyroid carcinoma: incidence, clinical-pathologic characteristics, molecular analysis, and biologic behavior. *Am J Surg Pathol* 2001;25:1478–1484.
3. Collini P, Mattavelli F, Pellegrinelli A, et al. Papillary carcinoma of the thyroid gland of childhood and adolescence: morphologic subtypes, biologic behavior and prognosis: a clinicopathologic study of 42 sporadic cases treated at a single institution during a 30-year period. *Am J Surg Pathol* 2006;30:1420–1426.
4. Troncone G, Russo M, Malapelle U, et al. Cytological and molecular diagnosis of solid variant of papillary thyroid carcinoma: a case report. *Cytojournal* 2008;5:2.
5. Nguyen GK, Lee MW. Solid/trabecular variant papillary carcinoma of the thyroid: report of three cases with fine-needle aspiration. *Diagn Cytopathol* 2006;34:712–714.
6. Cvejic DS, Savin SB, Petrovic IM, et al. Galectin-3 expression in papillary thyroid carcinoma: relation to histomorphologic growth pattern, lymph node metastasis, extrathyroid invasion, and tumor size. *Head Neck* 2005;27:1049–1055.
7. Nikiforov YE, Rowland JM, Bove KE, et al. Distinct pattern of *ret* oncogene rearrangements in morphological variants of radiation-induced and sporadic thyroid papillary carcinomas in children. *Cancer Res* 1997;57:1690–1694.
8. Trovisco V, Soares P, Soares R, et al. A new BRAF gene mutation detected in a case of a solid variant of papillary thyroid carcinoma. *Hum Pathol* 2005;36:694–697.
9. Lupi C, Giannini R, Ugolini C, et al. Association of BRAF V600E mutation with poor clinicopathological outcomes in 500 consecutive cases of papillary thyroid carcinoma. *J Clin Endocrinol Metab* 2007;92:4085–4090.
10. Zipkin P. Hyalinähnliche collagene kugeln als produkte epitelialer zellen in malignen strumen. *Virchows Arch* 1905;182:374–406.
11. Masson P. Cancers thyroidiens a polarite alternative. *Bull Cancer* 1922;11:350–355.
12. Ward JV, Murray D, Horvath E, et al. Hyaline cell tumor of the thyroid with massive accumulation of cytoplasmic microfilaments. *Lab Invest* 1982;46:88A.
13. Carney JA, Ryan J, Goellner JR. Hyalinizing trabecular adenoma of the thyroid gland. *Am J Surg Pathol* 1987;11:583–591.
14. Bronner MP, LiVolsi VA, Jennings TA. PLAT: Paraganglioma-like adenomas of the thyroid. *Surg Pathol* 1988;1:383–389.

15. Sambade C, Franssila K, Cameselle-Teijeiro J, et al. Hyalinizing trabecular adenoma: a misnomer for a peculiar tumor of the thyroid gland. *Endocr Pathol* 1991;2:83–91.
16. Molberg K, Albores-Saavedra J. Hyalinizing trabecular carcinoma of the thyroid gland. *Hum Pathol* 1994;25:192–197.
17. McCluggage WG, Sloan JM. Hyalinizing trabecular carcinoma of the thyroid gland. *Histopathology* 1996;28:357–362.
18. Katoh R, Jasani B, Williams ED. Hyalinizing trabecular adenoma of the thyroid. A report of three cases with immunohistochemical and ultrastructural studies. *Histopathology* 1989;15:211–224.
19. Rosai J, Carcangiu ML, DeLellis RA. Tumors of the thyroid gland. In: *Atlas of tumor pathology*. 3rd series, fascicle 5. Washington, DC: Armed Forces Institute of Pathology, 1992.
20. Cheung CC, Boerner SL, MacMillan CM, et al. Hyalinizing trabecular tumor of the thyroid: a variant of papillary carcinoma proved by molecular genetics. *Am J Surg Pathol* 2000;24:1622–1626.
21. Papotti M, Volante M, Giuliano A, et al. RET/PTC activation in hyalinizing trabecular tumors of the thyroid. *Am J Surg Pathol* 2000;24:1615–1621.
22. Li M, Carcangiu ML, Rosai J. Abnormal intracellular and extracellular distribution of base membrane material in papillary carcinoma and hyalinizing trabecular tumors of the thyroid: implication for deregulation secretory pathways. *Hum Pathol* 1997;28:1366–1372.
23. Boerner SL, Asa SL. Hyalinizing trabecular tumor of the thyroid gland: much ado about nothing? *Am J Clin Pathol* 2004;122:495–496.
24. Chan JKC, Tse CCH, Chiu HS. Hyalinizing trabecular adenoma-like lesion in multinodular goitre. *Histopathology* 1990;16:611–614.
25. Akin MR, Nguyen GK. Fine-needle aspiration biopsy cytology of hyalinizing trabecular adenomas of the thyroid. *Diagn Cytopathol* 1999;20:90–94.
26. Jayaram G. Fine needle aspiration cytology of hyalinizing trabecular adenoma of the thyroid. *Acta Cytol* 1999;43:978–980.
27. Kuma S, Hirokawa M, Miyauchi A, et al. Cytologic features of hyalinizing trabecular adenoma of the thyroid. *Acta Cytol* 2003;47:399–404.
28. Casey MB, Sebo TJ, Carney JA. Hyalinizing trabecular adenoma of the thyroid gland: cytologic features in 29 cases. *Am J Surg Pathol* 2004;28:859–867.
29. Baloch ZW, LiVolsi VA. Cytologic and architectural mimics of papillary thyroid carcinoma. Diagnostic challenges in fine-needle aspiration and surgical pathology specimens. *Am J Clin Pathol* 2006;125(suppl):S135–S144.
30. Hirokawa M, Carney JA, Ohtsuki Y. Hyalinizing trabecular adenoma and papillary carcinoma of the thyroid gland express different cytokeratin patterns. *Am J Surg Pathol* 2000;24:877–881.
31. Hirokawa M, Carney JA, Ohtsuki Y. Hyalinizing trabecular adenoma and papillary carcinoma of the thyroid gland express different cytokeratin patterns. *Am J Surg Pathol* 2000;24:877–881.
32. Fonseca E, Nesland JM, Sobrinho-Simoes M. Expression of stratified epithelial-type cytokeratins in hyalinizing trabecular adenomas supports their relationship with papillary carcinomas of the thyroid. *Histopathology* 1997;31:330–335.
33. Hirokawa M, Carney JA. Cell membrane and cytoplasmic staining for MIB-1 in hyalinizing trabecular adenoma of the thyroid gland. *Am J Surg Pathol* 2000;24:575–578.
34. Casey MB, Sebo TJ, Carney JA. Hyalinizing trabecular adenoma of the thyroid gland identification through MIB-1 staining of fine-needle aspiration biopsy smears. *Am J Clin Pathol* 2004;122:506–510.
35. Leonardo E, Volante M, Barbareschi M, et al. Cell membrane reactivity of MIB-1 antibody to Ki67 in human tumors: fact or artifact? *Appl Immunohistochem Mol Morphol* 2007;15:220–223.
36. Hirokawa M, Carney JA, Ohtsuki Y. Hyalinizing trabecular adenoma and papillary carcinoma of the thyroid gland express different cytokeratin patterns. *Am J Surg Pathol* 2000;24:877–881.

37. Carcangiu ML, Zampi G, Rosai J. Poorly differentiated ("insular") thyroid carcinoma. A reinterpretation of Langhans' "wuchernde Struma". *Am J Surg Pathol* 1984;8:655–668.

38. Sakamoto A, Kasai N, Sugano H. Poorly differentiated carcinoma of the thyroid. A clinicopathologic entity for a high-risk group of papillary and follicular carcinomas. *Cancer* 1983;52:1849–1855.

39. Papotti M, Botto Micca F, Favero A, et al. Poorly differentiated thyroid carcinomas with primordial cell component. A group of aggressive lesions sharing insular, trabecular, and solid patterns. *Am J Surg Pathol* 1993;17:291–301.

40. Volante M, Collini P, Nikiforov YE, et al. Poorly differentiated thyroid carcinoma: the Turin proposal for the use of uniform diagnostic criteria and an algorithmic diagnostic approach. *Am J Surg Pathol* 2007;31:1256–1264.

41. Hiltzik D, Carlson DL, Tuttle RM, et al. Poorly differentiated thyroid carcinomas defined on the basis of mitosis and necrosis: a clinicopathologic study of 58 patients. *Cancer* 2006;106:1286–1295.

42. Sironi M, Collini P, Cantaboni A. Fine needle aspiration cytology of insular thyroid carcinoma. A report of four cases. *Acta Cytol* 1992;36:435–439.

43. Guiter GE, Auger M, Ali SZ, et al. Cytopathology of insular carcinoma of the thyroid. *Cancer* 1999;87:196–202.

44. Pietribiasi F, Sapino A, Papotti M, et al. Cytologic features of poorly differentiated "insular" carcinoma of the thyroid, as revealed by fine-needle aspiration biopsy. *Am J Clin Pathol* 1990;94:687–692.

45. Ghofrani M, Sosa JA, Ocal IT, et al. Fine needle aspiration of poorly differentiated oxyphilic (Hurthle cell) thyroid carcinoma: a case report. *Acta Cytol* 2006;50:560–562.

46. Fischer S, Asa SL. Application of immunohistochemistry to thyroid neoplasms. *Arch Pathol Lab Med* 2008;132:359–372.

47. Garcia-Rostan G, Zhao H, Camp RL, et al. ras mutations are associated with aggressive tumor phenotypes and poor prognosis in thyroid cancer. *J Clin Oncol* 2003;21: 3226–3235.

48. Garcia-Rostan G, Camp RL, Herrero A, et al. Beta-catenin dysregulation in thyroid neoplasms: down-regulation, aberrant nuclear expression, and CTNNB1 exon 3 mutations are markers for aggressive tumor phenotypes and poor prognosis. *Am J Pathol* 2001; 158:987–996.

49. Kondo T, Ezzat S, Asa SL. Pathogenetic mechanisms in thyroid follicular-cell neoplasia. *Nat Rev Cancer* 2006;6:292–306.

50. Cheung CC, Ezzat S, Freeman JL, et al. Immunohistochemical diagnosis of papillary thyroid carcinoma. *Mod Pathol* 2001;14:338–342.

51. Santoro M, Papotti M, Chiappetta G, et al. RET activation and clinicopathologic features in poorly differentiated thyroid tumors. *J Clin Endocrinol Metab* 2002;87:370–379.

52. Mase T, Funahashi H, Koshikawa T, et al. HBME-1 immunostaining in thyroid tumors especially in follicular neoplasm. *Endocr J* 2003;50:173–177.

53. Choi YL, Kim MK, Suh JW, et al. Immunoexpression of HBME-1, high molecular weight cytokeratin, cytokeratin 19, thyroid transcription factor-1, and E-cadherin in thyroid carcinomas. *J Korean Med Sci* 2005;20:853–859.

54. Lam KY, Lui MC, Lo CY. Cytokeratin expression profiles in thyroid carcinomas. *Eur J Surg Oncol* 2001;27:631–635.

55. Santoro M, Papotti M, Chiappetta G, et al. RET activation and clinicopathologic features in poorly differentiated thyroid tumors. *J Clin Endocrinol Metab* 2002;87:370–379.

56. Sobrinho-Simoes M, Maximo V, Rocha AS, et al. Intragenic mutations in thyroid cancer. *Endocrinol Metab Clin North Am* 2008;37:333–362, viii.

57. Baloch ZW, LiVolsi VA. Neuroendocrine tumors of the thyroid gland. *Am J Clin Pathol* 2001;115(suppl):S56–S67.

58. Das K, Kendall C, Isabelle M, et al. FTIR of touch imprint cytology: a novel tissue diagnostic technique. *J Photochem Photobiol B* 2008;92:160–164.

59. Jimenez C, Hu MI, Gagel RF. Management of medullary thyroid carcinoma. *Endocrinol Metab Clin North Am* 2008;37:481–484, xi.

60. Reubi JC, Chayvialle JA, Franc B, et al. Somatostatin receptors and somatostatin content in medullary thyroid carcinomas. *Lab Invest* 1991;64:567–573.
61. Lamberts SWJ, Bakker WH, Reubi JC, et al. Somatostatin-receptor imaging in the localization of endocrine tumors. *N Engl J Med* 1990;323:1246–1249.
62. Lamberts SWJ, Krenning EP, Reubi JC. The role of somatostatin and its analogs in the diagnosis and treatment of tumors. *Endocr Rev* 1991;12:450.
63. Schimke RN, Hartmann WH. Familial amyloid-producing medullary thyroid carcinoma and pheochromocytoma: a distinct genetic entity. *Ann Intern Med* 1965;63:1027–1037.
64. Goodfellow PJ. Mapping the inherited defects associated with multiple endocrine neoplasia type 2A, multiple endocrine neoplasia type 2B, and familial medullary thyroid carcinoma to chromosome 10 by linkage analysis. *Endocrinol Metab Clin North Am* 1994;23:177–185.
65. Carson NL, Wu J, Jackson CE, et al. The mutation for medullary thyroid carcinoma with parathyroid tumors (mTC with PTs) is closely linked to the centromeric region of chromosome 10. *Am J Hum Genet* 1990;47:946–951.
66. Nelkin BD, Nakamura N, White RW, et al. Low incidence of loss of chromosome 10 in sporadic and hereditary human medullary thyroid carcinoma. *Cancer Res* 1989;49:4114–4119.
67. Mulligan LM, Kwok JBJ, Healey CS, et al. Germ-line mutations of the *RET* proto-oncogene in multiple endocrine neoplasia type 2A. *Nature* 1993;363:458–460.
68. Hofstra RMW, Landsvater RM, Ceccherini I, et al. A mutation in the *RET* proto-oncogene associated with multiple endocrine neoplasia type 2B and sporadic medullary thyroid carcinoma. *Nature* 1994;367:375–376.
69. Marsh DJ, Robinson BG, Andrew S, et al. A rapid screening method for the detection of mutations in the RET proto-oncogene in multiple endocrine neoplasia type 2A and familial medullary thyroid carcinoma families. *Genomics* 1994;23:477–479.
70. Castellone MD, Santoro M. Dysregulated RET signaling in thyroid cancer. *Endocrinol Metab Clin North Am* 2008;37:363–374, viii.
71. Brandi ML, Gagel RF, Angeli A, et al. Guidelines for diagnosis and therapy of MEN type 1 and type 2. *J Clin Endocrinol Metab* 2001;86:5658–5671.
72. Wolfe HJ, Melvin KEW, Cervi-Skinner SJ. C-cell hyperplasia preceding medullary thyroid carcinoma. *N Engl J Med* 1973;289:437–441.
73. DeLellis RA, Wolfe HJ. The pathobiology of the human calcitonin (C)-cell: a review. *Pathol Annu* 1981;16:25–52.
74. Albores-Saavedra J, Monforte H, Nadji M, et al. C-cell hyperplasia in thyroid tissue adjacent to follicular cell tumors. *Hum Pathol* 1988;19:795–799.
75. Biddinger PW, Brennan MF, Rosen PP. Symptomatic C-cell hyperplasia associated with chronic lymphocytic thyroiditis. *Am J Surg Pathol* 1991;15:599–604.
76. Scopsi L, Di Palma S, Ferrari C, et al. C-cell hyperplasia accompanying thyroid diseases other than medullary carcinoma: an immunocytochemical study by means of antibodies to calcitonin and somatostatin. *Mod Pathol* 1991;4:297–304.
77. Nosé V. Familial non-medullary thyroid carcinoma: an update. *Endocr Pathol.* 2008;19:226–40.
78. Santoro M, Rosati R, Grieco M, et al. The *ret* proto-oncogene is consistently expressed in human pheochromocytomas and thyroid medullary carcinomas. *Oncogene* 1990;5:1595–1598.
79. Zedenius J, Larsson C, Bergholm U, et al. Mutations of codon 918 in the RET proto-oncogene correlate to poor prognosis in sporadic medullary thyroid carcinomas. *J Clin Endocrinol Metab* 1995;80:3088–3090.
80. Moley JF, Brother MB, Wells SA, et al. Low frequency of *ras* gene mutations in neuroblastomas, pheochromocytomas, and medullary thyroid cancers. *Cancer Res* 1991;51:1596–1599.
81. Yang KP, Castillo SG, Nguyen CV. C-myc, N-ras, c-erb B: lack of amplification or rearrangement in human medullary thyroid carcinoma and a derivative cell line. *Anticancer Res* 1990;10:189–192.

82. Yana I, Nakamura T, Shin E. Inactivation of the p53 gene is not required for tumorigenesis of medullary thyroid carcinoma or pheochromocytoma. *Jpn J Cancer Res* 1992; 83:1113–1116.

83. Collins BT, Cramer HM, Tabatowski K, et al. Fine needle aspiration of medullary carcinoma of the thyroid. Cytomorphology, immunocytochemistry and electron microscopy. *Acta Cytol* 1995;39:920–930.

84. Forrest CH, Frost FA, de Boer WB, et al. Medullary carcinoma of the thyroid: accuracy of diagnosis of fine-needle aspiration cytology. *Cancer* 1998;84:295–302.

85. Papaparaskeva K, Nagel H, Droese M. Cytologic diagnosis of medullary carcinoma of the thyroid gland. *Diagn Cytopathol* 2000;22:351–358.

86. Valenta LJ, Michel-Bechet M, Mattson JC, et al. Microfollicular thyroid carcinoma with amyloid rich stroma, resembling the medullary carcinoma of the thyroid (MCT). *Cancer* 1977;39:1573–1586.

87. Harach HR, Williams ED. Glandular (tubular and follicular) variants of medullary carcinoma of the thyroid. *Histopathology* 1983;7:83–97.

88. Lam KY, Lui MC, Lo CY. Cytokeratin expression profiles in thyroid carcinomas. *Eur J Surg Oncol* 2001;27:631–635.

89. Nelkin BD, de Bustros AC, Mabry M, et al. The molecular biology of medullary thyroid carcinoma. A model for cancer development and progression. *JAMA* 1989;261: 3130–3135.

90. Mendelsohn G, Wells SA, Baylin SB. Relationship of tissue carcinoembryonic antigen and calcitonin to tumor virulence in medullary thyroid carcinoma. An immunohistochemical study in early, localized and virulent disseminated stages of disease. *Cancer* 1984;54:657–662.

91. Schröder S, Klöppel G. Carcinoembryonic antigen and nonspecific cross-reacting antigen in thyroid cancer. An immunocytochemical study using polyclonal and monoclonal antibodies. *Am J Surg Pathol* 1987;11:100–108.

92. Williams ED, Morales AM, Horn RC. Thyroid carcinoma and Cushing's syndrome. A report of two cases with a review of the common features of the non-endocrine tumours associated with Cushing's syndrome. *J Clin Pathol* 1968;21:129–135.

93. Birkenhäger JC, Upton GV, Seldenrath HJ, et al. Medullary thyroid carcinoma: ectopic production of peptides with ACTH-like, corticotrophin releasing factor-like and prolactin production-stimulating activities. *Acta Endocrinol (Copen)* 1976;83:280–292.

94. Goltzman D, Huang S-N, Browne C, et al. Adrenocorticotropin and calcitonin in medullary thyroid carcinoma: frequency of occurrence and localization in the same cell type by immunohistochemistry. *J Clin Endocrinol Metab* 1979;49:364–369.

95. LiVolsi VA. Mixed thyroid carcinoma: a real entity? *Lab Invest* 1987;57:237–239.

96. Holm R, Sobrinho-Simoes M, Nesland JM, et al. Concurrent production of calcitonin and thyroglobulin by the same neoplastic cells. *Ultrastruct Pathol* 1986;10:241–248.

97. Holm R, Sobrinho-Simoes M, Nesland JM, et al. Medullary thyroid carcinoma with thyroglobulin immunoreactivity. A special entity? *Lab Invest* 1987;57:258–268.

98. Mizukami Y, Michigishi T, Nonomura A, et al. Mixed medullary-follicular carcinoma of the thyroid occurring in familial form. *Histopathology* 1993;22:284–287.

99. Apel RL, Alpert LC, Rizzo A, et al. A metastasizing composite carcinoma of the thyroid with distinct medullary and papillary components. *Arch Pathol Lab Med* 1994;118: 1143–1147.

100. Fink A, Tomlinson G, Freeman JL, et al. Occult micropapillary carcinoma associated with benign follicular thyroid disease and unrelated thyroid neoplasms. *Mod Pathol* 1996;9:816–820.

101. González-Cámpora R, Lopez-Garrido J, Martin-Lacave I, et al. Concurrence of a symptomatic encapsulated follicular carcinoma, an occult papillary carcinoma and a medullary carcinoma in the same patient. *Histopathology* 1992;21:380–382.

102. Pastolero GC, Coire CI, Asa SL. Concurrent medullary and papillary carcinomas of thyroid with lymph node metastases. *Am J Surg Pathol* 1996;20:245–250.

103. Hsieh MH, Lin MC, Shun CT, et al. Fine needle aspiration cytology of mixed medullary-follicular thyroid carcinoma: a case report. *Acta Cytol* 2008;52:361–365.

104. LiVolsi VA. Branchial and thymic remnants in the thyroid and cervical region: an explanation for unusual tumors and microscopic curiosities. *Endocr Pathol* 1993;4: 115–119.

105. Asa SL, Dardick I, Van Nostrand AWP, et al. Primary thyroid thymoma: a distinct clinicopathologic entity. *Hum Pathol* 1988;19:1463–1467.

106. Chan JK, Rosai J. Tumors of the neck showing thymic or related branchial pouch differentiation: a unifying concept. *Hum Pathol* 1991;22:349–367.

107. Reimann JD, Dorfman DM, Nose V. Carcinoma showing thymus-like differentiation of the thyroid (CASTLE): a comparative study: evidence of thymic differentiation and solid cell nest origin. *Am J Surg Pathol* 2006;30:994–1001.

108. Dorfman DM, Shahsafaei A, Miyauchi A. Intrathyroidal epithelial thymoma (ITET)/ carcinoma showing thymus-like differentiation (CASTLE) exhibits CD5 immunoreactivity: new evidence for thymic differentiation. *Histopathology* 1998;32:104–109.

109. Cameselle-Teijeiro J. Mucoepidermoid carcinoma and solid cell nests of the thyroid. *Hum Pathol* 1996;27:861–863.

110. Baloch ZW, Solomon AC, LiVolsi VA. Primary mucoepidermoid carcinoma and sclerosing mucoepidermoid carcinoma with eosinophilia of the thyroid gland: a report of nine cases. *Mod Pathol* 2000;13:802–807.

111. Albores-Saavedra J, Gu X, Luna MA. Clear cells and thyroid transcription factor I reactivity in sclerosing mucoepidermoid carcinoma of the thyroid gland. *Ann Diagn Pathol* 2003;7:348–353.

112. Baloch ZW, LiVolsi VA. Unusual tumors of the thyroid gland. Endocrinol. *Metab Clin North Am* 2008;37:297–310, vii.

113. Vazquez RF, Otal SC, Argueta MO, et al. Fine needle aspiration cytology of high grade mucoepidermoid carcinoma of the thyroid. A case report. *Acta Cytol* 2000;44:259–264.

114. Geisinger KR, Steffee CH, McGee RS, et al. The cytomorphologic features of sclerosing mucoepidermoid carcinoma of the thyroid gland with eosinophilia. *Am J Clin Pathol* 1998;109:294–301.

115. LiVolsi VA. *Surgical pathology of the thyroid*. Philadelphia: WB Saunders, 1990.

116. Porcell AI, Hitchcock CL, Keyhani-Rofagha S. Use of immunohistochemistry in fine needle aspiration of thyroid nodules in patients with a history of malignancy. A report of two cases. *Acta Cytol* 2000;44:393–398.

117. Ryska A, Cap J. Tumor-to-tumor metastasis of renal cell carcinoma into oncocytic carcinoma of the thyroid. Report of a case and review of the literature. *Pathol Res Pract* 2003;199:101–106.

118. Koo HL, Jang J, Hong SJ, et al. Renal cell carcinoma metastatic to follicular adenoma of the thyroid gland. A case report. *Acta Cytol* 2004;48:64–68.

119. LaGuette J, Matias-Guiu X, Rosai J. Thyroid paraganglioma: a clinicopathologic and immunohistochemical study of three cases. *Am.J.Surg.Pathol.* 1997;21:748–753.

120. Yano Y, Nagahama M, Sugino K, Ito K, Kameyama K, Ito K. Paraganglioma of the thyroid: report of a male case with ultrasonographic imagings, cytologic, histologic, and immunohistochemical features. *Thyroid* 2007;17:575–578.

121. Maly A, Meir K, Maly B. Isolated carcinoid tumor metastatic to the thyroid gland: report of a case initially diagnosed by fine needle aspiration cytology. *Acta Cytol.* 2006;50:84–87.

12

SQUAMOID, SPINDLE, AND GIANT-CELL LESIONS

UNDIFFERENTIATED (ANAPLASTIC) CARCINOMA

Anaplastic or undifferentiated carcinoma accounts for 5% to 10% of all primary malignant tumors of the thyroid [1], but in many centers this number is decreasing, presumably due to earlier detection of antecedent disease. These are tumors of the elderly and show a slight female predominance. Their rapid growth and massive local invasion precipitate local symptoms that tend to clinically overshadow metastases to the lung, adrenals, and bone [2,3]. These are highly lethal malignancies with a 5-year survival rate of only 7.1% [4] and a mean survival period of 6.2 to 7.2 months following diagnosis [4,5].

The data suggest that anaplastic carcinoma most often originates in an abnormal thyroid gland. The tumor has a higher incidence in regions of endemic goiter, and a history of goiter is reported in over 80% of cases [4,6]. However, it is difficult to document transformation of a benign lesion to a highly malignant tumor. The reported association between well-differentiated thyroid carcinoma and anaplastic carcinoma ranges from 7% to 89% of cases. The lower figures are likely underestimates, attributable to failure to detect a well-differentiated component due to inadequate sampling [4–10]. The association of papillary carcinoma, particularly the more aggressive tall cell variant, with anaplastic tumors has been well described [6,10,11].

Thyroid carcinomas can exhibit an entire spectrum of differentiation through insular to anaplastic foci. The significance of microscopic insular or anaplastic change is controversial. Some people have suggested that focal microscopic dedifferentiation does not alter prognosis, but others have shown that this finding alone is statistically significant as a marker of aggressive behavior. Poorly differentiated carcinoma is intermediate in the spectrum, and may represent a transition form [10,12].

The factors underlying dedifferentiation in thyroid tumors remain to be established, although age and exposure to radiation have been implicated [13,14]. Clearly, the vast majority of well-differentiated thyroid lesions do not undergo transformation to anaplastic carcinoma. A pattern of genetic mutations resulting in oncogene activation or loss of tumor

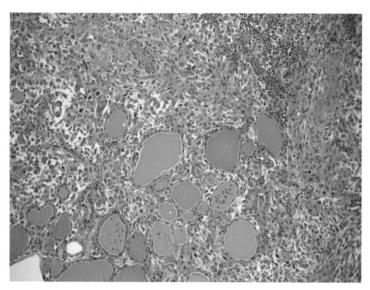

FIGURE 12.1 Anaplastic carcinomas of the thyroid are aggressively invasive malignancies showing intrathyroidal invasion as illustrated in this image, resulting in entrapment of normal thyroid follicles, as well as extrathyroidal extension into adjacent structures (hematoxylin & eosin stain).

suppressor gene activity has been proposed to correlate with the stepwise progression from adenoma to carcinoma and through the dedifferentiation process in thyroid [15–17]. p53 mutations are common in anaplastic thyroid carcinomas [15,16,18–22]. Since the mutated forms of this tumor suppressor gene have prolonged half-lives, the application of immunohistochemistry has yielded positive results in these tumors [23,24]. At the molecular level, the patterns of allelic loss show that the majority of cases have a core of conserved mutations in differentiated and undifferentiated areas with substantial increases in mutation rates in the anaplastic components [25], suggesting that additional genetic events promote tumor progression.

Anaplastic carcinomas are highly infiltrative tumors and on histology it is common to find the malignant cells entrapping normal thyroid elements (Fig. 12.1, e-Fig. 12.1). The tumor also invades into skeletal muscle, adjacent adipose tissue and other extrathyroidal structures. Blood vessel invasion and thrombosis are frequent, with or without tumor cell involvement.

On both cytology and histology, anaplastic carcinomas exhibit wide variations in appearance with several morphologic patterns recognized and many tumors manifesting a mixed morphology. A common morphologic presentation, and one that is most easily recognized as an anaplastic carcinoma of thyroid, is that of the biphasic spindle and giant-cell tumor (Fig. 12.2, e-Fig. 12.2). Other tumors are dominated by bizarre, malignant giant cells and still others may show a more pure population of spindle

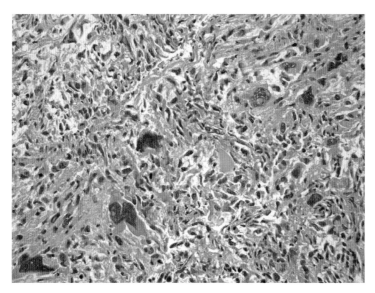

FIGURE 12.2 Anaplastic carcinomas of the thyroid frequently have a mixture of histologic patterns. In this example, there is a spindle cell background in which numerous giant malignant cells are seen with large, hyperchromatic and often frankly bizarre nuclei (hematoxylin & eosin stain).

cells (Fig. 12.3, e-Fig. 12.3). Occasionally, the tumor is simply a highly malignant, undifferentiated, large cell carcinoma resembling a lymphoepitheliomalike carcinoma (Fig. 12.4, e-Fig. 12.4). All variations of anaplastic carcinoma of the thyroid are highly proliferative with numerous mitotic

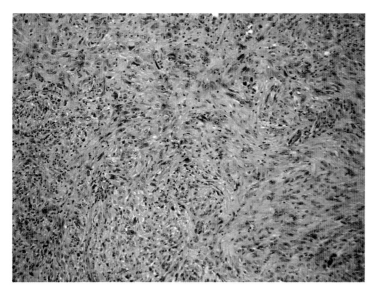

FIGURE 12.3 In the spindle cell variant of anaplastic carcinoma, spindle cells dominate the tumor (hematoxylin & eosin stain).

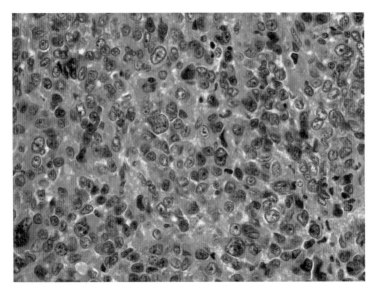

FIGURE 12.4 Some examples of anaplastic carcinoma of thyroid have the appearance of a poorly differentiated large cell carcinoma, resembling a lymphoepitheliomalike carcinoma (hematoxylin & eosin stain).

figures and atypical mitoses (Fig. 12.5, e-Fig. 12.5). There is usually extensive geographic necrosis (Figs. 12.6 and 12.7, e-Figs. 12.6–12.8) and in some cases, the necrosis may be so widespread that the only viable tumor is preserved around blood vessels. Inflammatory infiltrates are frequently

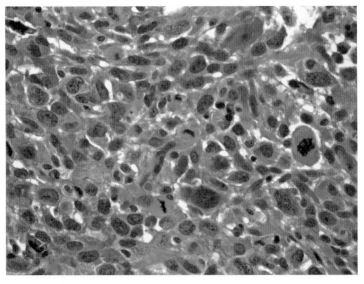

FIGURE 12.5 In keeping with their rapid growth, mitoses are frequent in anaplastic carcinomas and atypical mitoses are commonly found (hematoxylin & eosin stain).

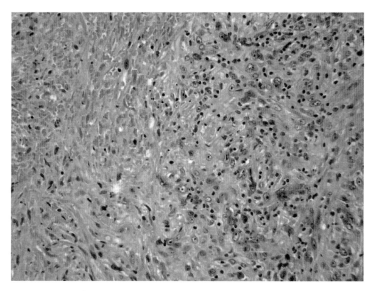

FIGURE 12.6 Necrosis is common in anaplastic carcinoma of the thyroid and as in this example may induce an inflammatory reaction (hematoxylin & eosin stain).

seen with the necrosis. Osteoclastlike giant cells may be present (Fig. 12.8, e-Figs. 12.9–12.10) and have been shown by immunohistochemical studies to be of the monocytic/histiocytic lineage [26,27]. Neoplastic bone and cartilage may also be identified.

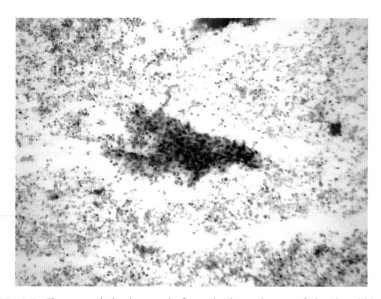

FIGURE 12.7 The necrotic background of anaplastic carcinoma of the thyroid is often apparent in fine needle aspiration samples admixed with a variable degree of inflammation (direct smear, Papanicolaou stain).

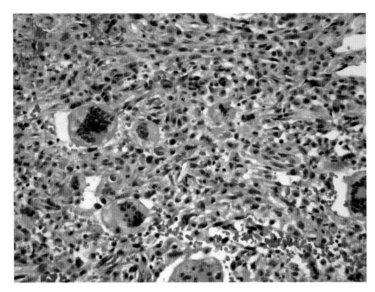

FIGURE 12.8 **Osteoclasticlike giant cells are found in some anaplastic carcinomas.** These giant cells are of monocyte lineage and show significant differences in nuclear morphology when compared to the carcinoma (hematoxylin & eosin stain).

On fine needle aspiration (FNA) or core biopsy, these tumors present a variety of differential diagnostic possibilities depending on the predominant morphologic pattern present in the sample. When tumor giant cells are numerous, the appearance is fairly characteristic and a high degree of certainty of an anaplastic carcinoma can be achieved. When the tumor presents in the form of a poorly differentiated, large cell carcinoma, the differential diagnosis includes medullary carcinoma, direct extension of a laryngeal carcinoma, metastatic carcinoma, metastatic melanoma, large cell lymphoma (both diffuse large cell lymphoma and anaplastic large cell lymphoma). When the spindle cell morphology dominates, or the tumor appears biphasic with both epithelial and spindle cell components, the differential diagnosis once again includes medullary carcinoma, metastatic carcinoma (in particular a sarcomatoid renal primary), and melanoma, but now must include sarcomas (both primary and metastatic) as well as involvement of the thyroid by a primary laryngeal sarcomatoid squamous carcinoma. Resolution of these diagnostic possibilities requires careful attention to the morphology, combined with immunohistochemical studies (which are often of limited help) and clinical information to arrive at the conclusion that the poorly differentiated malignancies are anaplastic carcinoma of thyroid.

Immunohistochemistry is useful in only a limited fashion in the diagnosis of these lesions. Most anaplastic carcinomas do not contain convincing reactivity for TTF-1 or thyroglobulin and the few that are positive have only a weak or focal reaction [5,8,27–31]. Positivity for TTF-1 or thyroglobulin must be interpreted carefully, since it may reflect trapped nontumorous follicles or follicular cells, or diffusion of thyroglobulin into nonfollicular cells. The epithelial nature of the tumor cells can be verified with stains for cytokeratins in some cases, but again most undifferentiated lesions are negative for this marker.

By electron microscopy [8,26,30,32,33], there may be formation of intercellular junctions, microvilli, and basal lamina, providing evidence of epithelial differentiation. However, many tumors do not exhibit evidence of any differentiation. Their large nuclei have prominent nucleoli and clumped chromatin; usually the cytoplasm contains only poorly developed rough endoplasmic reticulum, scattered dense bodies, lipid droplets, numerous free ribosomes, mitochondria, and lysosomes. Intermediate filaments (keratin or vimentin) may form filamentous whorls that correspond to the acidophilic hyaline globules seen by light microscopy. Secretory granules are not seen in these tumors. Some tumors do not exhibit immunohistochemical or ultrastructural markers that allow classification as epithelial malignancies. Nevertheless, the diagnosis of anaplastic carcinoma should be favored for pleomorphic lesions in older patients if they arise in the thyroid. Most anaplastic thyroid carcinomas are aneuploid on flow cytometry; this abnormality correlates with poor outcome [34].

Giant-Cell Variant of Anaplastic Carcinoma

The most common type of anaplastic carcinoma is the *giant-cell variant*. As the name suggests, these tumors are predominantly composed of large cells with abundant amphophilic or eosinophilic, typically granular cytoplasm and bizarre, often multiple, hyperchromatic nuclei (Fig. 12.9, e-Fig. 12.11). Some have round, densely acidophilic intracytoplasmic hyaline globules. These tumors grow in solid sheets, but artifactual tissue fragmentation may simulate an alveolar pattern (Fig. 12.10, e-Fig. 12.12). FNA of the giant-cell variant of anaplastic carcinoma is characterized by pleomorphic and often bizarre giant cells with multilobulated, single or multiple nuclei (Fig. 12.11, e-Figs. 12.13–12.15). The chromatin pattern is coarse with prominent parachromatin clearing and often multiple and bizarre nucleoli [35–37]. Necrotic material may be present in the background with a variable inflammatory reaction (Fig. 12.12, e-Fig. 12.16). The malignant giant cells can be identified as epithelial if they express CK7, CK8, and CK18 [38].

An unusual variant of anaplastic thyroid carcinoma is the *rhabdoid tumor* [39–41]. This is a very rare and aggressive thyroid tumor with few case reports appearing in the literature. These tumors are invasive, nonencapsulated solid lesions composed of large neoplastic cells supported by a delicate fibrovascular stroma. Areas of geographic necrosis and hemorrhage are seen (Figs. 12.13–12.15, e-Figs. 12.17–12.21). The neoplastic cells are large with abundant eosinophilic cytoplasm containing eosinophilic cytoplasmic inclusions and large eccentrically placed vesicular nuclei,

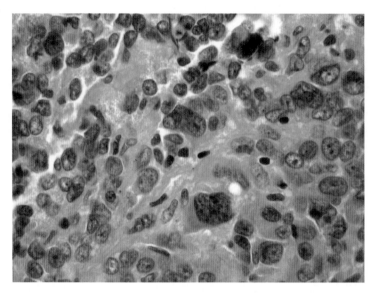

FIGURE 12.9 In the giant cell variant of anaplastic carcinoma of the thyroid, there are sheets of large malignant cells with abundant amphophilic or eosinophilic cytoplasm with large, often bizarre, hyperchromatic nuclei (hematoxylin & eosin stain).

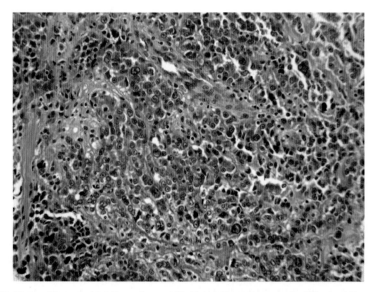

FIGURE 12.10 The combination of a nesting growth pattern and artifactual tissue fragmentation may simulate an alveolar pattern in giant cell anaplastic carcinomas (hematoxylin & eosin stain).

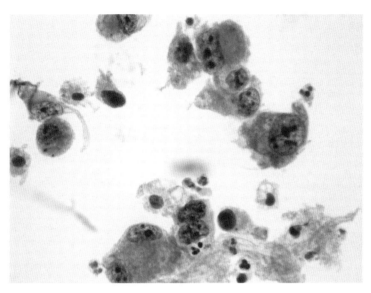

FIGURE 12.11   The giant cell variant of anaplastic carcinoma is readily recognized as malignant on fine needle aspiration, but, at times it may be difficult to establish the epithelial nature of the tumor. In such cases, immunoperoxidase staining for cytokeratin 7 or low molecular weight keratins 8 and 18 may prove helpful (ThinPrep Papanicolaou stain).

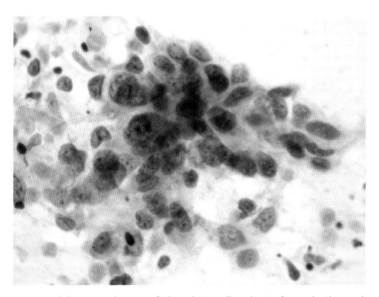

FIGURE 12.12   High power image of the giant-cell variant of anaplastic carcinoma of thyroid. Note the necrotic material in the background and the spindle morphology of some of the tumor cells (direct smear, Papanicolaou stain).

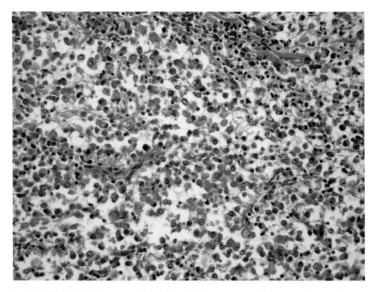

FIGURE 12.13 Rhabdoid tumor of the thyroid is a rare and aggressive malignancy composed of sheets of neoplastic cells supported by a fine fibrovascular stroma. Areas of geographic necrosis and hemorrhage are common (hematoxylin & eosin stain).

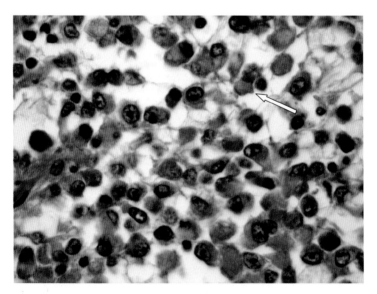

FIGURE 12.14 The neoplastic cells of the rhabdoid tumor are large with abundant, eosinophilic cytoplasm containing eosinophilic cytoplasmic inclusions (*arrow*) and large eccentrically placed vesicular nuclei, frequently demonstrating a prominent nucleolus (hematoxylin & eosin stain).

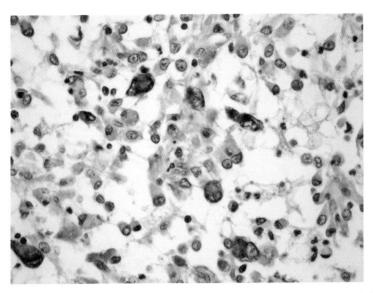

FIGURE 12.15   Expression of keratins may be found in some rhabdoid tumors of the thyroid as seen in this case in which there is focal staining with AE1:AE3 (immunoperoxidase stain AE1:AE3 & hematoxylin stain).

frequently demonstrating a prominent nucleolus. Immunohistochemically, the rhabdoid cells may have focal positivity for TTF-1, vimentin, sarcomeric actin, epithelial membrane antigen, and cytokeratin. They are negative for thyroglobulin, smooth muscle actin, desmin, myogenin, synaptophysin, chromogranin, and carcinoembryonic antigen [41,42]. The cytoplasmic aggregates in the rhabdoid cells are often positive for epithelial markers [41] and by electron microscopy are seen to be composed of masses of intermediate filaments [40]. To our knowledge, the cytologic morphology of this lesion on aspiration biopsy has not been reported.

Squamoid Variant of Anaplastic Carcinoma

The *squamoid variant* is composed of large, moderately pleomorphic epithelial cells that form nests, resembling squamous carcinoma. They may even form keratin pearls. Squamoid areas may exhibit reactivity for high molecular weight keratins and/or epithelial membrane antigen (EMA) [5,8,27,28]. They frequently express CK7, CK8, and CK18 [43].

Spindle Cell Variant of Anaplastic Carcinoma

On histology, *spindle cell anaplastic carcinomas* have a fascicular architecture of spindle-shaped tumor cells interwoven with varying degrees of stromal collagen [44] (Figs. 12.3, 12.16 and 12.17, e-Figs. 12.3, 12.22–12.24). They may resemble fibrosarcoma or when seen with an inflammatory infiltrate, may suggest malignant fibrous histiocytoma. When the vasculature becomes prominent the tumor may suggest hemangioendothelioma [3,6,45].

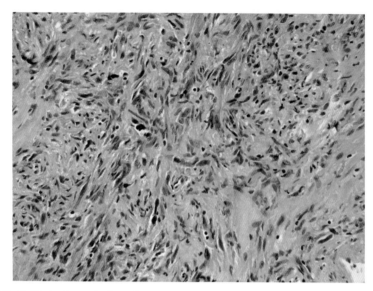

FIGURE 12.16 In the spindle cell variant of anaplastic carcinoma, fascicles of spindle-shaped tumor cells are interspersed within dense bands of stromal collagen (hematoxylin & eosin stain).

FNA of spindle cell anaplastic carcinomas generates samples of variable cellularity (Fig. 12.18, e-Fig. 12.25). Some spindle cell anaplastic carcinomas are markedly paucicellular or provide no sample at all due to a densely fibrotic stroma that refuses to yield any cellular material

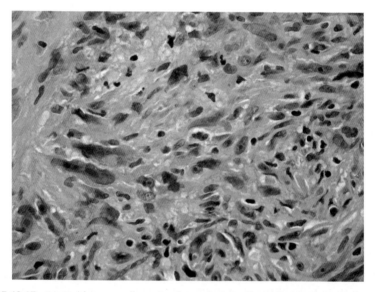

FIGURE 12.17 Large, bizarre, malignant cells are frequently evident in the spindle cell variant of anaplastic carcinoma and distinction from a sarcoma (either primary or metastatic) or sarcomatoid squamous carcinoma may be problematic (hematoxylin & eosin stain).

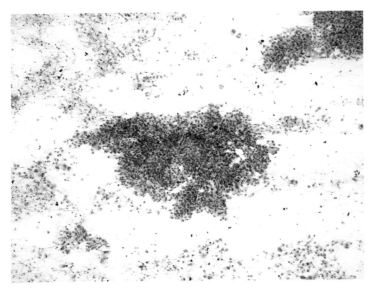

FIGURE 12.18 The cellularity of an aspirate obtained from a spindle cell anaplastic carcinoma is variable. The specimens may range from virtually acellular, in a densely fibrotic lesion, to abundantly cellular, as in this image. Note the necrotic material in the background (direct smear, Papanicolaou stain).

on aspiration. FNAs of less densely sclerotic spindle cell anaplastic carcinoma are highly cellular with numerous dissociated spindle cells and tissue fragments (Fig. 12.19, e-Fig. 12.26). These spindle cells may vary from relatively small, bland cells to frankly malignant cells (Fig. 12.20, e-Figs. 12.27–12.28). Mitoses may be numerous and the background may reveal necrotic material. When cellular, it is not uncommon to obtain large tissue fragments of spindle cells (Figs. 12.21 and 12.22, e-Figs. 12.29 and 12.30), often arranged around vascular structures. These may resemble the papillary structures seen in some papillary carcinomas, particularly the tall cell variant, but the tumor cells tend to be more pleomorphic and lack the nuclear features of papillary carcinoma of thyroid [46].

Paucicellular Variant of Anaplastic Carcinoma

This variant of anaplastic carcinoma is composed mainly of sclerotic stroma and infarcted tissue with spindle cells arranged in fascicular or storiform patterns [8,29,47]. This uncommon morphologic variant of anaplastic thyroid carcinoma histologically mimics Riedel's thyroiditis, which is a reactive condition with a very favorable prognosis. The distinguishing features that identify a case as an anaplastic carcinoma include the presence of necrosis, atypical spindle cells obliterating large blood vessels and immunoreactivity within the spindle cells for epithelial markers. The cytologic characteristics of this tumor have not been described, likely due to an inability to obtain a sample for evaluation on an aspiration.

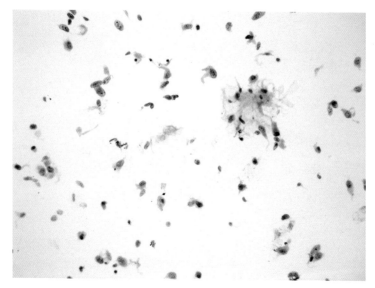

FIGURE 12.19 Cellular dissociation may occur in spindle cell anaplastic carcinoma, resulting in small cell clusters and individual spindle cells with some scattered nuclei stripped of their cytoplasm (ThinPrep, Papanicolaou stain).

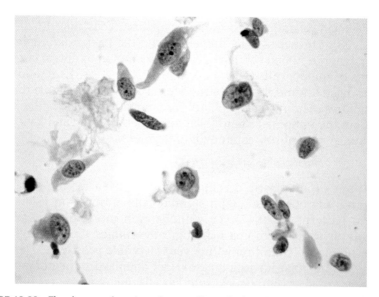

FIGURE 12.20 The degree of nuclear abnormality varies in spindle cell anaplastic carcinoma ranging from small bland nuclei to frankly malignant nuclei (ThinPrep, Papanicolaou stain).

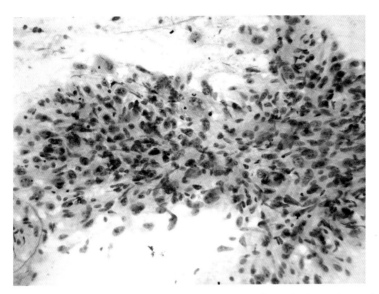

FIGURE 12.21 This large tissue fragment from a spindle cell anaplastic carcinoma is composed of malignant spindle cells arranged around a central vascular structure (direct smear, Papanicolaou stain).

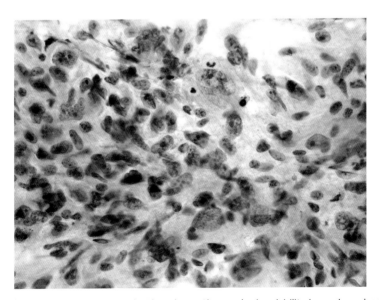

FIGURE 12.22 High power examination shows the marked variability in nuclear abnormalities in the spindle cell anaplastic carcinoma (direct smear, Papanicolaou stain).

GIANT-CELL MEDULLARY CARCINOMA

An unusual variant of medullary carcinoma of thyroid is characterized by the presence of large, bizarre giant tumor cells that may mimic anaplastic carcinoma found admixed with regions showing the typical histomorphology of medullary carcinoma. Aspiration of such a lesion yields a hypercellular specimen composed of polygonal and spindle-shaped cells in loosely cohesive groups. Eccentrically located nuclei have the coarse granular chromatin, giving them the characteristic "salt-and-pepper" appearance of neuroendocrine cells, but binucleate and multinucleate forms give rise to giant cells that are atypical [48]. Immunohistochemical localization of calcitonin, chromogranin, and carcinoembryonic antigen proves the diagnosis.

SQUAMOUS CELL CARCINOMA

Primary squamous cell carcinoma of thyroid is rare [49,49–51], accounting for less than 1% of thyroid malignancies. Occasional tumors have been associated with papillary carcinoma, suggesting that in some cases, the well-known squamous metaplasia of papillary carcinomas can progress to squamous carcinomas [11,52,53]. These tumors are frequently keratinizing squamous carcinoma and on cytology may reveal a necrotic background in which may be seen individual dyskeratotic malignant cells, tadpole cells, and rare keratin pearls [54,55] (e-Figs. 12.31–12.33). Syncytial clusters and sheets of malignant cells may also be found, composed of large cells with moderately abundant, dense cyanophilic cytoplasm and large nuclei with coarse chromatin and small nucleoli. The cytologic appearance of primary squamous carcinoma of the thyroid is not distinctive and its appearance is identical to squamous carcinoma arising elsewhere. Thus, the mandate that a metastatic squamous carcinoma must be excluded prior to making the diagnosis of a primary squamous carcinoma of thyroid becomes impossible by morphologic means on FNA.

As in cytologic preparations, the histology of squamous carcinoma of the thyroid is identical to the same tumor seen in other sites and ranges from well to poorly differentiated varieties. By definition, the entire tumor must be composed of squamous carcinoma and should not be in close association with another type of thyroid carcinoma. Primary squamous carcinoma must be distinguished from squamous metaplasia arising in benign thyroid lesions (lymphocytic thyroiditis), carcinoma showing thymuslike differentiation (CASTLE), direct extension or metastatic squamous carcinoma, and other thyroid carcinomas in which squamous differentiation has developed.

Immunoperoxidase studies have shown that primary squamous carcinoma of the thyroid expresses cytokeratin 19 and occasionally cytokeratin 7 [52,56–58], whereas it lacks expression of cytokeratin 10/13 [56]. Many cases studied have lacked expression of thyroglobulin and TTF-1 [57–60] and if detected, these markers tended to be focal and weak in staining [52,61].

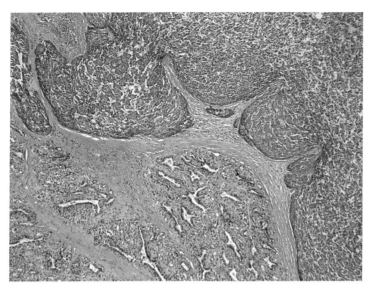

FIGURE 12.23 Spindle cell tumor with thymuslike differentiation (SETTLE) is typically a biphasic tumor with a lobulated appearance imparted by broad fibrous septae (hematoxylin & eosin stain).

SPINDLE EPITHELIAL TUMOR WITH THYMUSLIKE DIFFERENTIATION (SETTLE)

This rare malignant tumor occurs in the thyroid, mainly in children and young adults, and presents as a solitary circumscribed thyroid mass, occasionally associated with compressive symptoms. Like the related CASTLE (Chapter 11), the cell of origin is not of follicular epithelial or C-cell derivation, but rather is likely ectopic thymic tissue or branchial pouch developmental remnants in the thyroid [49,62–65]. It is a low-grade malignant neoplasm typified by the development of late hematogenous metastases. Few reports have appeared concerning the cytomorphology of this tumor on FNA [66–68]. The reports that have appeared have not provided a definitive diagnosis prospectively, and the tumor is classified as some form of spindle cell neoplasm as the spindle cell population frequently predominates. If the biphasic nature of the tumor is appreciated, an erroneous cytologic diagnosis of synovial sarcoma may be made.

Histologically, the tumor is biphasic with a monophasic variant recognized (Chapter 11). In the classical biphasic appearance, variable bands of fibrosis may be seen (Fig. 12.23, e-Fig. 12.34) with a spindle cell component forming interlacing fascicles of spindle cells with minimal cytoplasm, elongated nuclei, fine chromatin, and inconspicuous nucleoli (Figs. 12.24 and 12.25, e-Figs. 12.35–12.37). Mitoses are uncommon, although some tumors have been reported with increased mitotic activity and focal necrosis

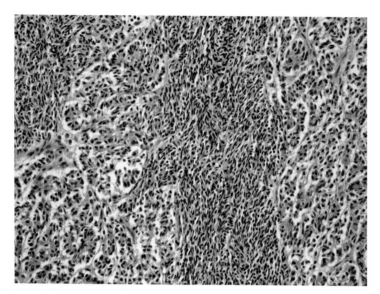

FIGURE 12.24   The spindle cell components of SETTLE tend to merge imperceptibly with tubulopapillary glandular components (hematoxylin & eosin stain).

[67]. The epithelial component is seen as cells arranged into tubules, papillae, cords and glandular spaces (Figs. 12.26–12.28, e-Figs. 12.38–12.42). The epithelial cells are cuboidal to columnar and become mucinous or ciliated with foci of squamous metaplasia occasionally seen.

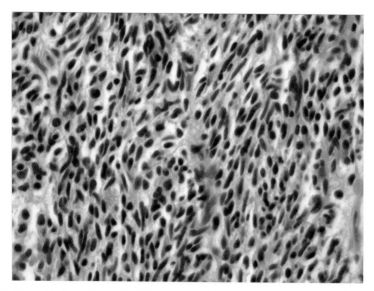

FIGURE 12.25   The spindle cells in SETTLE form interlacing fascicles with minimal cytoplasm, elongated nuclei, fine chromatin and inconspicuous nucleoli (hematoxylin & eosin stain).

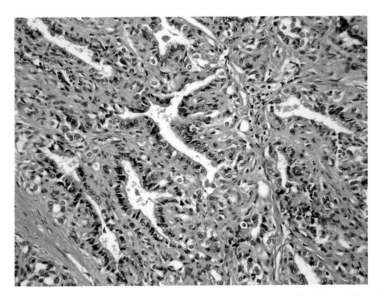

FIGURE 12.26 The glandular component of SETTLE forms small pale staining islands admixed with large epithelial-lined glands (hematoxylin & eosin stain).

The differential diagnoses of SETTLE include anaplastic carcinoma of thyroid, spindle cell variants of medullary carcinoma, other sarcomas, both primary and metastatic, with synovial sarcoma the most difficult to distinguish from SETTLE. The application of immunohistochemistry studies may

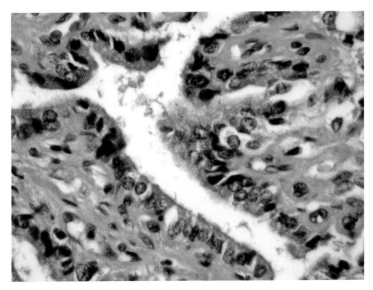

FIGURE 12.27 The glandular epithelium of SETTLE may show a variety of cell types including ciliated cells (hematoxylin & eosin stain).

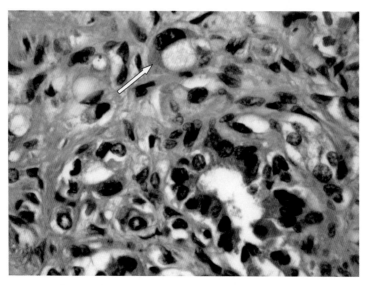

FIGURE 12.28   Mucinous differentiation (*arrow*) is also frequently evident in SETTLE (hematoxylin & eosin stain).

be helpful in distinguishing these possibilities. The cells of SETTLE are positive for cytokeratins, smooth muscle actin, muscle-specific actin, and MIC-2, but lack expression of thyroglobulin, calcitonin, chromogranin, S-100, and CD5 [49]. Given the similarities with synovial sarcoma both morphologically and by immunohistochemistry, it may be necessary to examine for the presence or absence of the *t*(X;18) translocation and its SYT/SSX fusion product associated with synovial sarcoma.

SPINDLE CELL METAPLASIA

Papillary carcinomas and even follicular adenomas can occasionally be associated with diffuse or nodular spindle cell proliferations that are considered to be metaplastic [69]. These proliferations are composed of bland spindle cells with fine chromatin and subtle nucleoli. Mitoses are rare, and inflammation is minimal. The spindle cells contain immunoreactivity for thyroglobulin, supporting origin from follicular epithelial cells. In some instances, these cells can comprise a significant proportion of the lesion and therefore may be identified on a biopsy. It is important to recognize these metaplastic proliferations and to distinguish them from aggressive malignant neoplasms.

NODULAR FASCIITISLIKE AND MYXOID STROMA

Papillary carcinomas have been described to have unusual stromal changes that can give rise to confusion and misdiagnosis on biopsy. The malignant epithelial cells form anastomosing tubules, clustered glands, or solid sheets with or without squamous metaplasia and exhibit the nuclear features of papillary carcinoma. The abundant stroma can be diffuse throughout the lesion or focal. It is composed of spindle cells within a mucoid matrix, collagen, and extravasated red blood cells. This stroma, which resembles fibroadenoma, phyllodes tumor, or fibrocystic disease of the breast, has been described as "myxoid" or "nodular-fasciitis-like" and is considered to be an exuberant mesenchymal reaction [70,71]. The importance of recognizing this change in papillary carcinoma is twofold. Firstly, if one encounters a fibroproliferative lesion of the thyroid, a diligent search should be made for papillary carcinoma. Secondly, this lesion must be distinguished from the vastly more aggressive papillary carcinomas with anaplastic transformation.

MESENCHYMAL SPINDLE CELL TUMORS

Primary mesenchymal tumors of the thyroid are rare. Reported cases include solitary fibrous tumor, fibrosarcoma, leiomyoma and leiomyosarcoma, granular cell tumor, vascular hemangioma, epithelioid hemangioendothelioma (Chapter 11), and angiosarcoma [44,49]. Because of the propensity for angiosarcoma, an immunohistochemical panel for the investigation of a mesenchymal tumor should include vascular markers even in the presence of immunoreactivity for epithelial markers. The diagnosis of these lesions is difficult on biopsy and usually resection is required for definitive diagnosis. When faced with these lesions, it is important to exclude a metastasis from a more common primary site.

Epithelioid Vascular Tumors

The most notable mesenchymal tumor of the thyroid is angiosarcoma that occurs in regions of endemic goiter such as the European Alps [6,49]. Although these lesions were originally considered to be anaplastic carcinomas, the immunoprofile and ultrastructural studies have proven the endothelial differentiation of tumor cells [72–77]. Aspiration of epithelioid angiosarcoma of the thyroid [78] has yielded cellular smears composed of single cells and small clusters of oval and round cells with indistinct cell borders and vacuolated cytoplasm. The nuclei are eccentric, with irregular nuclear membranes, a single prominent nucleolus and a coarse chromatin pattern. Features suggestive of intracytoplasmic lumens have been identified.

On histologic examination, the tumors are composed of large, round and abnormal epithelioid cells lining vascular spaces. As seen in the cytology, the malignant cells contain moderately abundant cytoplasm in which intracytoplasmic lumens may be appreciated. The nuclei are eccentric with a coarse hyperchromatic chromatin pattern and prominent nucleoli (Figs. 12.29–12.31, e-Figs. 12.43–12.47). The neoplastic cells may be immunoreactive for AE1:AE3, cytokeratin 7, and show expression of vimentin, CD31, and factor VIII. Epithelioid angiosarcoma should be considered in the differential diagnosis of epithelioid neoplasms of the thyroid.

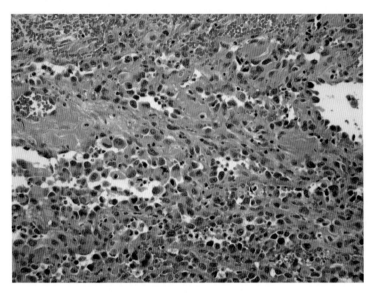

FIGURE 12.29 Angiosarcoma of the thyroid is composed of large, malignant, epithelioid endothelial cells lining vascular channels (hematoxylin & eosin stain).

Giant-Cell Sarcoma—Osteosarcoma

Primary osteosarcoma of the thyroid is an extremely rare tumor. The reported appearance on aspiration has been that of a high-grade tumor composed of spindle and epithelioid malignant cells with a background of

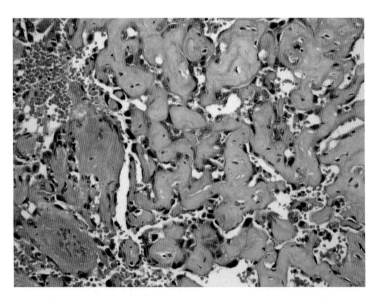

FIGURE 12.30 This complex anastomosing patterns of vascular spaces lined by malignant cells is typical of angiosarcoma (hematoxylin & eosin stain).

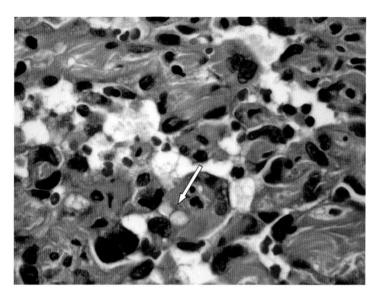

FIGURE 12.31 Intracytoplasmic lumens (*arrow*) may be seen in the malignant endothelial cells of epithelioid angiosarcoma (hematoxylin & eosin stain).

multinucleated giant cells. Dense, fibrillar metachromatic extracellular material was noted within cell clusters and surrounding some individual cells. The cytologic appearance generated a differential diagnosis of sarcoma, anaplastic carcinoma and medullary carcinoma. Histologically, the tumor is characterized by a pleomorphic sarcoma with malignant osteoid production, indicating osteosarcoma [79].

REFERENCES

1. Samaan NA, Ordoñez NG. Uncommon types of thyroid cancer. *Endocrinol Metab Clin North Am* 1990;19:637–648.
2. Murray D. The thyroid gland. In: Kovacs K, Asa SL, eds. *Functional endocrine pathology*. Boston: Blackwell Science, 1998:295–380.
3. Rosai J, Carcangiu ML, DeLellis RA. Tumors of the thyroid gland. In: *Atlas of tumor pathology*. 3rd series, fascicle 5. Washington, DC: Armed Forces Institute of Pathology, 1992.
4. Aldinger KA, Samaan NA, Ibanez M, et al. Anaplastic carcinoma of the thyroid. A review of 84 cases of spindle and giant cell carcinoma of the thyroid. *Cancer* 1978;41: 2267–2275.
5. Venkatesh YSS, Ordoñez NG, Schultz PN, et al. Anaplastic carcinoma of the thyroid. A clinicopathologic study of 121 cases. *Cancer* 1990;66:321–330.
6. LiVolsi VA. *Surgical pathology of the thyroid*. Philadelphia: WB Saunders, 1990.
7. Nishiyama RH, Dunn EL, Thompson NW. Anaplastic spindle-cell and giant-cell tumors of the thyroid gland. *Cancer* 1972;30:113–127.
8. Carcangiu ML, Steeper T, Zampi G, et al. Anaplastic thyroid carcinoma. A study of 70 cases. *Am J Clin Pathol* 1985;83:135–158.
9. Spires JR, Schwartz MR, Miller RH. Anaplastic thyroid carcinoma. Association with differentiated thyroid cancer. *Arch Otolaryngol Head Neck Surg* 1988;114:40–44.

10. Van der Laan BFAM, Freeman JL, Tsang RW, et al. The association of well-differentiated thyroid carcinoma with insular or anaplastic thyroid carcinoma: evidence for dedifferentiation in tumor progression. *Endocr Pathol* 1993;4:215–221.

11. Bronner MP, LiVolsi VA. Spindle cell squamous carcinoma of the thyroid: an unusual anaplastic tumor associated with tall cell papillary cancer. *Mod Pathol* 1991;4:637–643.

12. Sakamoto A, Kasai N, Sugano H. Poorly differentiated carcinoma of the thyroid. A clinicopathologic entity for a high-risk group of papillary and follicular carcinomas. *Cancer* 1983;52:1849–1855.

13. Yoshida A, Kamma H, Asaga T, et al. Proliferative activity in thyroid tumors. *Cancer* 1992;69:2548–2552.

14. Kapp DS, LiVolsi VA, Sanders MM. Anaplastic carcinoma following well-differentiated thyroid cancer: etiological considerations. *Yale J Biol Med* 1982;55:521–528.

15. Fagin JA. Genetic basis of endocrine disease 3. Molecular defects in thyroid gland neoplasia. *J Clin Endocrinol Metab* 1992;75:1398–1400.

16. Farid NR, Shi Y, Zou M. Molecular basis of thyroid cancer. *Endocr Rev* 1994;15:202–232.

17. Kondo T, Ezzat S, Asa SL. Pathogenetic mechanisms in thyroid follicular-cell neoplasia. *Nat Rev Cancer* 2006;6:292–306.

18. Fagin JA, Matsuo K, Karmakar A, et al. High prevalence of mutations of the p53 gene in poorly differentiated human thyroid carcinomas. *J Clin Invest* 1993;91:179–184.

19. Donghi R, Longoni A, Pilotti S, et al. Gene p53 mutations are restricted to poorly differentiated and undifferentiated carcinomas of the thyroid gland. *J Clin Invest* 1993;91:1753–1760.

20. Nakamura T, Yana I, Kobayashi T, et al. p53 gene mutations associated with anaplastic transformation of human thyroid carcinomas. *Jpn J Cancer Res* 1992;83:1293–1298.

21. Ito T, Seyama T, Mizuno T, et al. Unique association of p53 mutations with undifferentiated but not with differentiated carcinomas of the thyroid gland. *Cancer Res* 1992;52:1369–1371.

22. Wyllie FS, Lemoine NR, Williams ED, et al. Structure and expression of nuclear oncogenes in multi-stage thyroid tumorigenesis. *Br J Cancer* 1989;60:561–565.

23. Hosal SA, Apel RL, Freeman JL, et al. Immunohistochemical localization of p53 in human thyroid neoplasms: correlation with biological behavior. *Endocr Pathol* 1997;8:21–28.

24. Jossart GH, Epstein HD, Shaver JK, et al. Immunocytochemical detection of p53 in human thyroid carcinomas is associated with mutation and immortalization of cell lines. *J Clin Endocrinol Metab* 1996;81:3498–3504.

25. Hunt JL, Tometsko M, LiVolsi VA, et al. Molecular evidence of anaplastic transformation in coexisting well-differentiated and anaplastic carcinomas of the thyroid. *Am J Surg Pathol* 2003;27:1559–1564.

26. Gaffey MJ, Lack EE, Christ ML, et al. Anaplastic thyroid carcinoma with osteoclast-like giant cells. A clinicopathologic, immunohistochemical, and ultrastructural study. *Am J Surg Pathol* 1991;15:160–168.

27. Ordóñez NG, El-Naggar AK, Hickey RC, et al. Anaplastic thyroid carcinoma. Immunocytochemical study of 32 cases. *Am J Clin Pathol* 1991;96:15–24.

28. Hurlimann J, Gardiol D, Scazziga B. Immunohistology of anaplastic thyroid carcinoma. A study of 43 cases. *Histopathology* 1987;11:567–580.

29. LiVolsi VA, Brooks JJ, Arendash-Durand B. Anaplastic thyroid tumors. Immunohistology. *Am J Clin Pathol* 1987;87:434–442.

30. Pilotti S, Collini P, Del Bo R, et al. A novel panel of antibodies that segregates immunocytochemically poorly differentiated carcinoma from undifferentiated carcinoma of the thyroid gland. *Am J Surg Pathol* 1994;18:1054–1064.

31. Fischer S, Asa SL. Application of immunohistochemistry to thyroid neoplasms. *Arch Pathol Lab Med* 2008;132:359–372.

32. Gaal JM, Horvath E, Kovacs K. Ultrastructure of two cases of anaplastic giant cell tumor of the human thyroid gland. *Cancer* 1975;35:1273–1279.

33. Jao W, Gould VE. Ultrastructure of anaplastic (spindle and giant cell) carcinoma of the thyroid. *Cancer* 1975;35:1280–1292.

34. Klemi PJ, Joensuu H, Eerola E. DNA aneuploidy in anaplastic carcinoma of the thyroid gland. *Am J Clin Pathol* 1988;89:154–159.

35. Luze T, Totsch M, Bangerl I, et al. Fine needle aspiration cytodiagnosis of anaplastic carcinoma and malignant haemangioendothelioma of the thyroid in an endemic goitre area. *Cytopathology* 1990;1:305–310.

36. Guarda LA, Peterson CE, Hall W, et al. Anaplastic thyroid carcinoma: cytomorphology and clinical implications of fine-needle aspiration. *Diagn Cytopathol* 1991;7:63–67.

37. Mehdi G, Ansari HA, Siddiqui SA. Cytology of anaplastic giant cell carcinoma of the thyroid with osteoclast-like giant cells—a case report. *Diagn Cytopathol* 2007;35:111–112.

38. Miettinen M, Franssila KO. Variable expression of keratins and nearly uniform lack of thyroid transcription factor 1 in thyroid anaplastic carcinoma. *Hum Pathol* 2000;31:1139–1145.

39. Chetty R, Govender D. Follicular thyroid carcinoma with rhabdoid phenotype. *Virchows Arch* 1999;435:133–136.

40. Albores-Saavedra J, Sharma S. Poorly differentiated follicular thyroid carcinoma with rhabdoid phenotype: a clinicopathologic, immunohistochemical and electron microscopic study of two cases. *Mod Pathol* 2001;14:98–104.

41. Lai ML, Faa G, Serra S, et al. Rhabdoid tumor of the thyroid gland: a variant of anaplastic carcinoma. *Arch Pathol Lab Med* 2005;129:e55–e57.

42. Agarwal S, Sharma MC, Aron M, et al. Poorly differentiated thyroid carcinoma with rhabdoid phenotype: a diagnostic dilemma—report of a rare case. *Endocr Pathol* 2006;17:399–405.

43. Miettinen M, Franssila KO. Variable expression of keratins and nearly uniform lack of thyroid transcription factor 1 in thyroid anaplastic carcinoma. *Hum Pathol* 2000;31:1139–1145.

44. Papi G, Corrado S, LiVolsi VA. Primary spindle cell lesions of the thyroid gland; an overview. *Am J Clin Pathol* 2006;125(suppl):S95–S123.

45. Shvero J, Gal R, Avidor I, et al. Anaplastic thyroid carcinoma. A clinical, histologic, and immunohistochemical study. *Cancer* 1988;62:319–325.

46. Saunders CA, Nayar R. Anaplastic spindle-cell squamous carcinoma arising in association with tall-cell papillary cancer of the thyroid: a potential pitfall. *Diagn Cytopathol* 1999;21:413–418.

47. Wan SK, Chan JK, Tang SK. Paucicellular variant of anaplastic thyroid carcinoma. A mimic of Reidel's thyroiditis. *Am J Clin Pathol* 1996;105:388–393.

48. Rekhi B, Kane SV, D'Cruz A. Cytomorphology of anaplastic giant cell type of medullary thyroid carcinoma—a diagnostic dilemma in an elderly female: a case report. *Diagn Cytopathol* 2008;36:136–138.

49. Baloch ZW, LiVolsi VA. Unusual tumors of the thyroid gland. *Endocrinol Metab Clin North Am* 2008;37:297–310, vii.

50. Makay O, Kaya T, Ertan Y, et al. Primary squamous cell carcinoma of the thyroid: report of three cases. *Endocr J* 2008;55:359–364.

51. Sanchez-Sosa S, Rios-Luna NP, Tamayo BR, et al. Primary squamous cell carcinoma of the thyroid arising in Hashimoto's thyroiditis in an adolescent. *Pediatr Dev Pathol* 2006;9:496–500.

52. Sutak J, Armstrong JS, Rusby JE. Squamous cell carcinoma arising in a tall cell papillary carcinoma of the thyroid. *J Clin Pathol* 2005;58:662–664.

53. Kitahara S, Ito T, Hamatani S, et al. Thyroid papillary carcinoma recurring as squamous cell carcinoma: report of a case. *Surg Today* 2006;36:171–174.

54. Mai KT, Yazdi HM, MacDonald L. Fine needle aspiration biopsy of primary squamous cell carcinoma of the thyroid gland. *Acta Cytol* 1999;43:1194–1196.

55. Kumar PV, Malekhusseini SA, Talei AR. Primary squamous cell carcinoma of the thyroid diagnosed by fine needle aspiration cytology. A report of two cases. *Acta Cytol* 1999;43:659–662.

56. Lam KY, Lo CY, Liu MC. Primary squamous cell carcinoma of the thyroid gland: an entity with aggressive clinical behaviour and distinctive cytokeratin expression profiles. *Histopathology* 2001;39:279–286.

57. Booya F, Sebo TJ, Kasperbauer JL, et al. Primary squamous cell carcinoma of the thyroid: report of ten cases. *Thyroid* 2006;16:89–93.

58. Fassan M, Pennelli G, Pelizzo MR, et al. Primary squamous cell carcinoma of the thyroid: immunohistochemical profile and literature review. *Tumori* 2007;93:518–521.

59. Zhou XH. Primary squamous cell carcinoma of the thyroid. *Eur J Surg Oncol* 2002;28: 42–45.

60. Shvero J, Koren R, Shpitzer T, et al. Immunohistochemical profile and treatment of uncommon types of thyroid carcinomas. *Oncol Rep* 2003;10:2075–2078.

61. Sahoo M, Bal CS, Bhatnagar D. Primary squamous-cell carcinoma of the thyroid gland: new evidence in support of follicular epithelial cell origin. *Diagn Cytopathol* 2002;27: 227–231.

62. Weigensberg C, Daisley H, Asa SL, et al. Thyroid thymoma in childhood. *Endocr Pathol* 1990;1:123–127.

63. Chan JK, Rosai J. Tumors of the neck showing thymic or related branchial pouch differentiation: a unifying concept. *Hum Pathol* 1991;22:349–367.

64. LiVolsi VA. Branchial and thymic remnants in the thyroid and cervical region: an explanation for unusual tumors and microscopic curiosities. *Endocr Pathol* 1993;4:115–119.

65. Reimann JD, Dorfman DM, Nose V. Carcinoma showing thymus-like differentiation of the thyroid (CASTLE): a comparative study: evidence of thymic differentiation and solid cell nest origin. *Am J Surg Pathol* 2006;30:994–1001.

66. Su L, Beals T, Bernacki EG, et al. Spindle epithelial tumor with thymus-like differentiation: a case report with cytologic, histologic, immunohistologic, and ultrastructural findings. *Mod Pathol* 1997;10:510–514.

67. Kirby PA, Ellison WA, Thomas PA. Spindle epithelial tumor with thymus-like differentiation (SETTLE) of the thyroid with prominent mitotic activity and focal necrosis. *Am J Surg Pathol* 1999;23:712–716.

68. Tong GX, Hamele-Bena D, Wei XJ, et al. Fine-needle aspiration biopsy of monophasic variant of spindle epithelial tumor with thymus-like differentiation of the thyroid: report of one case and review of the literature. *Diagn Cytopathol* 2007;35:113–119.

69. Vergilio J, Baloch ZW, LiVolsi VA. Spindle cell metaplasia of the thyroid arising in association with papillary carcinoma and follicular adenoma. *Am J Clin Pathol* 2002;117:199–204.

70. Ostrowski MA, Moffat FL, Asa SL, et al. Myxomatous change in papillary carcinoma of thyroid. *Surg Pathol* 1989;2:249–256.

71. Chan JK, Carcangiu ML, Rosai J. Papillary carcinoma of thyroid with exuberant nodular fasciitis-like stroma. Report of three cases. *Am J Clin Pathol* 1991;95:309–314.

72. Beer TW. Malignant thyroid haemangioendothelioma in a non-endemic goitrous region, with immunohistochemical evidence of a vascular origin. *Histopathology* 1992;20: 539–541.

73. Eusebi V, Carcangiu ML, Dina R, et al. Keratin-positive epithelioid angiosarcoma of thyroid. A report of four cases. *Am J Surg Pathol* 1990;14:737–747.

74. Mills SE, Stallings RG, Austin MB. Angiomatoid carcinoma of the thyroid gland. Anaplastic carcinoma with follicular and medullary features mimicking angiosarcoma. *Am J Clin Pathol* 1986;86:674–678.

75. Tanda F, Massarelli G, Bosincu L, et al. Angiosarcoma of the thyroid: a light, electron microscopic and histoimmunological study. *Hum Pathol* 1988;19:742–745.

76. Tötsch M, Dobler G, Feichtinger H, et al. Malignant hemangioendothelioma of the thyroid. Its immunohistochemical discrimination from undifferentiated thyroid carcinoma. *Am J Surg Pathol* 1990;14:69–74.

77. Vollenweider I, Hedinger C, Saremaslani P, et al. Malignant haemangioendothelioma of the thyroid, immunohistochemical evidence of heterogeneity. *Path Res Pract* 1989;184: 376–381.

78. Lin O, Gerhard R, Coelho Siqueira SA, et al. Cytologic findings of epithelioid angiosarcoma of the thyroid. A case report. *Acta Cytol* 2002;46:767–771.

79. Tong GX, Hamele-Bena D, Liu JC, et al. Fine-needle aspiration biopsy of primary osteosarcoma of the thyroid: report of a case and review of the literature. *Diagn Cytopathol* 2008;36:589–594.

SMALL CELL LESIONS

Small cell carcinomas and lymphomas constitute a common source of diagnostic error, often misclassified as anaplastic carcinomas [1–4] (Figs. 13.1–13.3, e-Figs 13.1–13.8).

MEDULLARY CARCINOMA AND OTHER NEUROENDOCRINE CARCINOMAS

A variant of medullary carcinoma composed of poorly differentiated cells resembles small cell carcinoma of lung or neuroblastoma [5]. Immunohistochemical staining identifies these lesions as medullary carcinoma when they contain calcitonin and carcinoembryonic antigen (CEA). Difficulty arises when the lesion is negative for those markers. Metastases have been described from lung and other sites, including bladder [6]. Unfortunately, TTF-1 is not a helpful marker in this distinction, since it is also positive in small cell tumors of lung and even bladder [7].

LYMPHOMAS

A significant proportion of small cell tumors of thyroid are lymphomas [8]. These lesions are readily identified as lymphoid using immunohistochemistry [9]. This subject is reviewed in detail in Chapter 8.

NEUROBLASTOMA

Neuroblastoma (NB) occurs at any site containing sympathetic neural tissue, with retroperitoneal and adrenal lesions being the most common. A primary thyroid NB with regional lymph node and distant multiple subcutaneous metastases has been reported [10] and metastatic NB involving thyroid has been diagnosed on the basis of the cytologic features [11].

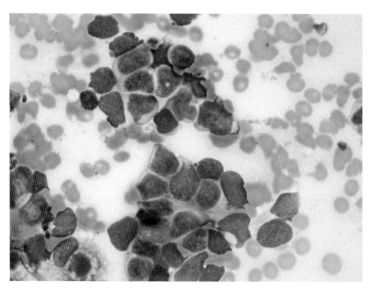

FIGURE 13.1 Small cell lesions of the thyroid engender a differential diagnosis that includes metastatic small cell carcinoma, small cell variant of medullary carcinoma, neuroblastoma, and lymphoma. In this example, the cohesive groups with nuclear molding point to a carcinoma (direct smear, Diff Quik stain).

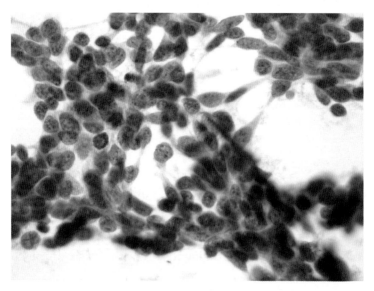

FIGURE 13.2 The presence of mitoses, apoptosis, and necrosis, combined with some spindle cell morphology may lead to a misclassification of small cell carcinoma as an anaplastic carcinoma of thyroid (direct smear, Papanicolaou stain).

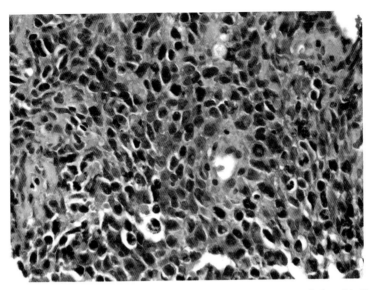

FIGURE 13.3 It may be impossible on morphologic examination to distinguish the small cell variant of medullary carcinoma from metastatic small cell carcinoma and thus require the demonstration of calcitonin by immunohistochemical staining (hematoxylin & eosin stain).

REFERENCES

1. LiVolsi VA. *Surgical pathology of the thyroid*. Philadelphia: WB Saunders, 1990.
2. Carcangiu ML, Steeper T, Zampi G, et al. Anaplastic thyroid carcinoma. A study of 70 cases. *Am J Clin Pathol* 1985;83:135–158.
3. Shvero J, Gal R, Avidor I, et al. Anaplastic thyroid carcinoma. A clinical, histologic, and immunohistochemical study. *Cancer* 1988;62:319–325.
4. Rosai J, Carcangiu ML, DeLellis RA. Tumors of the thyroid gland. In: *Atlas of tumor pathology*. 3rd series, fascicle 5. Washington, DC: Armed Forces Institute of Pathology, 1992.
5. Harach HR, Bergholm U. Small cell variant of medullary carcinoma of the thyroid with neuroblastoma-like features. *Histopathology* 1992;21:378–380.
6. Puente S, Velasco A, Gallel P, et al. Metastatic small cell carcinoma to the thyroid gland: a pathologic and molecular study demonstrating the origin in the urinary bladder. *Endocr Pathol* 2008;19:190–196.
7. Jones TD, Kernek KM, Yang XJ, et al. Thyroid transcription factor 1 expression in small cell carcinoma of the urinary bladder: an immunohistochemical profile of 44 cases. *Hum Pathol* 2005;36:718–723.
8. Heimann R, Vannineuse A, De Sloover C, et al. Malignant lymphomas and undifferentiated small cell carcinoma of the thyroid: a clinicopathological review in the light of the Kiel classification for malignant lymphomas. *Histopathology* 1978;2:201–213.
9. Kendall CH. Distinguishing lymphoma and small cell anaplastic carcinoma of the thyroid by immunocytochemistry. *J Clin Pathol* 1986;39:231.
10. Kumar M, Gupta P, Chaubey A. The thyroid: an extremely rare primary site of neuroblastoma. *Hum Pathol* 2006;37:1357–1360.
11. Ramljak V, Ranogajec I, Novosel I, et al. Thyroid tumour in a child previously treated for neuroblastoma. *Cytopathology* 2006;17:295–298.

LEGENDS OF ELECTRONIC FIGURES (E-FIGURES)

CHAPTER 2: THE NORMAL THYROID

1. Anatomy and histology of the normal thyroid gland.
2. Hematoxylin–eosin stain of the normal thyroid gland demonstrating the lobules composed of follicles defined by delicate fibrovascular stroma.
3. A hematoxylin–phloxine–saffron stain demonstrates the fine fibrous bands that separate each lobule of normal thyroid (Fig. 2.2).
4. The lobules of thyroid may be artifactually exaggerated due to tissue separation during processing and sectioning.
5. Follicles of normal thyroid lined by a single layer of small cuboidal epithelial cells.
6. Typical cuboidal epithelium lining of a normal follicle of thyroid with round regular nuclei, fine chromatin pattern, and inconspicuous nucleoli (Fig. 2.3).
7. Scalloping of colloid during resorption in active follicle. Notice that the surrounding follicles do not show the same effect.
8. High magnification of scalloped colloid and interface between absorptive cells and colloid (Fig. 2.4).
9. Hematoxylin–eosin stain of thyroid in a region with parafollicular C cells. The C cells are often indistinguishable, but occasionally may have a clear cytoplasm.
10. An immunoperoxidase stain for calcitonin marks the C cells (Fig. 2.5).
11. Higher magnification reveals the presence of the C cells adjacent to the basement membrane lining the follicles (calcitonin immunoperoxidase stain).
12. Solid cell nests represent remnants of the ultimobranchial body and are significant in that they must be distinguished from microcarcinomas (Fig. 2.6).
13. The cells of a solid cell nest typically have a squamoid or transitional cell appearance and may demonstrate nuclear grooves.
14. Cystic changes may be identified within solid cell nests. The cysts frequently contain eosinophilic material.

CHAPTER 4: CYTOLOGIC APPROACH TO DIAGNOSIS OF THYROID PATHOLOGY

1. Sample from FNA deposited on microscope slide for direct smearing with the slide held for smearing.
2. Compression of the sample droplet between the smearing slide held perpendicular to the sample slide on which the sample had been deposited.
3. A direct smear where the sample is well positioned and distributed on the slide.
4. When the sample droplet is too large, a touch slide is produced by first positioning a second slide as if to smear the sample, and gently contact the sample.
5. The second slide is then taken away removing a small portion of the sample by capillary action.
6. Monolayered sheet of follicular epithelium.
7. Monolayered sheet of follicular epithelium.
8. Monolayered sheet in which the cell boundaries are visible. Note the bland nuclear morphology.
9. Folding of a monolayered sheet.
10. Tissue fragment of macrofollicles held together by stroma. Each macrofollicle is composed of a single layer of epithelial cells that when ruptured form a monolayered sheet.
11. Tissue fragment of normal thyroid showing its delicate fibrovascular stroma in contrast to the thick fibrovascular stalks of papillae from papillary carcinoma (e-Fig 4.12).
12. Thick vascular stalk from a papillary carcinoma.
13. Monolayered sheets generated by denuding of the papillary stalks of a papillary carcinoma.
14. Increased nuclear crowding in the epithelium of a papillary carcinoma results in a monolayered sheet taking on more of an appearance of a syncytial cluster.
15. Comparison of epithelial architecture of a monolayered sheet to a syncytial cluster.
16. Microfollicular architecture.
17. Cytologic appearance of colloid.

CHAPTER 7: CYSTIC LESIONS

1. Gross photograph of the colloid from a colloid cyst as seen on a direct smear.
2. Gross photograph of the colloid from a colloid cyst as seen on a ThinPrep prepared slide.
3. FNA of a hemorrhagic cyst where the old erythrocytes resistant to erythrolysis are evident in the background of proteinaceous material and hemosiderin-laden macrophages.

4. Partially denuded thyroglossal duct cyst where the preserved epithelium includes squamous and ciliated cells.
5. Ciliated respiratory epithelium lining a thyroglossal duct cyst.
6. Thyroglossal duct cyst lined by squamous epithelium.
7. Thyroid parenchyma embedded within the wall of a thyroglossal duct cyst.
8. Higher magnification reveals benign features in the follicular epithelium of the thyroglossal duct cyst.
9. Low power image of a lymphoepithelial cyst of the thyroid gland.
10. The lymphoepithelial cyst is lined by squamous epithelium overlaying lymphoid tissue with numerous primary and secondary lymphoid follicles.
11. Frequently the epithelium is infiltrated by numerous lymphocytes.
12. Careful search will show the squamous nature of the lining epithelium.
13. Contents of a parapharyngeal (Zenker's) diverticulum showing mature squamous cells, bacteria, and vegetable matter.
14. Parapharyngeal (Zenker's) diverticulum with necrotic skeletal muscle reflecting ingested meat.

CHAPTER 8: INFLAMMATORY AND LYMPHOID LESIONS

1. FNA of acute inflammation of the thyroid shows an abundance of neutrophils with other inflammatory cells and occasionally granulation tissuelike capillary structures.
2. Abundant neutrophils in acute inflammatory lesion of thyroid.
3. Capillaries forming granulation tissuelike structures in acute inflammatory lesion.
4. Intimate association of the inflammatory cells with the vascular network.
5. "Sulfur granules" of *Actinomyces* sp. seen in an FNA of an acute inflammatory lesion.
6. FNA of an acute inflammatory lesion of the thyroid demonstrating fungal organisms morphologically compatible with *Aspergillus* sp.
7. Thyroid FNA showing necrotic material with scattered cysts of *Toxoplasma gondii*.
8. A fragment of a granuloma from granulomatous thyroiditis as seen on an air-dried smear stained with Diff Quik.
9. A fragment of a granuloma from granulomatous thyroiditis as seen on an air-dried smear stained with Diff Quik.
10. A fragment of a granuloma from granulomatous thyroiditis as seen on an air-dried smear stained with Diff Quik.
11. Multinucleated giant cell from granulomatous thyroiditis. Multinucleated giant cells may also be seen in papillary carcinoma and are not specific to granulomatous thyroiditis.
12. Multinucleated giant cell from granulomatous thyroiditis.

13. A fragment of a granuloma with associated multinucleated giant cells seen on a Papanicolaou-stained direct smear.
14. A complex mass of granulomas and multinucleated giant cells (Papanicolaou-stained direct smear).
15. Granuloma fragment on a Papanicolaou-stained direct smear.
16. High power image of the epithelioid histiocytes of a granuloma fragment.
17. Papanicolaou-stained ThinPrep FNA of thyroid showing granulomas.
18. Granuloma fragment seen in ThinPrep.
19. Histology of palpation thyroiditis is characterized by a focal folliculocentric process.
20. Granulomatous thyroiditis.
21. Higher magnification of a granuloma in granulomatous thyroiditis.
22. Intrathyroidal thymic tissue.
23. Hassle's corpuscles in intrathyroidal thymic tissue.
24. Low power appearance of a typical lymphoid infiltrate in lymphocytic thyroiditis on air-dried direct smears.
25. The lymphoid infiltrate of lymphocytic thyroiditis is composed of small lymphocytes, centrocytes, centroblasts, and plasma cells as seen in an air-dried direct smear stained with Diff Quik.
26. Low power appearance of the lymphoid infiltrate in lymphocytic thyroiditis as seen on alcohol fixed Papanicolaou-stained direct smears.
27. Again, the constituent cells of lymphocytic thyroiditis include small lymphocytes, centrocytes, centroblasts, and plasma cells as seen on an alcohol fixed Papanicolaou-stained direct smear.
28. Small lymphocytes, centrocytes, and centroblasts in a germinal center fragment seen on a ThinPrep slide from lymphocytic thyroiditis.
29. Germinal center fragments on a direct smear.
30. Tingible body macrophage from germinal center.
31. Binucleate follicular dendritic cell embedded within germinal center.
32. Bland follicular epithelium in a case of lymphocytic thyroiditis.
33. Epithelial cells clusters with a germinal center fragment. Care must be taken to ensure that the germinal center fragments are not mistaken for a group of epithelial cells.
34. High power image of germinal center fragment from e-Figure 78.
35. High power image of epithelial cells showing Hürthle cell (oncocytic) change from e-Figure 78.
36. Germinal center fragment on ThinPrep for comparison to a cluster of epithelial cells from the same case in e-Figure 82.
37. Epithelial cells on ThinPrep for comparison to germinal center fragment from the same case in e-Figure 81.
38. Colloid in a heavy lymphoid infiltrate of lymphocytic thyroiditis. The presence of the colloid confirms aspiration of thyroid and not adjacent lymph nodes.

39. Hürthle cell change with vacuolated and granular cytoplasm that appears eosinophilic due to the mitochondrial content.
40. Vacuolation in Hürthle cells.
41. Nuclear atypia in Hürthle cells occurring in lymphocytic thyroiditis.
42. Histology of lymphocytic thyroiditis in which a large region of lymphoid tissue is interposed between lobules of thyroid parenchyma.
43. Lymphoid follicles frequently develop in cases of lymphocytic thyroiditis.
44. The lymphoid tissue infiltrates among the thyroid follicles in lymphocytic thyroiditis.
45. Higher power magnification of the lymphoid infiltrate in lymphocytic thyroiditis.
46. Epithelial alterations in lymphocytic thyroiditis range from flattened and attenuated atrophic epithelium to Hürthle cell (oncocytic) change.
47. Higher magnification of the Hürthle cells.
48. Nodules composed entirely of Hürthle cells may develop in lymphocytic thyroiditis.
49. The cytology of relatively bland Hürthle cells.
50. Cytologic atypia in benign Hürthle cells in lymphocytic thyroiditis.
51. Fibrosing lymphocytic thyroiditis in which most of the thyroid has been replaced by fibrous tissue.
52. Foci of chronic inflammation in fibrosing lymphocytic thyroiditis, but with virtually no preservation of thyroid parenchyma.
53. In fibrosing thyroiditis, the residual epithelium may show Hürthle cell change and squamous metaplasia is common.
54. Higher magnification of a region of squamous metaplasia in fibrosis thyroiditis.
55. Low power image of Riedel's thyroiditis.
56. Interface between residual normal thyroid gland and the dense mass of fibrous tissue in Riedel's thyroiditis.
57. Obliteration of the thyroid gland by broad bands of dense fibrous tissue in Riedel's thyroiditis.
58. Residual colloid in the midst of fibrosis of Riedel's thyroiditis.
59. Extension of fibrosis into adjacent fat and vascular occlusion in Riedel's thyroiditis.
60. High power image of vascular obliteration in Riedel's thyroiditis.
61. FNA of large cell non-Hodgkin's lymphoma of the thyroid gland.
62. FNA of another case of large cell non-Hodgkin's lymphoma of the thyroid gland.
63. Cell surface immunophenotype obtained by laser scanning cytometry with a reactive population of T cells (blue) and two different B-cell populations. One small population of polyclonal B cells (red) with a larger population of lambda light chain restricted B cells (green).
64. Histology of diffuse large B-cell lymphoma involving the thyroid gland.

65. Sheets of centroblastlike cells in diffuse large B-cell lymphoma.
66. Cytology of the malignant centroblastlike cells in large cell lymphoma.
67. Follicular lymphoma involving the thyroid gland.
68. Neoplastic follicle of a follicular lymphoma composed of predominantly centroblastlike cells.
69. Extranodal margin zone lymphoma (MALT) of the thyroid showing a single preserved lymphoid follicle and scattered thyroid follicles.
70. Extranodal margin zone lymphoma with residual epithelial elements.
71. Neoplastic infiltrate in extranodal margin zone lymphoma in which the lymphoid cells appear plasmacytoid.
72. Neoplastic infiltrate in MALT lymphoma with more marked atypia and an increase in larger transformed cells.
73. Lymphoepithelial lesion in which the follicular epithelial cells are infiltrated by the lymphoma.
74. Immunoperoxidase stain for mixed keratins (AE1:AE3) to highlight the epithelial component of the lymphoepithelial lesion.
75. Colloid variant of a lymphoepithelial lesion in which the neoplastic lymphoid cells infiltrate the colloid of the thyroid follicles.
76. Mixed keratin immunoperoxidase stain (AE1:AE3) on the colloid variant of the lymphoepithelial lesion in thyroid MALT lymphoma.
77. FNA of Langerhans cell histiocytosis of the thyroid gland, air-dried Diff Quik-stained direct smear.
78. Higher power image of the Langerhans cells with a more epithelioid appearance.
79. Low power appearance of Langerhans cell histiocytosis on alcohol fixed, Papanicolaou-stained direct smear.
80. Langerhans cells in Langerhans cell histiocytosis are epithelioid, stellate, or spindleform with moderately abundant vacuolated cytoplasm.
81. Nuclear grooves and clefts characterizing Langerhans cells.
82. Core biopsy of Langerhans cell histiocytosis.
83. Eosinophils may be identified in addition to the histiocytic population.
84. Nuclear irregularities and grooves evident in the histology of Langerhans cell histiocytosis.
85. Immunoperoxidase staining for low molecular weight keratin to illustrate the presence of atrophic epithelial elements. The histiocytic infiltrate is negative of low molecular weight keratin, which stains the residual epithelial elements.
86. Focus of necrosis with adjacent mitosis in Langerhans cell histiocytosis.
87. Immunoperoxidase staining for CD1a in Langerhans cell histiocytosis.

CHAPTER 9: PAPILLARY LESIONS

1. Low power appearance of Graves disease with intrafollicular papillary projections of hyperplastic epithelium.

2. Papillary hyperplasia of Graves disease with reduce colloid content in the follicle.
3. Papillary hyperplasia of Graves disease.
4. The epithelial cells in Graves disease are frequently columnar and contain round and regular nuclei, lacking nuclear grooves and intranuclear inclusions.
5. Although nuclear crowding may occur in Graves disease, the nuclei are basally oriented and lack nuclear grooves and intranuclear inclusions. Notice the scalloping of colloid.
6. Lymphoid infiltrates are very scarce in Graves disease.
7. Treatment of Graves disease with antithyroid medication results in colloid reaccumulation.
8. Fibrosis may be seen in antithyroid medications, but is usually focal. More widespread fibrosis characterizes radioiodine therapy.
9. The fibrosis associated with radioiodine treatment with focal infiltration by lymphoid tissue.
10. Two characteristic changes induced by radioiodine treatment are large, hyperchromatin, and bizarre nuclei with scattered "smudge" nuclei.
11. Low power appearance of papillary hyperplastic nodule.
12. The papillae of papillary hyperplastic nodules contain fibrovascular cores.
13. The epithelium lining of the papillae in papillary hyperplastic nodules lacks the nuclear features of papillary carcinoma; particularly nuclear grooves and intranuclear inclusions.
14. FNA of papillary hyperplastic nodules may result in collection intact papillae.
15. The epithelium of papillary hyperplastic nodules lacks the diagnostic nuclear features of papillary carcinoma.
16. Papillary carcinoma with conventional papillary architecture.
17. Papillary carcinoma with follicular architecture.
18. Low power appearance of intact papillae from a papillary carcinoma.
19. The fibrovascular stalks of some papillae will be visible.
20. The papillae are subject to denudation of the epithelium, which in this case has resulted in patchy exposure of the underlying fibrovascular core.
21. Epithelium from the tip of a papilla that has retained its original shape despite a degloving injury during FNA and slide preparation.
22. Large denuded fibrovascular stalk as seen on an alcohol fixed, Papanicolaou-stained slides.
23. Denuded fragment of a fibrovascular stalk seen on an air-dried Diff Quik-stained slide.
24. Nuclear enlargement and elongation occur in papillary carcinoma with loss of basal orientation and nuclear crowding with overlapping.
25. Cytologically, the nuclear enlargement results in syncytial epithelial clusters.

26. Mild pleomorphism of elongated oval nuclei in papillary carcinoma.
27. Most nuclei have round and regular contours, but some nuclei will be found with markedly irregular nuclear contours.
28. Nuclear grooves in papillary carcinoma.
29. The nuclear groove represents a superficial invagination of the nuclear membrane and occasionally the edges of the invagination can be resolved.
30. Nuclear grooves seen on edge reveal the profile of the invagination as a "nuclear notch."
31. On air-dried Romanowsky-stained material, the nuclear groove appears as a thin pale line crossing the nucleus. Nuclear notches are harder to appreciate due to the flattening effect of air-drying.
32. In histologic sections, the nuclear grooves show all the same characteristics as in cytologic preparations.
33. Nuclear grooves in histology, note that the nuclear notches can be seen in some cells.
34. Nuclear grooves in papillary carcinoma.
35. Intranuclear inclusion on alcohol-fixed, Papanicolaou-stained direct smear.
36. Intranuclear inclusion with the numerous nuclear grooves and nuclear notches noted in the surrounding cells.
37. Intranuclear inclusion seen in a ThinPrep slide.
38. Intranuclear inclusion seen in a ThinPrep slide.
39. Intranuclear inclusion in air-dried Romanowsky-stained direct smear.
40. Intranuclear inclusion in air-dried Romanowsky-stained direct smear.
41. Intranuclear inclusion in histology.
42. Intranuclear inclusion in histology.
43. Intranuclear inclusion in histology.
44. Optically clear or "Orphan Annie-eye" nuclei.
45. Optically clear or "Orphan Annie-eye" nuclei.
46. "Bare" nucleoli seen in papillary carcinoma.
47. Psammoma body that has shattered during the sectioning process.
48. Aggregate of psammoma bodies. Note the preservation of the concentric laminations.
49. Intracytoplasmic psammoma bodies seen in a ThinPrep slide.
50. Classical psammoma body with intracytoplasmic psammoma bodies.
51. Intracytoplasmic psammoma bodies.
52. Variably sized follicles containing dense colloid with scalloping in papillary carcinoma.
53. Chewing gum or ropey colloid of papillary carcinoma on air-dried Romanowsky-stained direct smears.
54. Chewing gum or ropey colloid of papillary carcinoma on air-dried Romanowsky-stained direct smears.
55. Multinucleated giant cells amongst papillae of papillary carcinoma.
56. Immunoperoxidase stain for mixed keratins (AE1:AE3), marking the epithelium, but not the giant cells.

57. Immunoperoxidase stain for the macrophage marker KP-1 (CD68), marking the giant cells, but not the epithelium.
58. Multinucleated giant cell in FNA of papillary carcinoma.
59. Multinucleated giant cell adjacent to epithelium of papillary carcinoma.
60. High power view of multinucleated giant cell.
61. Monolayered sheets of papillary carcinoma adjacent to metaplasticlike cells.
62. Metaplasticlike cells seen in papillary carcinoma.
63. A region of squamous differentiation in papillary carcinoma.
64. High power view of the squamous differentiation in papillary carcinoma.
65. Epithelial cells with septate vacuoles seen on air-dried Romanowsky-stained direct smear.
66. Epithelial cells with septate vacuoles seen on alcohol fixed, Papanicolaou-stained direct smear.
67. High power view of septate vacuoles.
68. Histiocytoid epithelial cells are epithelial cells from papillary carcinoma with marked cytoplasmic vacuolation.
69. Aggregate of histiocytoid epithelial cells with associated psammoma body. Note the intranuclear inclusion.
70. Macrophages from a cystic papillary carcinoma in comparison to the histiocytoid epithelial cells in e-Figures 200 and 201.
71. Lymphoid infiltrate in thyroid parenchyma adjacent to papillary carcinoma.
72. Cytokeratin 19expression in papillary carcinoma and adjacent compressed thyroid tissue.
73. Galectin-3 expression in papillary carcinoma.
74. HBME-1 expression in papillary carcinoma.
75. Papillary microcarcinoma.
76. Papillary microcarcinoma.
77. Papillary microcarcinoma.
78. Oncocytic variant of papillary carcinoma.
79. Nuclear features of oncocytic variant of papillary carcinoma.
80. FNA of oncocytic variant of papillary carcinoma showing transgressing vessels.
81. FNA of oncocytic variant of papillary carcinoma in which the full nuclear features of papillary carcinoma are not apparent.
82. Warthin's-like tumor of thyroid.
83. Nuclear features of Warthin's-like tumor.
84. Tall cell variant of papillary carcinoma.
85. The nuclear features of the tall cell variant of papillary carcinoma.
86. Low power appearance of columnar cell variant of papillary carcinoma.
87. Note the nuclear pseudostratification of this columnar cell variant of papillary carcinoma.

88. Columnar cell variant of papillary carcinoma.
89. Columnar cell variant of papillary carcinoma.
90. Low power appearance of diffuse sclerosis variant or papillary carcinoma. Note a distinct tumor mass is not evident.
91. Intrathyroidal lymphatic permeation by the diffuse sclerosis variant of papillary carcinoma. Note the profusion of psammoma bodies.
92. Intrathyroidal lymphatic permeation by the diffuse sclerosis variant of papillary carcinoma.
93. The epithelium of the diffuse sclerosis variant of papillary carcinoma showing a squamous metaplastic appearance.
94. Epithelium of diffuse sclerosis variant of papillary carcinoma.
95. Architectural variations in the cribriform-morular variant of papillary carcinoma.
96. Architectural variations in the cribriform-morular variant of papillary carcinoma.
97. Papillary growth pattern in the cribriform-morular variant of papillary carcinoma.

CHAPTER 10: FOLLICULAR LESIONS

1. Low power appearance of sporadic nodular disease.
2. Low power appearance of sporadic nodular disease.
3. Sporadic nodular disease with poorly demarcated nodules, which in fact have been demonstrated to be clonal.
4. The variable size of follicles in sporadic nodular disease.
5. The bland morphology of the follicular epithelium in sporadic nodular disease.
6. Fine needle aspiration of a sporadic nodular disease with abundant colloid and bland follicular epithelium.
7. Fine needle aspiration of a sporadic nodular disease with abundant colloid and bland follicular epithelium.
8. Oncocytic change in sporadic nodular disease.
9. Well-spaced follicular epithelial cells without nuclear atypia, but showing oncocytic changes in sporadic nodular disease.
10. Bland follicular epithelium for sporadic nodular disease.
11. Bland follicular epithelium for sporadic nodular disease.
12. Paravacuolar granules in sporadic nodular disease.
13. Secondary changes with hemosiderin-laden macrophages in sporadic nodular disease.
14. Core biopsy of sporadic nodular disease.
15. Bland histomorphology of the follicles in a core biopsy of sporadic nodular disease.
16. Full thickness capsular invasion in a minimally invasive follicular carcinoma.
17. Invasion of follicular carcinoma into adjacent thyroid parenchyma in a minimally invasive follicular carcinoma.

18. Low power view of invasion into the capsule.
19. Invasion into the capsule may be mimicked by fibrous entrapment of islands of neoplastic cells and is not accepted as equivalent to full thickness penetration of the capsule.
20. Vascular invasion identified along the outer circumference of a tumor.
21. The identification of tumor cells invading through a vessel wall and thrombus adherent to intravascular tumor is required to distinguish true vascular invasion from artifact.
22. Healing needle tract with early granulation tissue.
23. Mature fibrous tissue defining previous needle tract.
24. Low power view of an infracted oncocytic tumor presumably resultant from previous needle biopsy.
25. Higher power view of the infracted tumor showing fibrous reaction at the edge of the lesion.
26. Residual oncocytic tumor island adjacent to infracted tumor.
27. Oncocytic variant of follicular adenoma of thyroid.
28. Oncocytic variant of follicular adenoma of thyroid.
29. Clear cell variant of follicular adenoma.
30. Clear cell variant of follicular adenoma.
31. Clear cell variant of follicular adenoma.
32. Low power appearance of follicular variant of papillary carcinoma.
33. Psammoma body within a follicular variant of papillary carcinoma.
34. Nuclear features of follicular variant of papillary carcinoma.
35. Low power appearance of follicular variant of papillary carcinoma.
36. Nuclear features of follicular variant of papillary carcinoma.
37. Needle tract injuries to the capsule of an infracted thyroid lesion.
38. Notice disruption of the fibrous capsule with development of granulation tissue.
39. High power of the granulation tissue with associated inflammation and hemosiderin deposition.
40. Second needle tract in capsule seen in cross section.
41. Nuclear alterations adjacent to needle tract generating Worrisome Histological Alterations Following FNA of Thyroid (WHAFFT). The nuclear alterations approach those of papillary carcinoma, but fall short.
42. WHAFFT alterations. Only unequivocal nuclear feature of papillary carcinoma may be accepted as diagnostic when the changes are seen adjacent to a needle tract.
43. Low power appearance of oncocytic follicular variant of papillary carcinoma.
44. Low power appearance of oncocytic follicular variant of papillary carcinoma.
46. Microfollicles of an oncocytic follicular variant of papillary carcinoma.
46. Nuclear features of oncocytic follicular variant of papillary carcinoma.
47. Nuclear features of oncocytic follicular variant of papillary carcinoma.

CHAPTER 11: SOLID AND TRABECULAR LESIONS

1. Solid variant of papillary carcinoma.
2. Nuclear features of solid variant of papillary carcinoma.
3. Insular carcinoma, low power.
4. Nuclear features of insular carcinoma.
5. Low power image of hyalinizing trabecular tumor (HTT).
6. Sharp demarcation of hyalinizing trabecular tumor from the adjacent normal thyroid.
7. Characteristic solid trabecular, cords and nesting architecture of hyalinizing trabecular tumor.
8. High power appearance of HTT epithelial cells.
9. Nuclear features and cytoplasmic bodies in HTT.
10. Hyaline stroma of HTT.
11. Psammoma body in hyalinizing trabecular tumor.
12. FNA of hyalinizing trabecular tumor showing hyaline stroma with radial arrangement of epithelial cells.
13. The hyalinized stroma of HTT on FNA.
14. Smearing artifact may disrupt the stroma aggregates and cause the loss of the radial architecture.
15. The epithelial cells surrounding the hyalinized stroma are elongated/spindle cells and often have indistinct cell borders.
16. Epithelial cell groups may be seen without adjacent stroma with small cell groups and individual cells scattered in the background.
17. Nuclear features of HTT with elongated nuclei, altered chromatin, micronucleoli with perinucleolar clearing, nuclear grooves, and intranuclear inclusions.
18. Nuclear features in HTT.
19. Focal expression of cytokeratin 19 in hyalinizing trabecular tumor.
20. High power image shows it is clear the tumor cells expressing CK19 within the HTT.
21. Membranous staining of HTT by MIB-1.
22. Membranous staining for MIB-1 without nuclear staining.
23. Low power appearance of poorly differentiated (insular) carcinoma.
24. Solid nest of tumor invading into the surrounding normal parenchyma in a poorly differentiated (insular) carcinoma.
25. Solid regions of a poorly differentiated (insular) carcinoma.
26. Poorly differentiated (insular) carcinoma in which the tumor has more of a trabecular architecture.
27. Mitotic activity in a poorly differentiated (insular) carcinoma.
28. Mitotic activity in a poorly differentiated (insular) carcinoma.
29. Low power appearance of a FNA of a poorly differentiated (insular) carcinoma on an air-dried, Diff Quik-stained direct smear. Not the hypercellularity and the absence of colloid.
30. Epithelial group in a poorly differentiated (insular) carcinoma on an air-dried, Diff Quik-stained direct smear.

31. Nuclear features of a poorly differentiated carcinoma on an air-dried, Diff Quik-stained direct smear.
32. Low power appearance of poorly differentiated carcinoma on ThinPrep with necrotic material apparent in the background.
33. Epithelial groups of a poorly differentiated carcinoma on a ThinPrep.
34. Nuclear features of an insular carcinoma on ThinPrep.
35. Oncocytic poorly differentiated carcinoma.
36. Low power of clear cell carcinoma of thyroid.
37. High power of clear cell carcinoma of thyroid.
38. Low power image of C-cell hyperplasia with clusters of C cell exceeding seven cells.
39. High power of C-cell hyperplasia
40. C-cell hyperplasia.
41. Prototypic biphasic FNA appearance of medullary carcinoma with epithelioid and spindle cells.
42. Epithelioid component of medullary carcinoma seen on low power.
43. Higher power of epithelioid cells with numerous binucleated cells.
44. Granular chromatin pattern of medullary carcinoma imparting the typical "salt and pepper" or "neuroendocrine" appearance to the chromatin.
45. Lower power appearance of spindle cell component of medullary carcinoma.
46. High power view of spindle cells of medullary carcinoma. Note the similarity of the chromatin pattern with the epithelioid cells in e-Figures 11.42-43.
47. Isolated bizarre neoplastic cells are encountered in a FNA of medullary carcinoma.
48. Red cytoplasmic granules in the epithelioid component of medullary carcinoma. These are uncommon and are best seen in May–Grünwald–Giemsa-stained air-dried direct smears.
49. Note the variation in size of the granules in comparison to e-Figure 11.47 and 11.49.
50. Cytoplasmic granules in medullary carcinoma.
51. Epithelioid and spindle cell cluster in medullary carcinoma. Note the intranuclear inclusion.
52. High power of the intranuclear inclusion.
53. Intranuclear inclusion as seen on May–Grünwald–Giemsa staining.
54. Psammoma bodies are rarely found in medullary carcinoma.
55. Neoplastic vascularization is seen in many cases of medullary carcinoma. Note the numerous capillary-sized vessel present in these tissue fragment.
56. Large thick-walled neoplastic vascular may be appreciated.
57. Note the adherence of the spindle cell component of the medullary carcinoma to the vessel wall.
58. Neoplastic vasculature as seen on air-dried Diff Quik-stained direct smears.

59. Higher power of the neoplastic vasculature.
60. Epithelial cell rosette on FNA of medullary carcinoma.
61. Large fragments of amyloid in medullary carcinoma. Note the epithelial cells appear to be embedded within the amyloid.
62. Separate fragment of amyloid in medullary carcinoma. It appears more waxy than colloid.
63. Amyloid of a medullary carcinoma mimicking follicles with colloid.
64. Low power image of solid sheets of medullary carcinoma.
65. Nesting pattern of medullary carcinoma with pseudofollicular structures.
66. Plasmacytoid epithelioid cells of medullary carcinoma with pseudofollicle.
67. Plasmacytoid epithelioid cells of medullary carcinoma.
68. Biphasic epithelioid and spindle cell region in medullary carcinoma.
69. Spindle cells of medullary carcinoma.
70. High power of pseudofollicles in medullary carcinoma.
71. Peripheral palisading in medullary carcinoma.
72. Cellular pleomorphism with bizarre cells.
73. Cellular pleomorphism with bizarre cells.
74. Amyloid stroma of medullary carcinoma.
75. e-Figure 11.73 (H & E stained slide) seen with polarized light.
76. Virtually acellular region of amyloid deposition.
77. Small nests of medullary carcinoma cells entrapped in amyloid stroma.
78. Nodular deposit of amyloid in medullary carcinoma.
79. e-Figure 11.77 (H & E stained slide) seen with polarized light. Note the apple green birefringence of the amyloid even though the slide has not been stained with Congo Red.
80. Same region of nodular amyloid as in e-Figure 11.77, but with Congo Red staining.
81. e-Figure 11.79 seen with polarized light.
82. Calcification of amyloid stroma.
83. Intranuclear inclusions in medullary carcinoma.
84. Intranuclear inclusions in medullary carcinoma.
85. Immunoperoxidase staining of medullary carcinoma with low molecular weight keratins (Cam 5.2).
86. Immunoperoxidase staining of medullary carcinoma with low molecular weight keratins (Cam 5.2).
87. Immunoperoxidase staining of medullary carcinoma with mixed keratins (AE1:AE3). While the follicular epithelium surrounding the tumor stains well, the medullary carcinoma shows only weak staining.
88. Medullary carcinoma typically is well stained with cytokeratin 7.
89. Immunoperoxidase staining of medullary carcinoma with TTF-1.
90. Immunoperoxidase staining of medullary carcinoma with chromogranin.

91. Immunoperoxidase staining of medullary carcinoma with synaptophysin.
92 Immunoperoxidase staining of medullary carcinoma with calcitonin. Note weak and focal staining of the epithelial cells.
93. Immunoperoxidase staining of amyloid with calcitonin in a medullary carcinoma.
94. Immunoperoxidase staining of medullary carcinoma with carcinoembryonic antigen (CEA).
95. Lower power of primary mucoepidermoid carcinoma of the thyroid.
96. Mixture of mucinous and epidermoid elements of a mucoepidermoid carcinoma of thyroid.
97. Squamous (epidermoid) and intermediate cells of a primary mucoepidermoid carcinoma of thyroid.
98. Mucinous elements of a mucoepidermoid carcinoma.
99. Juxtaposition of mucinous and squamoid elements of mucoepidermoid carcinoma.
100. Metastatic colonic carcinoma in FNA of thyroid with necrotic debris and malignant columnar epithelium.
101. Malignant columnar epithelium of a colonic carcinoma.
102. Histologic section of metastatic colonic carcinoma within the thyroid gland.
103. Classical "dirty necrosis" of metastatic colonic carcinoma with garlandlike arrangement of malignant epithelium.

CHAPTER 12: SQUAMOID, SPINDLE, AND GIANT-CELL LESIONS

1. Infiltration of normal thyroid follicles by anaplastic carcinoma of thyroid.
2. Combined spindle and giant cell variants of anaplastic carcinoma in with frankly bizarre giant cells.
3. Spindle cell variant of anaplastic carcinoma of thyroid.
4. Anaplastic carcinoma of thyroid resembling lymphoepitheliomalike carcinoma.
5. Mitotic activity in anaplastic carcinoma of thyroid.
6. Large region of geographic necrosis in anaplastic carcinoma.
7. Necrotic region of anaplastic carcinoma with associated inflammation.
8. Necrotic material and inflammation in a FNA of anaplastic carcinoma of thyroid.
9. Osteoclasticlike giant cells in anaplastic carcinoma of thyroid.
10. Osteoclasticlike giant cells in anaplastic carcinoma of thyroid. Note the difference in nuclear morphology between the carcinoma and the giant cell.
11. Giant cell variant of anaplastic carcinoma of thyroid.
12. Artifact clefting generating somewhat of an alveolar pattern in a giant cell variant of anaplastic carcinoma of thyroid.

13. FNA of giant cell variant of anaplastic carcinoma of thyroid.
14. The epithelial nature of the giant cell variant of anaplastic carcinoma of thyroid may be evident in cohesive clustering, but staining for low molecular weight keratins may be necessary.
15. Abnormal mitotic figure is frequently identified in FNA of anaplastic carcinoma of thyroid.
16. High power image of giant cell variant of anaplastic carcinoma. Note the necrotic material and some cells showing spindle morphology.
17. Low power image of rhabdoid tumor of thyroid showing delicate fibrovascular stroma and sheets of neoplastic cells.
18. Rhabdoid tumor of thyroid.
19. High power appearance of the rhabdoid cells with cytoplasmic inclusion.
20. Focal expression of keratins (AE1:AE3) in a rhabdoid tumor of thyroid.
21. Expression of sarcomeric actin in rhabdoid tumor of thyroid.
22. Low power image of spindle cell anaplastic carcinoma.
23. Fascicular arrangement of spindle cells in spindle cell anaplastic carcinoma.
24. Cytologic abnormality in spindle cells of anaplastic carcinoma.
25. Low power appearance of spindle cell anaplastic carcinoma on FNA.
26. Dissociated spindle cells from anaplastic carcinoma of thyroid.
27. Variability of nuclear abnormalities seen in spindle cell anaplastic carcinoma of thyroid.
28. More marked cytologic abnormality in spindle cell anaplastic carcinoma.
29. Tissue fragment from spindle cell anaplastic carcinoma.
30. High power appearance of cells in spindle cell anaplastic carcinoma.
31. FNA of primary squamous cell carcinoma of thyroid. Note the necrotic background with individual malignant cell.
32. FNA of a primary squamous carcinoma of thyroid.
33. FNA showing dyskeratotic cell in primary squamous cell carcinoma of thyroid.
34. Fibrous septate and biphasic appearance of spindle cell tumor with thymuslike differentiation (SETTLE).
35. Merging of spindle cell and glandular cells of SETTLE.
36. Spindle cell component of SETTLE.
37. Spindle cell component of SETTLE.
38. Glandular component of SETTLE.
39. Pale staining islands of glandular cells with large glandular spaces in SETTLE.
40. High power of glandular component of SETTLE.
41. Ciliated cells lining glandular spaces in SETTLE.
42. Mucinous differentiation in glandular component of SETTLE.
43. Low power appearance of epithelioid angiosarcoma of thyroid.
44. Anastomosing vascular channels of angiosarcoma of thyroid.

45. High power of angiosarcoma of thyroid.
46. Intracytoplasmic lumens identified in epithelioid angiosarcoma of thyroid.
47. Expression of the endothelial cell marker CD31 in an angiosarcoma of thyroid.

CHAPTER 13: SMALL CELL LESIONS

1. Small cell carcinoma on an air-dried direct smear stained with Diff Quik.
2. High power appearance of small cell carcinoma.
3. ThinPrep appearance of small cell carcinoma.
4. Greater cell dissociation may occur with ThinPrep slides on small cell carcinoma.
5. Alcohol fixed, Papanicolaou-stained direct smear of small cell anaplastic carcinoma.
6. High power appearance of small cell carcinoma.
7. Histologic appearance of small cell carcinoma.
8. Small cell carcinoma with large areas of tumor necrosis.

INDEX

Page numbers followed by "f" denote a figure; page numbers followed by "t" denote a table.